# Athletic Movement Skills

## Training for Sports Performance

### Clive Brewer

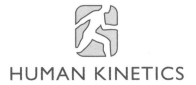

**HUMAN KINETICS**

**Library of Congress Cataloging-in-Publication Data**

Names: Brewer, Clive, author.
Title: Athletic movement skills : training for sports performance / Clive
  Brewer.
Description: Champaign, IL : Human Kinetics, [2017] | Includes
  bibliographical references and index.
Identifiers: LCCN 2016026947 (print) | LCCN 2016058398 (ebook) | ISBN
  9781450424127 (print) | ISBN 9781492543954 (ebook)
Subjects: LCSH: Athletes--Training of. | Physical education and training. |
  Movement, Aesthetics of. | Sports--Physiological aspects. | Physical
  fitness--Physiological aspects.
Classification: LCC GV711.5 .B76 2017 (print) | LCC GV711.5 (ebook) | DDC
  613.7/1--dc23
LC record available at https://urldefense.proofpoint.com/v2/url?u=https3A__lccn.loc.gov_ 2016026947&d=DwI-
FAg&c=R1lkIB1gpi-haQptoL4D6CEfNLBiDeRQp4faUYSM_Mw&r=bKaWuPKK1p-n8iw5JTnyQg3bBvzZDcn3NwGG9DP-
MAaA&m=pxmNN_pkCefMvrulyB5ym47YyiBZjAHXwZxGJomTB3w&s=s150MUqM2afrIWxRHvckLezDog4IOw9ik3-By-
FpjusI&e=

ISBN: 978-1-4504-2412-7 (print)

This publication is written and published to provide accurate and authoritative information relevant to the subject matter presented. It is published and sold with the understanding that the author and publisher are not engaged in rendering legal, medical, or other professional services by reason of their authorship or publication of this work. If medical or other expert assistance is required, the services of a competent professional person should be sought.

The web addresses cited in this text were current as of October 2016, unless otherwise noted.

**Senior Developmental Editor:** Cynthia McEntire; **Managing Editor:** Nicole Moore; **Copyeditor:** Bob Replinger; **Indexer:** Andrea Hepner; **Permissions Manager:** Martha Gullo; **Graphic Designer:** Denise Lowry; **Cover Designer:** Keith Blomberg; **Photograph (cover):** Human Kinetics; **Photographs (interior):** © Human Kinetics or Clive Brewer unless otherwise noted; **Visual Production Assistant:** Joyce Brumfield; **Photo Production Manager:** Jason Allen; **Art Manager:** Kelly Hendren; **Illustrations:** © Human Kinetics unless otherwise noted; **Printer:** Sheridan Books

Printed in the United States of America     10  9  8  7  6  5  4  3  2  1

The paper in this book is certified under a sustainable forestry program.

**Human Kinetics**
Website: www.HumanKinetics.com

*United States:* Human Kinetics, P.O. Box 5076, Champaign, IL 61825-5076
800-747-4457
e-mail: info@hkusa.com

*Canada:* Human Kinetics, 475 Devonshire Road Unit 100, Windsor, ON N8Y 2L5
800-465-7301 (in Canada only)
e-mail: info@hkcanada.com

*Europe:* Human Kinetics, 107 Bradford Road, Stanningley, Leeds LS28 6AT, United Kingdom
+44 (0) 113 255 5665
e-mail: hk@hkeurope.com

*Australia:* Human Kinetics, 57A Price Avenue, Lower Mitcham, South Australia 5062
08 8372 0999
e-mail: info@hkaustralia.com

*New Zealand:* Human Kinetics, P.O. Box 80, Mitcham Shopping Centre, South Australia 5062
0800 222 062
e-mail: info@hknewzealand.com

E5649

# Contents

# Foreword

Throughout my coaching career of over 40 years, I have motivated myself to pursue an improved understanding of and continual engagement with all aspects of athletic performance. Being able to understand the *why* when it comes to helping athletes reach their ultimate athletic potential, regardless of the sport, has enabled me to push athletes to new levels of performance. To that end, through my educational pursuits and applied work, I have developed a philosophy whereby I encourage coaches and athletes to strive for an improved understanding and mastery of all aspects of athletic development.

This philosophy has led me to coaching not only athletes but also coaches, teams, international federations and Olympic committees in a multitude of sports. From my early days as a high school coach at my alma mater, Madison East, I leveraged the leadership of my professors and coaches to influence athletes in ice hockey and girls' track and field, which resulted in state championship performances. This approach of doing my best to understand everything to do with sport performance moved me to the collegiate ranks at the University of Wisconsin, University of Tennessee and Louisiana State University. At LSU, I was fortunate to lead an extraordinary group of coaches and athletes to five NCAA team championships as head women's track and field coach in a programme that produced 140 All-American female athletes. These principles helped athletes like Dawn Sowell (10.78 and 22.03) and Sheila Echols (10.83 and 6.94 metres [22 feet, 9 1/4 inches]) garner accolades and achieve medal-winning performances.

During this period I was sometime criticized by other coaches for speaking with my athletes in terms that were too scientific. One day I confronted one of these coaches. I called an athlete over and asked her to explain a performance concept in biomechanics. To the surprise of the now-confounded coach, the athlete replied with a correct, eloquent and succinct explanation. One of my proudest accomplishments as a coach is seeing many of the athletes with whom I worked choose to pursue a career or avocation in coaching and watching them apply principles they had learned.

In 1989 I 'turned pro' and stepped away from the collegiate environment to work in the arena of the professional athlete. Names in track and field include Gwen Torrence, double silver medallist in the 100 and 200 metres in the 1991 IAAF World Championships. More recently, athletes in all three disciplines—the sprints, hurdles and jumps—have had great success. Donovan Bailey, Dwight Phillips, Angelo Taylor, LaShawn Merritt and Tianna Bartoletta eagerly learned while achieving stellar performances and picking up hardware. I am proud that Dwight Phillips has joined our coaching staff at IMG Academy.

Team-sport athletes will equally benefit from the knowledge you will gain and put into practice after pouring over Clive Brewer's newest publication. I was able to help the Atlanta Falcons when I joined their staff as a speed and performance consultant in 1989, long before many teams had this position. That year the Falcons went to the Super Bowl, partly because they had the fewest number of games missed by starters and the greatest point differential in the fourth quarter. They were fitter, faster and healthier. I have spent time consulting with the Chicago Bulls, Detroit Lions, Jacksonville Jaguars and players such as Hershel Walker, Dorsey Levens, Marco Coleman and Glenn 'Big Baby' Davis, just to mention a few.

*Athletic Movement Skills: Training for Sports Performance* by Clive Brewer, a world-recognized expert in high-performance sport conditioning and applied sport science, presents readers with a comprehensive guide to such applied knowledge. I believe that coaches should have the widest possible database to draw on for the eventualities that may come their way. Coaches should be knowledgeable in all fields relevant to performance enhancement, whilst actively seeking new and innovative advancements. This book provides just that type of applied information—material that will engage, educate and inspire readers to prioritize the development of athletic movement skills for widespread success.

I have always believed that the first role of any athletic development practitioner is to be a movement coach. Athletes must be able to get their joints in the right position, at the right time, so that the muscles can work in an optimal manner. Poor movement mechanics lead not only to inefficient actions, but also to injury because muscles, ligaments and joints are subjected to high force or repetitive actions that they are not designed to withstand. After all, what sport doesn't require athletes to move well? Competent movement techniques therefore form the basis not only for conditioning work but also for physical education programmes and sport-specific coaching. Movement techniques are at the heart of a sound performance development programme.

Throughout this pursuit for knowledge and experience in the field of performance coaching across the developmental spectrum, I have worked with colleagues who share the same passion. We have shared our experiences and expertise to aid our collective understanding of the *why* behind the *what* and the *how*. Throughout my career, I have attempted to do the same for coaches and scientists who have the same thirst for learning so that they can help others achieve more than they thought possible as independent learners. *Athletic Movement Skills* provides just that learning opportunity.

Clive Brewer and I have been friends and colleagues for more than a decade. Our first meeting in Dublin, Ireland, where I was presenting at the European Athletics Coaches Association Symposium, was memorable. I immediately recognized Clive's keen interest

in and understanding of some of the most complex aspects of strength and power development, especially as it related to speed and movement. Clive's path has blended the practical with the scientific, a combination I believe is vital when expressing and justifying what works from an evidence-based and field application perspective. Clive has published numerous articles and peer-reviewed papers on wide and varied subject matter in the areas of human performance that have significantly contributed to the body of knowledge. I have consistently relied on Clive to assist me in the vetting of new ideas and to lend ideas for crafting presentations. Most recently in Birmingham, England, we collaborated again on the stage in a presentation on strength and power as they relate to speed across the athlete's career from youth and novice levels to the elite international level. This past year Clive has worked with me in Florida, providing strength and conditioning to the national team track athletes I was coaching as they prepared for the Rio Olympics.

*Athletic Movement Skills* sees Clive take his work to a new level. He shares content on how the body optimally functions and explores the importance of physical literacy and a finely tuned movement vocabulary in chapter 1. This book shows in detail how different sports have commonalities and can draw from a body of evidence and expertise through the use of movement skills to solve a variety of challenges posed. The book delves into how the neuromotor system works and, even more important, how the athlete's systems change through the stages of age-related development in chapters 2 and 3, respectively.

Chapter 4 focuses on the mechanical functions of athletic movement skills and the effect that forces have on successful execution. Understanding these concepts will aid readers as they guide athletes through a developmental journey towards movement mastery.

An in-depth view on posture and its importance and effect on movement efficiency in chapter 5 is followed by a comprehensive discussion of how to analyse such physical alignment from a static and dynamic point of view. Chapter 6 emphasizes the evaluation and monitoring of movement skill development, in particular when seeking to correct commonly seen challenges along a development pathway.

Armed with this foundational information, readers learn in chapter 7 how to construct an applied and progressive curriculum that generates a designed and personalized stage rather than an age-appropriate progression. This chapter incorporates fundamentals in the areas of speed and agility development and reactive strength that encompass effective take-off and landing movements. Chapters 8, 9 and 10 show how functional strength can be seamlessly integrated into a programme. Readers will benefit from an array of exercises and technique-specific guidance that allow progression towards more advanced drills and exercises that build functional movement skill mastery.

No book would be complete without real-world examples from a variety of sporting disciplines that readers can relate to and learn from. *Athletic Movement Skills* presents several case studies in chapter 11 that give readers practical insight into the process of identifying what is needed to solve the challenges through a comprehensive, tailored movement education programme. Links to the foundational principles that the book sets out are recalled to help readers comprehend and fine-tune their delivery of support.

Working with Clive first hand enabled me to experience personally how the content and philosophy advocated by *Athletic Movement Skills* plays out in coaching sessions. In keeping with my personal philosophy of sharing concepts, ideas and practice, I commend Clive on sharing his expertise so that we as a community can grow together and support the athletes and clients we work with.

By reading *Athletic Movement Skills*, you will gain further insight on how to help your athletes and clients reach their potential in any of their physical endeavours.

**Loren Seagrave**
Director of speed and movement and
Director of track and field and cross country
IMG Academy, Bradenton, Florida

# Preface

When I discuss my role with the Toronto Blue Jays of Major League Baseball, I am often asked when I stopped thinking of myself as a coach and began to think of myself as a scientist. The answer is that this transformation has never happened. Coaching is a people business, a problem-solving opportunity to enable athletes to get the best out of themselves. I am first a coach, but I am a coach who practises science.

Most people who work with athletes do so because their fundamental desire is to make the athlete better. I wanted to write a book inspired by my passion to help others by providing the *why* and *what* of how to coach core movement skills to athletes of different ages and standards. You will find this book useful for identifying where the athlete is in his or her movement development and what he or she might need to do to progress. I have incorporated a practical blend of the *what, how* and, most important, the *why* of movement skill development.

This book can be used at any stage of the training programme design. Chapters 1 through 5 provide a practical understanding of how the body works and how it can be improved. Chapters 6 and 7 pull this information into progressive programmes based on observations. Chapters 8 through 10 are full of technical guidance for developing multidirectional speed and power with athletes in any context. The book concludes with a series of examples of integrated programmes in chapter 11.

If you are a coach who wants practical ideas but also wants to understand why these methods are important, or an athletic trainer who understands how the body works but is looking for ways to progress and challenge clients, this book has something for you. Similarly, if you are a student who is looking for examples of how to engage with science and bring it to life in a meaningful way, this book is an invaluable resource. It provides a shared language that will build bridges between the knowledge of various professionals.

Science is based on organizing and restructuring principles and knowledge to explain, predict or influence certain phenomenon. In my professional life, that phenomenon is movement. Movement is the common theme that underpins every successful sporting performance. It is the basis for the quality we know as athleticism, because athletes use movements to solve problems posed to them in sporting situations. We can identify many forms of movement, and we should study all of them, but when I was the national programme manager for athlete development in Scotland, almost all the sports I worked with required fundamental qualities relating to the ability to run (acceleration, deceleration, change of direction), jump and exert forces rapidly. This understanding has formed the basis of my work with international performers in soccer, American football, rugby, track and field, tennis and baseball ever since. I have worked not just at the elite level; I have delivered coaching programmes for academies such as the IMG Academy in Florida and sport-specific children's programmes in the United Kingdom to develop movement vocabularies and physical literacy.

Many people collaborate to develop an athlete to his or her potential, and they need to share a common language and principles to support the athlete. One thing that guides my philosophy every day is that the athlete needs to be at the centre of any coaching process. The support professional (scientist, strength and conditioning coach, athletic trainer) or sport coach must not put his or her body of knowledge above the needs of the athlete.

Everyone working with the athlete should be able to access and understand basic principles of how the body works, responds and learns (training always equates to learning) and apply these to the practices we design. This book will empower you to evaluate your current athletic development techniques and methods and consider how you can further personalize the design and delivery of your training sessions.

The body is a complex interaction of different yet interrelated systems, and training must take into account how the motor control system works. This basic principle guides the early chapters of the book. I identify the basic principles of how the body works in sport, how a child grows and develops into adulthood and how the athlete manages forces in three dimensions (front to back, side to side, up and down). We need to be able to communicate this knowledge. Scientists are notorious for writing in a way that is understood only by other scientists. Therefore, the knowledge remains inaccessible to many. My goal is to engage coaches, students, parents, teachers and medical professionals and empower their understanding without dumbing down the science or misrepresenting it in any way. When we understand why something should be done, we are better able to determine how to improve required responses in the athlete. Similarly, if we understand the developmental process an athlete has gone through (or is going through), we are better informed about how we can optimize the athlete's progression.

I bring concepts to life and illustrate them with real-life examples and case studies across a wide spectrum of sports. This method is an important part of coaching education. A coach who understands that impulse (chapter 4) is the key physical quality to teach his or her athletes also understands the need to optimize strength and power training to cause adaptive change in various body systems (chapter 2). Armed with this understanding, the coach can critically evaluate training methods and ask whether they will develop the desired qualities. If they will not, why should the athlete use them? Ultimately, the objectives we are trying to achieve in coaching will determine the methods we should use. Therefore, this book teaches the practitioner what the requirements are, how they build into objectives and what can be done to achieve these objectives individually.

Quality movement training develops correct postures and body positioning during any movement to allow effective force transfer and the powerful expression of force through a movement or sport-specific skill. Early in my career, I learned the importance of working with other bodies of knowledge. I studied anatomy with medical students, and my daily work with physiotherapists about injury causes and return-to-training progressions led me to realize that technique is all about getting the right joint positions at the right time so that the muscles can operate with optimal efficiency. This realization transformed the way I approached coaching. I changed my focus from the outcome (How fast did the athlete go?) to the process (How does the athlete move? How can I make the athlete move more efficiently?). By trusting the process and by applying the right amount of effort, the athlete can achieve a better outcome. This message is described in detail throughout chapters 5 and 6, which discuss the importance of posture and describe evaluating posture to identify areas to improve through a coaching plan.

We share a common goal. Sound movement education is based on progressing generic movement competencies into sport-specific movement qualities. Ultimately, rehabilitation from injury is exactly the same process. By building bridges between professional knowledge bases, we enhance the outcome for the athlete. This approach is seen throughout the book. When the athlete's needs are at the centre of the process, we shouldn't be able to identify who provides the solution because we have a more holistic perspective to athletic development. I am confident that this text contains an equal distribution of applied learning opportunities and contextual insights for coaches, academics, athletic trainers, athletes and parents.

My aim is to foster an understanding of why things should be done and to use examples to demonstrate how these activities can be delivered with purpose. A wise man once said,

'Exercise is a doing thing; movement is a feeling thing.' Every exercise, drill and activity has a goal. Identifying that goal for the athlete gives him or her a target. A goal directs behaviour and helps the athlete move with purpose and focus on what matters. In movement, feeling is essential. A common theme through the book is the importance of the central nervous system as the governor of the musculoskeletal system to produce movement. Athletes who know this can enhance the quality of how they do things.

Chapter 7 builds on the concept of developing competence. This chapter looks at structuring learning progressions when developing athletic movement skills and building on competences. Learned techniques become skills that become part of an overall movement strategy that the athlete can deploy in any sporting context as part of a diverse and independent movement vocabulary. The chapter offers advice about coaching education programmes, such as what to consider when setting up a demonstration and how to use questions to develop understanding in a learner. Another key concept presented in this chapter is differentiation, that is, how a skill can be presented to a group of athletes but be structured to develop both confidence and competence in each individual. This issue goes to the centre of good physical education in any context.

In chapters 8 through 10, the concepts of how the motor system works and how forces can be effectively transferred in and by the athlete come to life in the applied learning of movement skills. Readers will be inspired by the links made between science and coaching.

Chapter 8 applies the scientific principles identified in earlier chapters as aspects of speed, a core component of athletic movement. For acceleration, deceleration and change of direction, what does good technique look like? What are the core drills that develop these techniques? More important, how can practitioners who understand the principles behind the drills further develop them when an athlete reaches competence? This approach will enhance the coach's ability to design and adapt drills.

I find that many people approach jumping and rebounding skills with imaginative drills and practices but without a fundamental understanding of the relationship between ground contact time and the ability to create and express ground reaction forces. The higher the resultant jump needs to be, the longer the ground contact time needs to be. Many coaches know the buzzwords for jumping (shorter ground contact time), yet they prescribe drills that require exactly the opposite. Coaches need to understand the physio-mechanical qualities that underpin jumping, recognize safe and effective technique and then look at progressing or regressing techniques to challenge the athlete's competence to achieve specific outcomes. Uniquely, chapter 9 does this and provides a guided progression for different intensities and complexities of plyometric skills, based on the relative challenge they provide.

The application of strength and power forms the basis of all sporting and movement skills. The athlete's ability to harness and apply power at critical moments is a determining factor in success. Strength is the basis of athletic performance, injury reduction and healthy living. Chapter 10 explores the concept of developing functionality in strength training, which is actually about deploying the spectrum of fundamental movements and challenging the athlete's neuromuscular system to access and employ strength usefully. I select several key movements central to this idea and illustrate how to progress or regress them to challenge the athlete's postural and mechanical systems, a fundamental move away from the 'just lift more and faster' way of strength training. Yes, traditional strength training has a time and place in an athlete's programme, and the book does not shy away from it. But the development of athleticism is related to the ability to undertake quality practice of quality movement patterns. Indeed, the first role of any strength coach is to be a movement coach.

One of the hardest things to do in training is to bring all the factors together into a balanced, structured programme that considers the fundamental principles of movement and is effective in enabling the athlete to achieve his or her goals. The final chapter consolidates the principles and practice of movement skill development into several theoretical case studies. This chapter is important for anyone involved in the development of an athlete. It provides a chance to understand the problem, read an evidence-based rationale for the intervention and see a structured and fully integrated training programme (including sport-specific practices). Most important, the chapter leads the reader to ask the fundamental question, 'What could I do differently?'

Regardless of your role in the training process, the age of the athletes or your background, this book will help you understand the importance of movement skills and provide fundamental knowledge and ideas to empower you to enhance movement skill capabilities. The best sport performers have one thing in common—they are all great athletes and have at some point been taught the basis of athleticism by someone who knew what to do and when to do it.

# CHAPTER 1

# Movement Skill Development

Athletes (sport performers in any context) are ultimately judged on their performances. Whether these performances are on the training field, in the weight room or in competitive arenas from the school field to international competition, the resulting and observable actions are a consequence of a complex series of interactions that occur within the body. A reasonable supposition is that a coach's overall objective is to improve observable performance.

Sport is a problem-solving activity in which much detailed planning needs to occur over both the long term and short term to optimize performance of an athlete (or a group of athletes, in a team-sport context) at predetermined points in time. Indeed, the specific intent of a training or educational programme is to enhance performance.[1] This objective may be geared towards long-, medium- and short-term plans.

- **Long term:** Developing the performance potential of a child towards a lifetime participation in sport requires the achievement of appropriate training, competition and recovery throughout the athlete's career, particularly in relation to the important growth stages in young people. This process involves not just developing a curriculum that matches the developmental stage of the athlete, but also managing the transitions that the athlete will undertake when moving from one programme to another or from one level of performance to the next (figure 1.1). This progression may incorporate multi-year programmes that see athletes progress from collegiate to national to international performance levels or the time frame between major events (for example, the quadrennial, or four-year, plans that run between Olympic cycles).

- **Medium term:** Developing performance capacity within a specific year or season may be about winning a championship, a cup or an Olympic medal. Medium-term planning may also be about achieving certain personal performance or competency attainment targets that mark key stages in a longer-term progression towards a longer-term aim.

- **Short term:** Planning in the short term (days or weeks) is about structuring precise training interventions (methods, volume loads) to target specific outcomes that build on each other to fulfil longer-term objectives.

The key to successful planning is understanding which elements of training are to be emphasized at a particular time. Although training programmes should not exclusively focus on specific abilities, a programme should have a specific emphasis. For example, in general preparation (preseason) phases, a basketball player may focus on developing physical qualities, whereas in-season, the emphasis is on maintaining physical capacities to enable a focus on playing well in games. Similarly, in preparation phases, the objective may be related to developing anaerobic power with some focus on anaerobic capacity or to developing strength with some aspects of speed as a precursor to specific power work.

The defined objective will drive the predominant training methods employed during this period (the emphasis load), and the sequence must build on what has been in place before hand, thus highlighting the concept that planning is about sequencing prerequisites or building on foundations.

For example, strength is the ability to exert forces and power is the ability to exert forces quickly. Therefore, power cannot be developed without speed, but the foundation on which power is built is strength. Similarly, if the programme undertakes to build speed endurance before speed, ultimately this approach will limit the athlete's ability to develop speed, the prerequisite for speed endurance. As will be alluded to throughout the book, a strong building is built on a well-laid foundation, and building human sporting talent is no different.

Performance outcomes are such a focus for many that what is often missed are the underlying contributors to the factors that made those performances possible. For many years, training programmes have been developed with long- and short-term fluctuations in training stimuli, designed to develop the performances of athletes towards a desired objective. These training interventions typically have been designed to target one or more functionally interrelated aspects of training aimed ultimately to influence the athlete's performances.[2]

The process emphasizes the role of quality preparation and delivery mechanisms, matched to key criteria based on individual development and focused on episodes and performance over the short, medium and long term.

Traditionally, coaching and coach education programmes have focused on training inputs designed to foster the technical, tactical, physical and mental aspects of a programme. This approach, however, significantly oversimplifies the process and arguably misses one of the aspects of programme development vital to sporting performance: the area of movement (motor) skills. As the Russian sport scientist Verkoshansky identified, the fundamental phenomenon central to all sporting tasks is

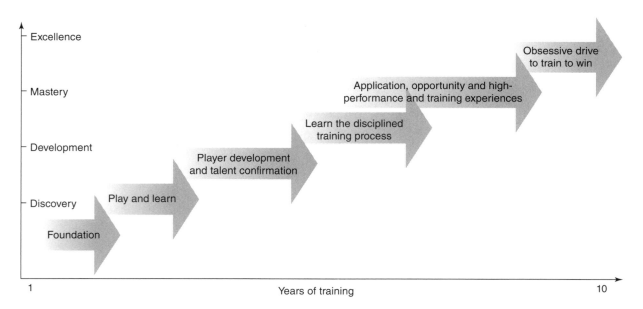

**Figure 1.1**   Planning for the long-term development of an athlete requires an understanding of the environments through which the athlete might pass.

movement: Sport is a problem-solving activity in which movements are used to produce the necessary solutions.[3]

All great sport performers have one common and definable quality: They are all great athletes! Athleticism is a simple term that everyone understands and recognizes, but athleticism can be broken down into a number of key characteristics related to movement effectiveness and motor control that form the basis in developing biomotor abilities (figure 1.2).

In educational fields, people have long accepted that foundation movement skills (e.g., catching, throwing and running) are prerequisites or building blocks for participation in all popular forms of sports and games.[4] Indeed, the theory of motor control provides a frequently referenced link between fundamental motor skill proficiency and its application to sport-specific situations. Fundamental motor skills are common motor activities that have specific observable patterns (such as running, jumping, throwing, and so on). Most sport-specific or movement skills are advanced variants of a fundamental movement or skill. Motor learning principles are based on a progression that builds on previously learned movements that prepare the athlete to master more advanced

or situation-specific skills. As this book explores in depth, the ability to move well with stability and well-developed object-control skills underpins most sport-specific skills and actions.

Observable performance in sport is based on the athlete's ability to move well. Movement proficiency is the basis of all skill, and it must therefore be developed in accordance with, and not in isolation of, other aspects of sport performance. This approach to programme development enables the athlete to integrate all parts of a movement into well-coordinated, mechanically correct and efficient acts.

Table 1.1 illustrates the basic components of movement skills. Note that an integrated approach is not always common in youth sport programmes, in which the emphasis is often on observable skill outcome rather than mastery of the motor skill and posture control processes that underpin the sport-specific skills.

Of these components, stability is arguably the bedrock skill to be developed, because all forceful locomotive and object-control movements are based on the foundations that a stable posture provides. This point is illustrated well in figure 1.3; the basis for the effective execution of the skill (return of serve) is the balanced position and postural integrity (a concept explored in chapter 5) of the tennis player:

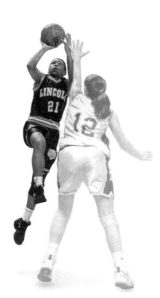

Spatial awareness

Sensory awareness

Produce energy to enable repeat performances

Control total-body movements to execute skills

Maintain joint alignment to preserve joint integrity

Exert necessary force in minimum time to execute desired skill

Dynamically change body position to ensure posture is always in position to exert or resist force

Control forces to external objects

Conserve energy through efficient mechanics

Maintain balance by controlling the centre of mass

**Figure 1.2** Physical qualities of successful athletes.

**Table 1.1**   Fundamental Movement Skill Themes

| Skill classification | Definition | Specific skill examples |
|---|---|---|
| Stability | Ability to sense a change in the relationship of the body parts that alter balance and to adjust rapidly and accurately for these changes with appropriate compensating movements. May be seen in static (stationary) or dynamic (active) situations in which gaining or maintaining balance is essential. | Posture, static balance, dynamic balance, falls and landings (forwards, backwards, sideways, on feet), rotation (forwards, backwards, sideways) |
| Multiplanar locomotion | Total-body movements in which the body is propelled from one point to another, usually with an upright posture, in a direction that has vertical, horizontal or rotational components. | Walking, running, vertical and horizontal jumping, hopping, galloping, skipping |
| Bilateral object control | Manipulation skills that use large body movements in which force is applied to or absorbed (received) from external objects. These skills are essential, not just as the basis for successfully playing many sports but also for allowing a child to interact purposefully with objects in the environment in a controlled manner. | Underarm and overarm throwing, catching, kicking, bouncing, striking static or moving objects, trapping (intercepting) |

- Stability: The centre of mass is within the base of support, creating a balanced position as the trunk rotates and providing a stable base from which power is generated. Ankle, knee, hip, spine and shoulder alignment provides a stable platform from which power can be generated and transferred.

- Movement: The feet move to the point at which the player can intercept the ball as it moves rapidly at a tangent to the player. The trunk rotates to generate rotational power, and the upper limbs orient themselves to align the racket with the ball.

- Object control: The muscles coordinate to manoeuvre each joint and apply forces through the body to the specific motor task of striking the ball with the racket (i.e., returning the serve) to place the opponent under pressure. The technique should transfer enough force to send the ball across the net under control so that the player can manipulate the direction of the ball, such as by imparting spin to the ball as required (topspin, backspin, and so on).

All athletic training programmes, regardless of the age, stage of development or level of performance to which they are targeted, require the correct balance of each movement skill element to develop successful

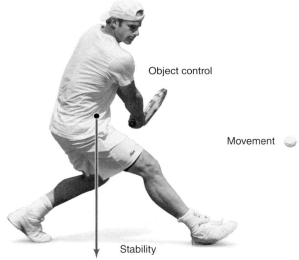

Object control

Movement

Stability

Gravity acting through the centre of mass

**Figure 1.3**   Foundation movement skills are the basis for the application of sport-specific skills.

performance. Experience tells us that the older the athlete is, the harder it becomes to teach these basic components. Therefore, these basics need to be the foundation for development and training programmes, rather than a remedial necessity at later stages of a person's sporting career.

Peak performance is hard to achieve. At elite levels, peak performance means being more committed, more focused, and more physically and mentally prepared than the competition. Indeed, the transfer of training to benefit performance has been one of the central challenges to coaching and physical education throughout the ages. Integrating all these training factors so that they come together to create optimal performance at the required time takes a great deal of planning and skill by the coach, as well as drive, dedication and skill on the part of the athlete.

Within a training progression, specific elements of the curriculum apply to all athletes, regardless of their age, experience or performance level. The athlete needs a balance of technical, tactical, mental, physical, and movement skills and lifestyle inputs. As illustrated in figure 1.4, if one of these aspects is out of synchronization with the other elements of the programme, the coach will not be able to optimize athletic performance in his or her charges.

Practitioners should note that this difference between training programme content is not simply related to athletes of different training and performance levels. Indeed, two people within the same training group may have similar performance levels but require very different training approaches to develop their performances. For example, one Olympic triple jumper may have a springy technique, whereas another may have a technique based on forceful impacts. Similarly, world-class tennis players such as Justine Henin or Serena Williams are vastly different physical athletes who need different training stimuli. This concept, known as differentiation, is explained in detail in chapter 7.

The aim of this book is to restructure some of the language of science and medicine and build bridges among the disciplines of coaching, teaching, sport science and sports medicine to answer some of these questions for practitioners, empowering them with tools for practical applications that will improve the athleticism of the athletes with whom they work.

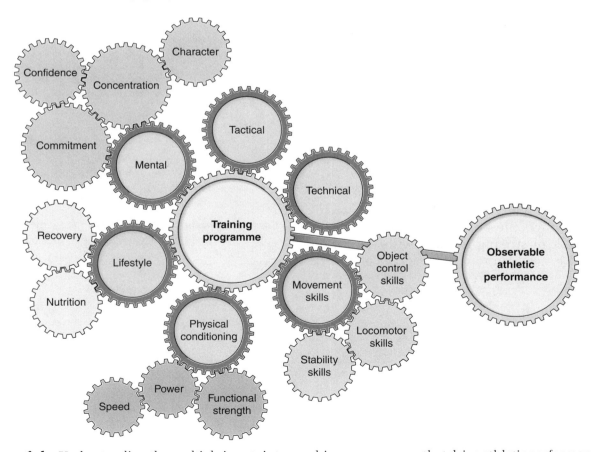

**Figure 1.4** Understanding the multiple inputs into coaching programmes that drive athletic performance.

# High Jump

The purpose of the high jump is to produce sufficient force to raise the centre of mass high enough so that the trunk and limbs can clear the bar. The high jump is a closed skill; the performance outcome is under the direct control of the athlete (a concept explored in more detail in chapter 7). The objective of the skill does not change regardless of whether the athlete is a novice (for example, athlete 1 in table 1.2) or a performance athlete (athlete 2). Similarly, all the elements of the coaching programme need to be included in the training plan devised for the athlete regardless of the performance level. As illustrated in table 1.2, however, the contents of each training element within the programme are very different, depending on the training age of the athlete and the performance objectives being sought. This idea applies whether the athlete is working in a singular event such as the high jump or in a dynamic and multiskilled context such as a team sport with many skill requirements.

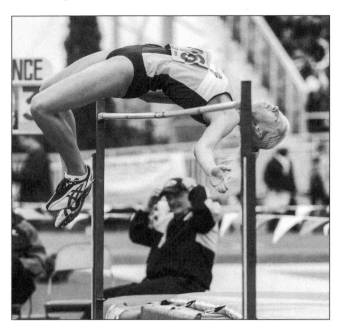

**Table 1.2**  Approaches to the Training Programme Inputs for Two Female High Jumpers With Different Training Histories

| Programme input | Athlete 1: age 12, learning to high jump | Athlete 2: age 22, personal best 1.80-metre high jump |
|---|---|---|
| Technical | Using jumping and movement into jumping combinations to move around a space<br>Moving body parts in an effective order to aid jumping height and efficiency; basic triple extension of hip, knee and ankle | Accelerating approach with an efficient and optimum conversion of horizontal velocity into vertical velocity<br>Actively drawing the heels towards the buttocks in midflight to cause the back to arch more, placing the centre of mass outside and below the body, enabling clearance of a greater height |
| Tactical | Choosing the height at which to enter the competition | Choosing the height at which to enter the competition and deciding when to pass on an attempt |
| Physical conditioning | Single- and double-support body-weight exercises (e.g., single-leg squats)<br>Multiple speed and power activities in multiple directions (e.g., jumping, hopping and skipping)<br>Range of small-sided games and multiple terrain activities to develop basic endurance | Advanced weightlifting programme of complex multimuscle, multijoint exercises with loaded extensions through ankles, knees and hips<br>Advanced plyometrics exercises incorporated into total jumping volume load |
| Movement skills | Maintaining centre of mass over base of support from dynamic situations<br>Foot and body positioning to enable the transitioning of horizontal movements into vertical movements | Advanced rotational gymnastics |

| Programme input | Athlete 1: age 12, learning to high jump | Athlete 2: age 22, personal best 1.80-metre high jump |
|---|---|---|
| Psychological skills | Clearly defined process and outcome goals to guide practice and competition | Consistent execution of well-defined (vivid) prejump mental rehearsal of the approach and jump<br>Highly developed focus and concentration on relevant cues (shutting out interference) throughout the competition |
| Lifestyle factors | Introduction to good nutritional practice; learning that healthy food is enjoyable<br>Maintaining a balance in sports, school and social life | Maximizing and taking full responsibility for personal approaches to nutrition, hydration, recovery and regeneration, lifestyle management<br>Strict liability for antidoping compliance |

# Physical Literacy

The key to successful coaching is to programme the appropriate coaching progressions to match sequential and developmental progressions. Planning for long-term performance development involves the logical and systematic sequencing of training factors to optimize specific training outcomes at predetermined times.[2] Accomplishing this requires the athlete to be able to achieve prerequisite movement (physical) competencies, which can be identified and monitored.

In short, the process is about developing physical education. This process can be related to the academic process of learning to write. A child first learns to write words (single skills, e.g., run, jump, throw, catch). Then he or she learns to put these words into sentences (linking skills, e.g., run and throw, run and jump, catch and run). By putting together sentences, a child can produce simple paragraphs (using the skills in a specific context, e.g., catch, pass and move into space). After a while, the child is able to produce increasingly complex and imaginative stories and adapt the use of prose to a range of academic and everyday challenges.

Sport performance is similar in that as increased physical capabilities develop, so does the child's ability to express the skills he or she has. The child becomes more physically literate! Similarly, an inability to execute simple skills can significantly reduce a child's confidence to take part in a range of sporting activities. This deficiency has massive implications for

a coach to recognize, because without confidence a child will not choose to participate in sporting tasks. Large implications for health and well-being will occur in the longer term. Indeed, research has shown that an inability to perform a simple catching task will reduce a child's confidence significantly enough for him or her to be deterred from taking part in over 40 different sporting activities![5]

Elite athletic performance always appears efficient, effective and effortless. People often wrongly assume that elite athletes and performers understand these movements and can perform them correctly, but evidence shows many cases to the contrary. For example, research has highlighted the frustration felt by young basketball players who are able to read the game and determine where a play will go but are unable to respond to these decisions because their motor skills are inadequate.[6] Coaches of elite gymnasts are often frustrated by the inability of their highly skilled performers to produce more force through the take-off in a vaulting action, a function of their learned inability (or rather their lack of developed running technique) to run efficiently and effectively in the approach to the springboard.

A well-developed movement vocabulary is associated with an ability to perform skills in a range of novel or dynamic situations. For example, a golfer may need to adapt to different types of golf courses (e.g., links courses in the United Kingdom versus championship courses in the United States). Similarly, tennis players who have grown up playing exclusively on clay courts may be extremely successful in tournaments played on clay or even on similar hard-court surfaces, but they are often not able to respond well to the fast and low bounces of grass-court surfaces.

Those without a well-developed movement vocabulary often develop movement limitations or compensations. These deficiencies are explored in more detail throughout the book, but at a conceptual level the coach should appreciate that the limitations should not be overlooked, or, more seriously still, should not be reinforced by a programme that allows—or does not challenge—inappropriate technique. Movement limitations lead to imbalances in muscle patterning, which can also lead to movement compensations. These in turn can distort motor learning, body awareness and movement mechanics. Besides reducing the efficiency of the movement, these movement patterns can also lead to increased risk of injury.

Many injuries in sport can be attributed to incorrect mechanics, joint positions or movement patterns within the athlete. For example, running at top speed and repeatedly contacting the ground with the foot in the wrong place (toe pointing downwards, as illustrated in figure 1.5) may lead to an increased incidence of hamstring or adductor injury because these muscle groups compensate for the nonactivation of other muscles and perform tasks (express forces at inappropriate times in the movement) for which they have not evolved.

Developing appropriate motor patterning requires the development of a progressive curriculum that has the appropriate rate of challenge and variance in stimulation to promote learning (a concept explored in detail in chapter 7). These progressions can take many weeks, months or even years, and they should not be cut short or circumvented to achieve performance outcomes in the short term. The ability to execute basic, skilled athletic techniques at optimum speed and under pressure with power and precision is key to successful physical performances.

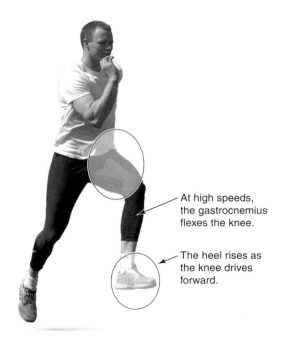

At high speeds, the gastrocnemius flexes the knee.

The heel rises as the knee drives forward.

Ankle dorsiflexion: As the stiff foot hits the ground, ground reaction and internal forces from the gluteals drive the centre of mass forward.

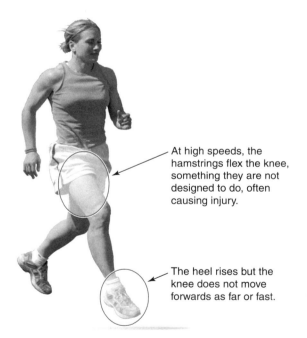

At high speeds, the hamstrings flex the knee, something they are not designed to do, often causing injury.

The heel rises but the knee does not move forwards as far or fast.

Ankle plantarflexion: As the pointed foot hits the ground toe first, the athlete lowers to the ball of the foot. Forces are absorbed (lost). The athlete has a longer ground contact time. The athlete's hips drop then rise again as the hip flexors drive the centre of mass forward.

**Figure 1.5**   Poor movement skills can lead to movement compensations that might increase the risk of injury.

As the contents of the following chapters will outline, these competencies are progressive in nature, building on prerequisite physio-mechanical capabilities. Sound movements enable the athlete's posture to be always in a position to withstand and exert optimum forces against both internal (muscles) and, more important, external forces (such as gravity and potentially contact with opponents).

When performance demands exceed the movement capabilities of the athlete, performance suffers and injuries occur more often. In these instances, a remedial programme is required to both rehabilitate the athlete and eradicate the cause of the injury problem. Not surprisingly, most rehabilitation programmes are based on motor patterning and joint positioning through a movement range.

Strength and conditioning, or athletic development programmes as they should more properly be called, should positively influence the physical development of athletes. Athletic development is a key term to understand. It differentiates the practitioner's role from simply getting the athlete stronger or fitter (i.e., having more endurance) into a role that emphasizes increasing the functional capacity of the athlete's motor system. The term *functional* has been misplaced in many contexts; it should not mean that anything else is dysfunctional by literal translation. The term should relate to using progressive methodologies (as exemplified in figure 1.6 and discussed in chapter 10) that develop the athlete's ability to

- control posture dynamically to create efficient movement patterns throughout the kinetic chain,
- exert and resist forces through a controlled posture,
- increase the magnitude of these forces,
- reduce the time taken to exert high-magnitude forces and

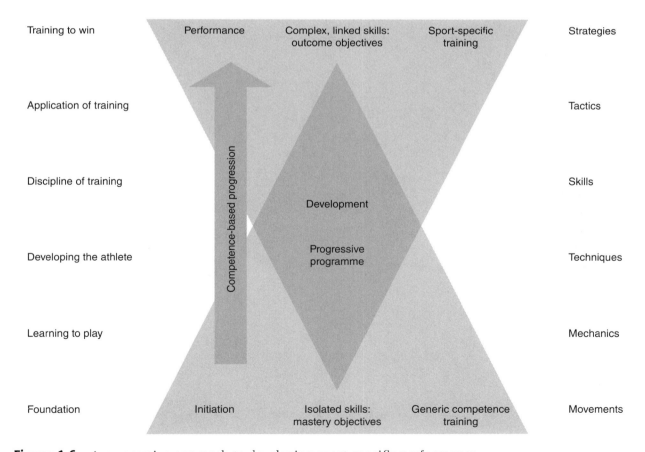

**Figure 1.6**  A progressive approach to developing sport-specific performance.

- produce the required forces through mechanically efficient sport-specific techniques.

All this involves developing the athlete's motor system: the brain (as the executive director of the athlete's movement programme); the spinal cord and the motor nerves, which transfer chemical signals from the brain to the muscles; the muscles themselves that contract to exert a pulling force; and the cardiorespiratory system, which enables ATP to be produced to fuel the work undertaken within the body.

Many resources have presented exercise regimes for people to follow. Conceptually, however, exercise is a doing thing; the focus is usually on the outcome (Did you lift more? Did you run faster?).

Conversely, the athletic development programme should focus on training movements, and movements are a feeling thing (Where was the bar relative to your body when you

lifted it? What did your foot do when it left the floor that enabled you to run faster?), and this cannot be developed without a focus on all aspects of the motor system.

Therefore, the motor system should be considered a prime focus for practitioners seeking to improve the performances of athletes. Indeed, as shown in figure 1.7, the aim of any physical development programme is to improve the capacity of the athlete's motor (movement) system to perform work. This may mean being able to do more work (faster, stronger, longer) or being able to work more efficiently (i.e., do the same amount of work for less energy cost). Efficient movement is a manifestation of an athlete's ability to exert and control forces. Doing this requires a focus on developing movement skills before, during and after a focus on performance.

To have a positive influence on skills, the practitioner needs to understand how to

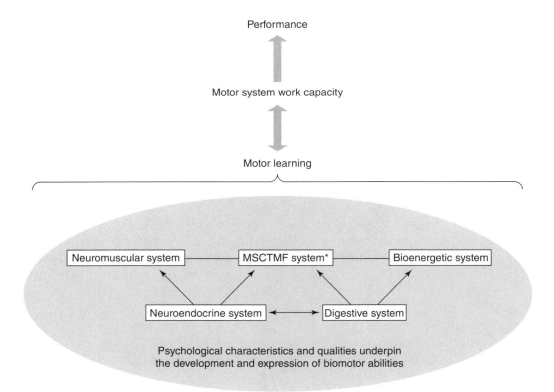

* The integrated system which connects muscles with the skeleton (musculoskeletal) with connective tissue, supported in the energetic transfer by myofascial tissue and the system of locomotive slings which surrounds the musculoskeletal system

**Figure 1.7**    The motor system comprises a number of component systems that can be manipulated to enhance performance.

develop an athlete's neuromuscular system as a primary source of motor capacity improvement. The athlete will then be able to activate motor units more effectively (see chapter 2) within and between muscles to perform mechanical work in a coordinated manner. The number of motor units, the sequencing of the nervous stimulus to fire motor units in particular sequences and the phasic recruitment and coordination of different muscles during an action can all be enhanced by neuromuscular system improvement.

Similarly, the transmission of forces through the posture relies on the fact that muscles are connected to bones through connective tissues that wrap around, and run within, the muscles. An activated muscle is able to exert a force on the bones attached to it by an inelastic tendon, and this force can be transmitted through the postural chain to result in movement. The body has other connective tissues, such as the fascial slings (for example, the thoracolumbar fascia around the trunk and back, and the iliotibial band in the thigh), that enable groups of muscles that may not be *structurally* linked but which are *functionally* linked to have a tissue connection that is relatively continuous. This enables efficient and effective energy and force transfer through a linked system.

Other chapters look at how to evaluate and coach specific movement competencies themselves and provide a progressive curriculum to develop them. Before this is considered, an understanding of how the biomotor abilities combine to contribute to performance is important, because this knowledge enables an appreciation of the movement qualities and the way they can be advanced. Some understanding of anatomy, physiology and biomechanics is needed here.

Anatomy and physiology are the areas of study that combine to provide an understanding of the physical factors contributing to performance. Anatomy relates to the structure and organization of the body, whereas sport physiology is concerned with how the body functions and responds to the demands of the environment, training and competition. Biomechanics explores the laws of mechanics as applied to biological systems, in this case in the context of gaining a greater understanding of athletic performance.

Many sport science programmes have attempted to explore these subject areas as discreet entities. The best programmes, however, are led by those who look at the problem rather than the discipline, realizing that making movements more efficient ultimately will spare energy so that more work can be done for the same energy cost or the same work can be done for less energy cost.

In essence, a working knowledge of an athlete's anatomy, biomechanical efficiencies and physiological processes underlying exercise responses allows those working with athletes (coaches, programme directors, support staff and so on) to become better at evaluating the physical competencies, capacities and potential responses of an athlete. This knowledge will assist in the planning and implementation of improved training programmes that link objectives to the development of physical qualities in young athletes, resulting in higher quality preparation either through to high-performance sporting excellence or more commonly for a lifetime of participation in sport.

As this book will illustrate, the human body is a highly evolved and complex organism that will adopt and adapt to the demands of its environment. Dynamic changes will occur in all systems of the body to respond to the tasks demanded of it. The body is able to produce adaptive movements in response to challenges of the situation. The working movements of the body are produced by a system of linkages (muscular–skeletal attachments and articulations) that we refer to as the kinetic chain. Like any chain, a series of linkages forms the connective structure, and, like any series of attachments, the weak point in the chain will limit the functional capacity of the structure.

The articulations within the body change repeatedly with respect to their orientation to each other. The relative angles between joints change simultaneously and in combination, enabling the human body to transfer rotational joint movements to linear or angular movements. The practitioner's role is to guide adaptations within the kinetic chain in a positive manner, that is, to develop the athlete's capacity towards efficiently meeting the challenges of sporting situations. For athletic development aspects (physical conditioning and movement skill) of the athlete's training, programme variables must be manipulated to achieve a positive adaptation of the motor system to undertake physical work.

# Human Adaptation to the Environment

A training programme is a means through which a coach organizes a process of planned exposure to training workloads by manipulating mode, volume and intensity of the training stimuli.[2]

The ability of the human organism to recognize and adapt to an environmental challenge of increasing demand (figure 1.8) is a fundamental principle that needs to be recognized in the development of basic movement skills. Just as an athlete can adapt positively to a well-presented training load, the body can also maladapt to an inappropriate training load or stimulus. For example, as illustrated in figure 1.5, poor movement patterns that are not corrected can become learned maladaptations and lead to movement compensations and injury problems later in an athlete's career.

Similarly, excessive stimuli without any variation may lead to adapted imbalances within the athlete. Conversely, excessive variation without any period of consolidated learning will mean that the athlete is unable to adapt. Both of these potential maladaptations will lead to a decrease in the observable performance or a slowed rate of learning and improvement. Short-term or chronic exposure to a stimulus of excessive volume or intensity (volume × intensity = volume load) may mean that the stressor is not one that the body can tolerate or adapt to, and injury will occur.

Training adaptations are the sum of transformations brought about by repeated exposures

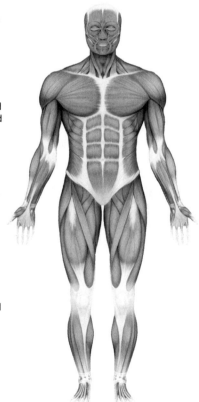

Neuro-transmitters have a threshold effect, meaning a muscle fibre is either contracted or not; there is no partial contraction of a motor unit. Multiple motor units can be contracted depending on the work required to be done.

The axial skeleton (trunk) is connected to the appendicular skeleton (limbs) via muscles and connective tissues that cross the shoulder and pelvic girdles.

A muscular and connective tissue cube of support increases pressure around organs mostly unprotected by skeletal structures.

Many first-class levers in the body act as pulleys to change direction of forces. For example, the line of pull of the quadriceps is altered by the action of the patella on the condylar groove of the femur.

Connective tissue forms a communication and energy transfer channel through the body.

When the ankle plantarflexes, the gastrocsoleus muscle complex, which runs in series with the Achilles tendon, connecting to the calcaneous, acts as a force multiplier, an example of a second-class lever system.

The body will adapt positioning to a continuously-present stimulus.

Good posture shows many examples of first-class levers. For example, the antagonistic arrangement of muscles acts to simultaneously balance forces around a joint.

The biceps brachii is an example of a biarticular muscle.

The flexed arm is an example of a third-class lever. A large force is applied to gain mechanical advantage in terms of increased speed of motion.

All major muscles cross more than one joint.

Muscle fibres run into connective tissue that combines into a common tendon attachment, enabling the efficient transfer of forces and energy from the muscle to the skeleton.

Skeletal muscle is striated. The fibres are angled to influence the function.

**Figure 1.8**   The evolved athletic qualities of the human kinetic chain.

to stimuli.[2] Adaptations may occur through informal play, deliberate practice or repeated exposure to specific training events. In seeking to take athletes (regardless of stage of development or experience) from where they are to where they have never been (the role of any coaching or personal development programme), the practitioner must recognize what biomotor ability needs to be influenced and then provide the relevant training stimulus to cause positive adaptation.

# Development of the Motor System

It takes many years of training to be world-class at anything. A systematic approach to developing athletes over a longer term would ensure that the athletes and those involved in programme delivery and development are equipped with the knowledge and skills needed to maximize the potential of athletes at the appropriate stages of their development through appropriately structured and monitored programmes. As chapter 3 details, these programmes should match periods in the developmental life of a young person with training methods that will maximize the effects of this training.[7]

If long-term adaptation in the motor capacity of an athlete is the longer-term goal, then it is important to consider how the systems that underpin the biomotor abilities (the neuromuscular, musculoskeletal, bioenergetic and neuroendocrine systems) develop. Those equipped with the necessary knowledge and skills to structure and monitor training programmes that match the anatomical and physiological development processes of athletes will be able to maximize their potential.

Conversely, because children show considerable and important differences in their bodily responses to exercise (compared with adults), coaches should be aware of the more important differences to avoid imposing undue physical stress on their young charges. In its simplest form, delivery of the athlete development programme requires relating the structure and nature of training to the performer's

developmental pathway so that he or she is doing the right thing at the right time for long-term, not necessarily immediate, development. This concept underpins almost all the physical and psychosocial models of athlete development that have underpinned sport development programmes in recent years.[8]

Although not all sport programmes are aimed at children, all are based on developing someone who was once a child. Later chapters in this book discuss the concept of profiling athletes based on their physical competencies. But if the process of how the child (or athlete) develops can be better understood, practitioners can arguably better understand how the end product is (or could be) evaluated.

Development, or coaching, of the athlete should reflect an inclusive process that encourages people to get involved in lifelong physical activity. The process should connect and integrate generic movement (physical) education programmes with specific sport preparation programmes (as identified in figure 1.6). Indeed, the aim of such activities should be child (athlete) centred, based on taking an individual and educational approach, and based on a desire to make a long-term difference to the participants. This objective will be reflected in the programmes that are delivered. This understanding applies not only to the physical aspects of the programme development but also to all areas of delivery. For example, executing many core skills within a sport requires physical size, strength or decision-making ability.

A cursory observational analysis of coaching practices and associated resources reveals that many sport programmes focus on ways in which the same sport-specific skills are delivered and developed with players across the full spectrum of participation (from the playground to the podium). Chapters 7 through 11 look at how progression can be achieved within many movement skills. But delivering the same skills across all age ranges in the same way is developmentally inappropriate, and coming to that understanding is a big step forward.

All human development is facilitated and constrained by an interactive dynamic of biological, psychological and sociological factors that change as children grow older. Participation motives, for example, likely change over time. Younger children seek excitement and pleasure, whereas older children may strive for achievement and satisfaction. As chapters 2 and 3 show, children's skeletal, muscular and nervous systems develop at different rates throughout childhood. The variance in rate of development has significant implications for each individual child's physical development and, consequently, his or her sporting performance and improvement.

Therefore, each child's perceptions of getting better will have associated psychological implications that need to be monitored and positively influenced. Further, this biological development will have obvious connotations for children's psychomotor development. That is, each child's capacity to demonstrate the movement skills fundamental to sport participation (e.g., balancing, travelling, controlling objects) will vary according to the maturity of his or her physical makeup. Hence, because developing these psychomotor behaviours is critical to all children, whether they progress to elite-level sport or lifelong participation, consideration should be given to each child's individual needs. These needs guide the development and delivery of movement and sport-skill programmes.

The developmental process towards performance-based training therefore needs to reflect individual needs. An organized and progressive approach should be used to achieve optimal training, competition and recovery throughout an athlete's career. The recognition that the developmental process takes many years and is based on the interplay of a number of components is a core feature of many models of athlete development that have been proposed in recent years.[8] Many people in sport have pointed out that much of what makes up many of these approaches is not new. Most of the research on which it is based is widely accepted and has been used to underpin quality physical education teaching and coaching practice for many years.

This observation may seem like common sense, but as with many truths, until it is stated, it is apparently less obvious. In addition, we need to reflect on whether common sense is actually common practice. The obvious point in this case is that any person who commences a sport or physical activity programme, regardless of performance level, has different needs and capabilities for training than someone who has been doing it longer. This contention is true no matter what age an athlete comes into a sport.

One commonality about all successful systems of athlete development is that they acknowledge that athlete development is not, in reality, a simple linear and staged process because events in each person's life will affect *his or her* rate of progress. For this reason, many peaks and troughs will occur along the way, so the long-term process will appear chaotic. The role of the skilled practitioner is to manage the athlete through this transitional and chaotic process to optimize the athlete's potential.

In the athletic development context, the practitioner must realize that these markers of progress take place within different environments and that various influencing agents need to be considered when planning the athlete's programmes. These transitions mark important physical, social, emotional and experiential opportunities for the athlete. The practitioner must also realize that the athlete will progress through these transitions, or stages of development (although some of these may be definite stages as defined by social or programme delivery contexts).

For example, the progression towards puberty is a gradual process, as is the transition away from being reliant on parents. In contrast, academic domains are clearly defined, in that a child is either in the elementary or secondary school system. Learning in the early stages is very much about associating outcomes with a stimulus or reward. This type of learning gradually progresses towards behaviour choices being determined by conscious decisions made before a logical process of sequencing specific behaviours within specific environments becomes apparent.

Coaches should also consider the different types of ages of athletes when planning a programme. The age of athletes needs to be considered in terms of years since birth, developmental age (children mature at different rates) and the number of years they have been training, either in athletics or in another sport.

In terms of the physical conditioning of a child, the biological age is the most important consideration. In terms of applied movement skill development, however, the athlete's training age is the predominant consideration. The biological age determines the anatomical and physiological limitations within which the programme should be developed, whereas the training age may provide an indicator of the movement experiences of a child (i.e., his or her potential physical competence). Regardless of a child's biological development and potential readiness for certain training stimuli, he or she should not be progressed beyond movement competency in executing a task for a wide variety of performance-enhancing and injury-reducing factors that will become clear throughout this book.

For example, as shown in table 1.3, a child who is an early developer may be anatomically and physiologically more able to tolerate certain training intensities but may (depending on the programmes he or she has experienced) have a smaller movement vocabulary than a child who is less biologically mature but who has more experience within a range of sports.

This concept is important when working with athletes of all ages, not simply children. For example, a 33-year-old professional soccer player retires and wishes to take up recreational marathon running because of its health benefits and competitive challenge. He may have a 25-year training age within soccer but 0 years in distance running. But his sporting training age (indicative of his ability to tolerate the imposition of a reasonable training volume load) may be considered in excess of 10 years for the coach who is beginning to work with the athlete. Compare this person with a 20-year-old who wishes to take up recreational distance running (maybe within the same running club) having not done any real physical exercise since leaving grade school 4 years previously, when he took part in physical education classes. The 20-year-old's biological age is lower and his training age may be much closer to 4 years than anything else (we can consider the accrued experiences of school physical education, but many of those gains will have been reversed by time away from physical activity).

Similarly, a coach may inherit a physically gifted triple jumper who is 14 years old and can triple jump 13 metres after 3 years of specific training. Although the performance potential of the athlete may be in a bracket with those who have been jumping for 10 years, the person should not use the same training programme as those advanced athletes, because his training age and background will not enable him to have sufficient physical experiences to cope with the imposed training volume load. In short, he would be highly likely to overtrain quickly and be at risk of injury. In this instance, the coach would recognize and nurture the performance potential of the athlete (recognized in technical and tactical progressions, but not with high-volume loading). The emphasis in conditioning training would be on developing a significant base to cope with the imposition of a higher training volume at later stages.

# Understanding Biological Age

A central theme of effective training systems is that children do not develop at even rates throughout their development. Some of these changes are obvious and easy to measure. Others are less visible and require some consideration if a child's potential is to flourish rather than be threatened by inappropriate training volumes or intensities.

**Table 1.3**  Maturation in Children: Hypothetical Comparison of Two Children

|  | Child 1 (years) | Child 2 (years) |
| --- | --- | --- |
| Chronological age | 13 | 13 |
| Biological age | 11 | 16 |
| Developmental age | 13 | 12 |
| Training age | 5 | 3 |

Understanding the development of the motor system is important if programmes and practices are to be modified to match the maturation of the participant children and maximize the opportunities that coaching sessions present them. This knowledge, when linked with some understanding of the physiological, social and behavioural development aspects of the child, will guide the choice of programme objectives that provide efficient and effective athletic development, regardless of the age and experience of the athlete.

Incorporating such knowledge into the development process enables the identification of practices and areas for targeted development and times in a child's life when training volume needs to be adapted to avoid hindering physio-mechanical development. How these generalized guidelines are adapted and incorporated into individualized delivery is a key theme within successful athletic development programmes.

As many researchers have identified, all young people follow the same basic pattern of growth from infancy through adolescence, but significant individual differences occur in both the timing and magnitude of the change in structure. These differences are particularly evident after puberty: the biological process of physical transition from childhood to adulthood, marked by the person reaching sexual maturation. This knowledge also enables practitioners to counter many of the pop-science tales that abound within sport, based on conjecture rather than empirical evidence. Some of these are addressed in the following chapters.

Note that many other important factors, such as the social and psychological development of the child, may be incorporated into specific programme designs. Where possible, these factors will be incorporated, but fully exploring these ideas in this text is impossible.

In the following chapters, the biomotor abilities and the developmental process that the motor system follows will be explored, encompassing the principle that people do not develop at the same uniform rate. The potential implications for this development within a coaching and especially athletic development context will also be presented. Ideas for how growth and development can be monitored will also be explored, thus presenting the best possible opportunity to influence coaching practice relative to the physical and movement skill development of the athlete.

## Summary

This chapter has introduced and positioned the importance of two foundational principles that should govern the practice of those involved in athletic development programmes for athletes at any level. These principles will continue to be central tenants in the rest of the book.

First, to achieve a level of progression in a physical task, mastery of prerequisite skills is important. This point builds on the notion of competency; the athlete should be able to execute the physical task properly.

The second major proposition is that the training stimulus provided to athletes to progress their level of competency requires knowledge of both how to progress the task (from a technical perspective) and how the athletes' motor systems will best respond to the stimulus at a given stage of biological development and level of training experience.

The following chapters address knowledge relevant to understanding how the body adapts with growth and to specific training stimuli. This topic will be linked to information about how important it is for the athlete to be able to move effectively in a sporting context and how this can be assessed to guide programme development. Chapters 8 through 10 discuss the progressive development of competence by focussing on some of the foundational movement qualities highlighted in this chapter as being the cornerstone of athletic movements: the ability to run, jump (linked with specialized rebound training methods known as plyometrics) and functionally exert forces. The book concludes by bringing all this information together into a series of case studies. The reader can view the reality of athlete programme development in context and reflect on the information presented throughout the book to determine whether understanding of the material reflects the detail presented in the practical application.

# CHAPTER 2

# Understanding Biomotor Abilities

The skeleton comprises bones and joints, which provide a framework and leverage for the body. But the joints cannot provide movement on their own. All functions of the body involving movement (or any unsupported action, such as standing) require muscle activity. Muscle action occurs because muscles change chemical energy into mechanical energy to generate force, perform work and produce movement.

The integrated action of the muscles, bones and joints enables the body to move, and skeletal muscle contractions in the body (within and between body segments) enable the body to stabilize in a number of static or dynamic situations. This interaction is complex. The human body is a multisegmented system, which means that movement in one segment (for example, the trunk) can influence all the other segments of the body. Movement requires a coordinated interaction throughout the kinetic chain. This movement is enabled by the various fascial slings and nervous system components of the body.

Skeletal muscle is so called because it is attached to bones and moves parts of the skeleton. Skeletal tissue is also called striate because of its alternating light and dark bands (a function of its contractile structure). Of more importance to the athletic development professional, skeletal muscle is known as voluntary muscle tissue, because it has a regulatory mechanism that means it can be made to contract under conscious control.

Each muscle group has a series of unique biomechanical characteristics (force, velocity and range of movement) that require coordination throughout the multijoint, multimuscle system to produce a common movement function. These characteristics will be explored in more detail from chapter 5 onwards. The executive control structure governing the movement process is within the brain. Movement is a feeling thing, a coordinated musculoskeletal response to the actions of the sensory and motor nervous systems (figure 2.1).

To understand the regulation of human movement, the practitioner needs a working understanding of the central nervous system and the motor unit as an operational structure within the body. This topic will be explained within this chapter. This knowledge leads to the realization that, if the central nervous system has a regulatory function in muscle action and therefore movements, athletes should be training the central nervous system to produce movement more effectively.

A fundamental tenant of developing athletes, then, is to train movements, not muscles. This approach differs widely from that of other similar industries, in which the aesthetic size and quality of muscle may be an objective. Developing the central nervous system is the cornerstone to the development of athletic movement qualities. Not surprisingly, this concept also forms the basis for rehabilitation (movement function re-education) programmes as well.

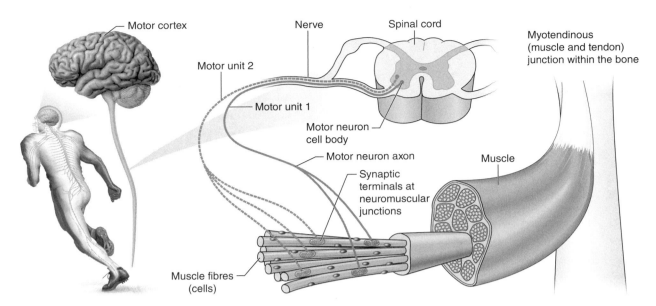

**Figure 2.1**   Movement is a brain thing! The central nervous system regulates muscular responses to the environment at any one time.

As with any programme objective, in educating (or training) the central nervous system, practitioners are seeking to move it from where it is (in terms of capabilities) to where it has never been. Effective training leads to improved physical abilities, skilled actions and movement capabilities through changes in the organism. This change occurs not only in the processes that cause movements to occur but also to the senses that detect the need for the movements to be initiated in the first place. To study this dynamic system is an extensive process.[1] The major considerations and their application to training development are outlined in this chapter.

## Musculoskeletal System

The skeletal and muscular systems work together to produce movement. Collectively, they are referred to as the musculoskeletal system. For a basic review of the major functions of each of these systems, see Kenney et al.[2]

As its name suggests, skeletal muscle anchors to bones and is responsible for movement and control of the skeleton. In mechanics, form dictates function. Therefore, studying the form (structure and shape) of the muscle leads to a greater understanding of how it functions and how training can influence it.

## Form and Function of Skeletal Muscle

Skeletal muscles attach to bone at either end of the muscle. Connective tissue runs throughout the collection of individual muscle fibres that come together to make a muscle. This connective tissue forms the tendons, which join muscle to bone. The myotendinous junction enables a pulling force to be created between the bones (i.e., if a muscle attaches to different bones at each of its ends, the muscle can exert a pull between bones, creating movement of one bone relative to the other).

This concept is simple when viewed in isolation. To illustrate this point, let's look at the biceps brachii, which attaches to the scapula and the humerus (upper arm bone) at one end and the ulna and radius bones of the forearm at the other end (figure 2.2a). With the shoulder fixed, contraction in the biceps brachii moves the hand towards the shoulder, and the elbow flexes (figure 2.2b); the ulna and radius are moved relative to the humerus. If the hands are fixed (for example, when hanging from a bar in a chin-up) and the biceps are contracted, the humerus is moved closer to the ulna and radius, again through elbow flexion (figure 2.2c).

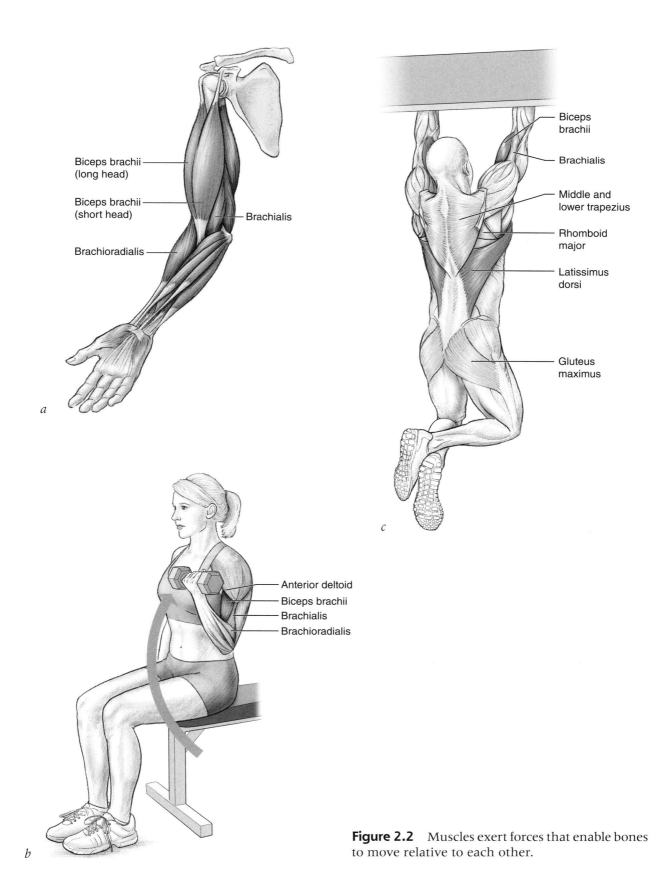

Biceps brachii
(long head)

Biceps brachii
(short head)

Brachioradialis

Brachialis

*a*

Anterior deltoid
Biceps brachii
Brachialis
Brachioradialis

*b*

Biceps
brachii

Brachialis

Middle and
lower trapezius

Rhomboid
major

Latissimus
dorsi

Gluteus
maximus

*c*

**Figure 2.2** Muscles exert forces that enable bones to move relative to each other.

Although this explanation is designed to illustrate how bones move relative to each other, the example is oversimplified. Movement doesn't really occur as an isolated action; for example, executing a chin-up requires the work of many muscles. Completely understanding movement means accepting that muscle actions rarely occur in isolation. A complex interaction between muscles exerting differential forces on bones produces the phenomenon that we observe as movement.

For example, to flex (bend) the arm at the elbow from a normal carrying position (assuming a relatively heavy mass) to a position in which the palm of the hand faces the shoulder joint at full flexion, the primary force is created by contracting the biceps brachii and the brachialis, with assistance from the brachioradialis as resistance increases. In this action, the primary stabilizer of the elbow joint is the anconeus. The position of the shoulder—the humeral head is in position against the glenoid fossa of the clavicle—is fixed by contraction of the rotator cuff muscles (infraspinatus, teres minor, subscapularis and supraspinatus). The triceps brachii (the primary extensor muscle of the elbow) also acts as a synergist to fix the position of the humerus relative to the shoulder (figure 2.3).[3]

Another example of how antagonistic muscle groups work in synchronization to bring about coordinated movement can be seen in the vertical jump. The practical considerations for developing and programming this activity are explored in detail in chapter 9.

The vertical jump involves the near simultaneous extension of the hip, knee and ankle joints from the flexed starting position at the beginning of the vertical component of the action (figure 2.4a). The prime extensor group for the knee is the quadriceps muscle group: vastus medialis, vastus intermedius, vastus lateralis and rectus femoris. Within this group, the rectus femoris crosses both the hip

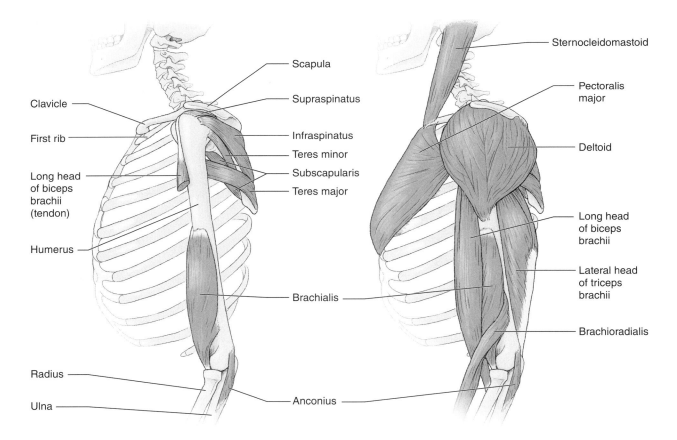

**Figure 2.3**    Muscle arrangement around the glenohumeral (shoulder) joint.

and knee joint and is responsible for flexion of the hip in standing (i.e., raising the femur until it is perpendicular to the floor) as well as extension of the knee. The conjoined muscles of the iliopsoas are also powerful hip flexors that bring the upper body forward when the feet are on the floor.

Therefore, if the desired hip extension is to occur, the hamstrings (biceps femoris, semi-membranosus and semitendinosus) and the gluteus maximus must concentrically contract to extend the hip joint from the leg to counter the hip-flexing actions of the rectus femoris and iliopsoas. This action brings the trunk into an upright position as the hip extends forcibly at the same time as the knee and ankle (figure 2.4b). The resultant force enables the body to leave the floor (figure 2.4c). The gluteus medius and gluteus minimus stabilize the hip joint in this action.

Note that the respective movements of the joints and the relative positioning of the bones to each other throughout the actions bring about the muscle activation patterns. This observation reinforces a fundamental training philosophy emphasized throughout this book: When athletic development programmes emphasize that technique is based on placing the joints in the right positions by developing

the correct movements, muscles are trained functionally. In other words, train movements, not muscles!

A principle central to this idea is that the arrangement (positioning) of the joints directly influences the functioning of the muscles, a concept explained by the gross structure of the muscles themselves (figure 2.5).

## Musculoskeletal System Responses to Training

Although many of the architectural features (for example, limb length) of the musculoskeletal system are not influenced by training, two specific adaptations can be targeted. The first is related in large part to the neuromuscular system in that it involves learning correct technique. Correct technique places the joints in the correct positions and moves them in the correct sequence to optimize the anatomical arrangement of the muscles.

Correct technique means that the correct muscles (i.e., those muscles that have evolved to best undertake this task) will be recruited and in position to perform the work required (i.e., to cause or assist in the motion of the joint). As this book continuously highlights, because joint position determines muscle function,

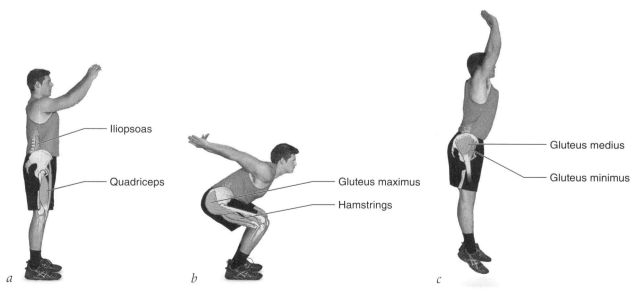

**Figure 2.4** Coordinated muscle actions in a vertical countermovement jump: *(a)* starting position; *(b)* hip, knee and ankle extend; *(c)* jump.

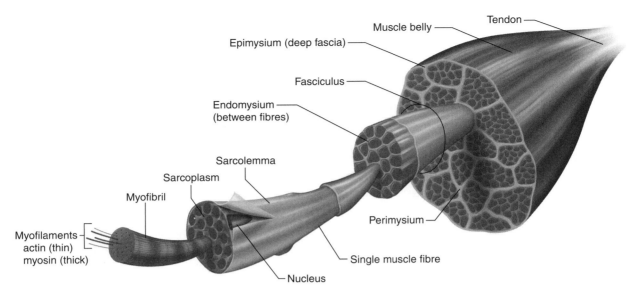

**Figure 2.5** Gross structure of muscle. The tendon connects to the bone.

an athletic development programme should emphasize the correct movement technique (dynamic joint positioning) to develop muscles.

The second training response is specific to the application of a resistive load. This response is an increase in the cross-sectional area of the muscle, or hypertrophy. Although the specific mechanisms for how this occurs are often debated,[3] an increase in muscle size is clearly caused by the addition of myofibrils (contractile proteins) to the muscle fibre. This result can be seen as advantageous to the athlete because muscle cross-sectional area is directly proportional to the maximum force-generating capability of the muscle.[4] A more detailed exploration of the concept of necessary (or functional) hypertrophy can be found in chapter 3.

## Neuromuscular System

Although skeletal muscle has a number of qualities, it has only one action. It can contract to cause or resist a force in response to a command from the central nervous system (formed by the brain and spinal column). The executive control structure governing the movement process is within the brain.

It has been established that movement is a feeling thing, a coordinated response to the actions of the sensory and motor nervous systems. Therefore, to develop effective movements, it is necessary to understand the role of the central nervous system and the motor unit structure in regulating human movement (figure 2.6).

If the central nervous system has a regulatory function in muscle action, and therefore movements, those involved in athletic development should be educating (training) the central nervous system to produce movement more effectively. This goal differentiates the athletic development professional from related professionals who have other objectives related to body sculpting purely for aesthetic reasons.

Anyone who is involved in the analysis and development of sporting performances should realize that the performer who can execute the most forceful skills usually wins; that is, the strongest and fastest prevails! Another important understanding is that the production and increased application of forces is the result of neuromuscular processes. In 1687, Isaac Newton wrote that the brain governed movement. Therefore, the fundamental principle of strength training is more than 400 years old. All muscle actions are initiated by neural stimulation, and therefore training (teaching) the neuromuscular system is the first object of the athletic development coach.

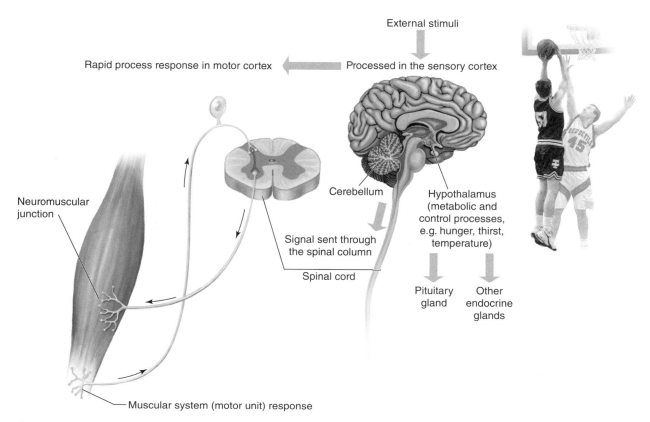

**Figure 2.6**   Interaction between the central nervous system and muscular and endocrine control.

Motor learning is the process of programming the brain and the central nervous system to undertake specific movement tasks under various complex conditions in terms of environmental demand. For example, consider shooting at goal in a game of soccer. A player can develop this technique by shooting at a goal in a practice context with no fatigue. Skill (which can be considered the forceful application of technique under pressure) can be better developed if the player shoots at a goal when pressured by a defender. Learning is tested even more fully if the player shoots at a goal while being pressured by a defender in the last few minutes of an exhausting game of high importance.

Functional application relating to the principles of motor learning and progression is a key theme for building any programme or curriculum. This topic is explored in more detail in chapter 7.

The central nervous system is responsible for processing information received from the environment (through the sensory cortex) and commanding a response from the rest of the body. This book focuses on movement responses involving a signal from the motor cortex, but the response could equally be a metabolic one (e.g., increased rate of respiration, increased heart rate or temperature regulation). These signals would be processed through the hypothalamus, which regulates primary hormonal responses as well as the autonomic nervous system (ANS). The ANS is largely responsible for involuntary systems that control normal functions, such as making the heart beat, which fortunately can't be regulated by voluntary thought processes!

As with all organs in the body, the brain develops progressively and in response to its environment. At times of peak growth, or transition in circumstances, the brain undertakes a rewiring process, whereby neural pathways that are well used and developed are retained and promoted, whereas those that are less needed in the present will be pruned or shut down to enable the release of brain capacity.

This phenomenon is important for anyone working with children to understand, because an inappropriate focus on highly specialized movements at too early a stage in an athlete's development may shut down neural pathways that could be important at a later stage of development, particularly in chaotic and multidirectional sports such as soccer, American football and basketball.

## Motor Units and Movement

The collective term for a motor neuron and all the muscle fibres that it innervates is a *motor unit* (figure 2.7). One motor neuron can make contact with an average of 150 muscle fibres. When stimulated, one motor unit will cause all the muscle fibres it connects with to contract. Remember that skeletal muscle is either activated (contracted) or not.

Muscles that control precise movements have one motor unit supplying small numbers of fibres, maybe as few as 2 or 3. Muscles responsible for powerful, gross movements (for example, a quadriceps muscle) have one motor unit supplying approximately 2,000 muscle fibres.

A motor neuron (nerve) delivers an electrical stimulus from the central nervous system to a muscle fibre, a cell within the muscle, which causes the fibre to contract. Note that the nerve stimulus is to the muscle fibre, not the whole muscle. Therefore, a percentage of fibres within a muscle can be activated, not necessarily the whole muscle. Motor units within a muscle fasciculus (see figure 2.5) can be differentially recruited according to the demand of the task; the greater the level of force required, the larger the number of motor units activated.

Messages are transferred along neural pathways through a motor action potential, a wave of depolarization (action potential) that is propagated from the central nervous system along the axon of the nerve.

The frequency of motor action potentials (MAPs) greatly influences the activation of motor units. The greater the frequency with which the motor action potential arrives at the motor end plate, the greater the force of contraction stimulated within both the motor unit and the muscle as a whole. Therefore, the more MAPs that are sent through the central nervous system along the axon of the nerve within a defined period, the greater the contractile response is within the muscle. This response is trainable, and stimuli to achieve this result can and should be integrated within training programmes to enhance the ability to recruit motor units more efficiently.

Around the axon of a motor nerve is a protein covering called myelin. This substance is often referred to as the white matter in the central nervous system. Myelin is crucial to human movement control. It is the regulatory protein that determines the speed of the motor action potential from the central nervous system to the muscle fibre. Myelin accelerates the motor action potential along the axon of the nerve, and therefore regulates movement control. As with most adaptations that occur within the human body, myelin is produced in response to repeated stimuli. If a signal is received with

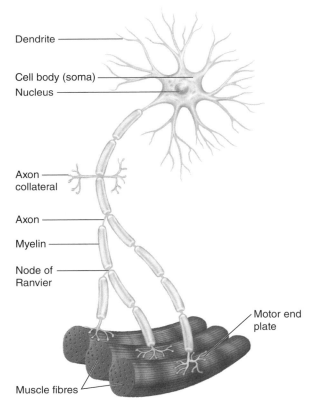

Dendrite

Cell body (soma)
Nucleus

Axon collateral

Axon

Myelin

Node of Ranvier

Motor end plate

Muscle fibres

**Figure 2.7**    Structure of a motor unit.

sufficient strength and frequency that the brain recognizes the movement pattern that needs reinforcing, myelin will be created in response to the increased need. This outcome is related to the concept of neural plasticity (the dynamic, experience-dependent development of the nervous system); that is, the neurological mechanisms within the body can change with use or disuse.

Why is it important to grasp this concept? We often hear that practice leads to perfect. This maxim has been reconceptualized to state that perfect practice makes permanent (learning equates to a more or less permanent change in behaviour). Part of this proposition can be argued against strongly, however, because one of the key features of learning theory is that to learn, a person must be able to make mistakes and receive feedback that can be used as a basis for adaptation. This idea is especially relevant when it comes to tactical learning, or the development of game sense, that is, how and when to use particular motor skills in a given sporting context.

But in terms of learning movement patterns and developing neural pathways, the coach should think of the proposition in a slightly different way: Perfect practice makes myelin; myelin makes permanent.[5] Looking at how the athlete moves is essential, because myelin should be laid down in a positive way to develop useful and coordinated movements with synchronous firing of motor units in a coordinated manner, as opposed to being laid down in a manner that promotes inappropriate movement patterns or those that lead to movement compensations. Put another way, repetition of incorrect or undesirable motor patterns will cause them to become ingrained and habitual, and therefore difficult to unlearn, especially when the movement skill has to be performed under pressure or fatigue.

Between the axon of the nerve and the sheath of the muscle is the motor end plate. This element has a junction, known as a synapse, that has a critical function in regulating movement. As the motor action potential reaches the end of the nerve, the signal has to cross the synapse so that the signal can initiate the contraction within the fibre. The communication mechanism between the nerve and muscle fibre is the neurotransmitter acetylcholine. The amount of neurotransmitter released is directly proportional to the strength of the neural signal. The greater the motor action potential is, the larger the release of acetylcholine is. Acetylcholine crosses the synapse and binds with a receptor site. This process continues until the motor action potentials cease to be transmitted along the axon.

This process is continuous. In a living human, a situation never occurs in which a neurotransmitter isn't being released. But to prevent motor units from being permanently activated, evolution has created a threshold effect. When enough neurotransmitter binds to the muscle fibre membrane, the electrical potential of the fibre membrane changes. If insufficient neurotransmitter is present, the electrical signal will not be passed to the muscle fibres attached to the motor nerve, and therefore the motor unit will not contract. This outcome is known as the all-or-nothing principle of motor unit contraction; that is, motor units are either activated or not.

## Motor Unit Classification

Motor units are classified according to the histochemical properties of the muscle fibre, which influence the speed of contraction of the fibres and therefore their function within human movement. The classification is predominantly determined by the enzyme profiles within the protein myofilaments of the fibre. But the volume and density of the sarcoplasmic reticulum also influence calcium release and other dynamic components of the muscular contraction mechanism.[2]

Motor units can consist of only one type of fibre: Type I, IIa or IIx. Besides signifying contractile speed, the fibre type also indicates the predominant metabolic pathway of the fibre (aerobic or anaerobic) and therefore the motor unit's resistance to fatigue. The synchronization between these motor units is crucial to producing skilled movement.

Type I fibres are predominantly known as slow-twitch, or endurance, fibres. Muscles required to be fatigue resistant are predominantly made up of slow-twitch fibres. For example, the gastrocnemius and soleus, the calf muscles, are predominantly slow twitch in nature because they allow humans to stand and walk for relatively long periods without muscle fatigue. Because of the endurance nature of these fibres, they rely predominantly on energy produced aerobically, a process known as slow glycolysis, which is explained later in this chapter.

As such, these fibres have a relatively slow contraction speed. Type I fibres need a good supply of oxygen, which in turn requires a good supply of blood. These fibres also have a large number of mitochondria (where ATP is produced by slow glycolysis) that are larger in size than the fibres of other muscles.

Type IIa are intermediate muscle fibres. They are known as fast-twitch oxidative-gly-colytic (FOG) fibres. Because these fibres contain large numbers of mitochondria, they tend to be reasonably resistant to fatigue and can recover quickly from bouts of intense exercise. Type IIa fibres are therefore ideal for athletes in multiple high-intensity (multiple sprints or collision) sports or events such as slalom skiing or the 800 to 1,500 metres, in which athletes perform explosive actions for longer periods.

Type IIx* muscle fibres have a fast contraction speed (i.e., they are fast-twitch fibres) and react up to 10 times faster than slow-twitch fibres. These fibres are responsible for powerful, high-intensity movements. They have an enzyme profile designed to produce energy by anaerobic glycolysis. As such, they are not resistant to fatigue and can operate maximally for only short periods.

Because Type IIx motor units do not require oxygen to produce ATP, they have a relatively poor blood supply. These fibre types also have fewer, smaller mitochondria than slow-twitch fibres do. Relatively speaking, athletes who excel in explosive movements (e.g., sprinters, throwers, weightlifters) can have a large number of type IIx muscle fibres. Motor units that have predominantly fast-twitch fibres are characterized by a large number of fibres for each motor neuron, so large forces can be achieved quickly by recruiting a relatively small number of motor units.

The contractile force achieved by a muscle can be increased through two mechanisms. First, more motor units can be recruited to perform the work. Force production is related to the recruitment sequence of fibres, which depends on the intensity of exercise. This concept is known as the size recruitment principle, illustrated in figure 2.8.

*In some texts, Type IIx muscle fibres are referred to as Type IIb fibres. Technically speaking, Type IIb fibres are found only in rodent tissue. But this small technicality should not change the context of referral.

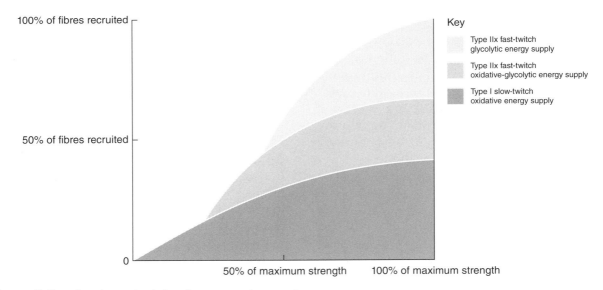

**Figure 2.8**    The size principle of motor unit recruitment.

Type I fibres are recruited first. Type IIa fibres are recruited next, either because of more force being required or because of fatigue in the Type I fibres. At near maximal levels of force requirement, the largest motor units, the Type IIx fibres, are recruited. But these fibres are not resistant to fatigue and will not perform work for long periods, even in highly trained athletes. Understanding the size recruitment principle is important. Type IIa or IIx fibres can be recruited (and therefore trained) only with loads or velocities that demand the appropriate contractile forces or intensities.

## Proprioception and the Stretch Reflex

The cerebellum is a key component of the central nervous system, because it is primarily responsible for coordinating the proprioceptive mechanisms within the body. Proprioception is the sense that determines the relative position of body parts to other parts of the body (or the ability to reposition a joint to a predetermined position) and the strength of effort being employed when moving or when resisting an externally imposed load.

A related (but distinct) sense is kinaesthesia, the sensation that a body part has moved. Proprioceptive organs exist within the muscles, the connective tissue, the joints and the skin.

They provide information back to the central nervous system about aspects of movement such as muscle length, muscle tension, contractile velocities and contact with external objects, often described by sport performers as touch or feel (i.e., 'feel of the ball'). Kinaesthesia allows the neuromuscular system to send motor action potentials to other muscles, enabling fine (or gross) adjustments to be made. This and other mechanisms provide feedback to the central nervous system and enable the brain to receive feedback about whether and how a consciously controlled movement was completed and then prepare for any subsequent actions.

Proprioception, object control and locomotor skills all require a well-defined sense of proprioception and kinesthesis. The ability to strike an object—for example, to kick a ball or hit a baseball pitch with a bat—requires a finely tuned sense of the position of the joints. With appropriately progressed training, this sense can become automatic and consolidated, which has a profound influence on skill development and sporting performance. Muscle spindle fibres and golgi tendon organs are proprioceptors that have a major influence on the functional performance of muscles, because they regulate one of the key mechano-physiological responses for the neuromuscular system in a sporting context: the stretch reflex.

Understanding the stretch reflex is important in developing physical qualities in a performer, because the stretch reflex is both a protective mechanism for the athlete and the key physio-mechanical action underpinning much movement control within the body. It is certainly the basis of the most powerful actions such as running, jumping and forceful training techniques such as plyometrics, as presented in chapters 8 and 9.

Muscle fibres have elastic properties that enable them to elongate. The action is similar to an elastic band, which can be stretched to store potential energy until it reaches a critical point. The critical point may be related to how far the stretch has elongated the muscle, sensed by proprioceptive organs called muscle spindle fibres.

Muscle spindles are encapsulated intrafusal fibres that lie in series (lengthwise) within the fasciculus (see figure 2.5). If the rate of change in length is excessive, then before the muscle fibre tissue is injured, the muscle spindle fibres will send a message to the spinal cord through Type 1a afferent nerves.[6] These nerves synapse with alpha motor neurons in the spinal cord to send a preprogrammed and rapid (typically 1 to 2 milliseconds) motor action potential back to the motor unit to initiate a strong reflex contraction in the muscle fibres.[7]

Synergistic muscles, those that produce or support the same movement, are also innervated when the stretch reflex is activated, further strengthening the protective (and powerful) reflex action. The stretch reflex (also known as a myotatic reflex) is important in both producing powerful sporting movements and maintaining postural integrity.

# A Practical Explanation of the Stretch Reflex

Stand with your hand on your thigh. Using your index finger, hit your thigh as hard as possible. Then, using your other hand, pull the index finger back until you feel a stretching sensation and then let it go. Pulling back the finger and releasing it causes the finger to hit the thigh much harder than hitting the thigh without the prior stretch of the finger. The quicker the finger is pulled back, the quicker the finger will release and hit the thigh. But even a pull back and pause action will elicit a slow stretch-shortening cycle response, and stored elastic energy will cause a high-force impact on the thigh compared with a voluntary contraction.

The proprioceptive senses enable a constant process of adjusting and maintaining dynamic postural control throughout the kinetic (movement) chain, the importance of which will be emphasized throughout this book. A practical means of explaining the stretch reflex is shown in the sidebar.

Golgi tendon organs are located within the muscle–tendon junction. These organelles respond to the rate of increase in muscular tension that occurs because of external loading. Stimulation of the golgi tendon organ causes muscle inhibition and overrides the neural stimulus to the motor unit to protect against excessive loading of the muscle.

Because sporting tasks often require the rapid development of high levels of tension within muscle groups because of external loadings, one of the things that programmes need to develop gradually is golgi tendon organ inhibition. The muscle can then resist rapid rates of force production in both training and sporting tasks without become deactivated. This outcome can be achieved through general strengthening and specific power activities such as plyometrics, which are the focus of chapter 9.

## Neuromuscular System Responses to Training

Many possible adaptations to training within the neuromuscular system are transferable to sporting actions.

First, when teaching skilled actions, the coach should emphasize joint positioning within techniques. At early stages of learning, joint positioning is more important than the speed or power of technical execution, because joint positioning determines muscle functioning. By reinforcing the movement patterning of the joints, the athlete will train the muscles that are recruited. Repetition of these actions also enables the development of proprioception and kinaesthetic awareness, enabling the athlete to execute the position in increasingly novel and complex tasks. This training will enhance intermuscular coordination, which refers to the ability of the agonist, antagonist and synergist muscles to contribute fully to the target activity, and involves minimizing coactivation and maximizing synergistic contribution.[8]

Training will increase the inhibition of certain organs (for example, the golgi tendon organs) or facilitate other actions (such as the activation of muscle spindle fibres), leading to increased ability to use a stretch-shortening cycle to produce powerful movements.

These adaptations will contribute to enhanced intramuscular coordination, which relates to the excitation and inhibition patterning of the agonist muscles.

Appropriate training also causes increased myelination to occur within the axon of the motor nerve (neuron), enabling much more effective transmission of the motor action potential from the central nervous system to the muscle. Learned patterns within the central nervous system also improve the sequencing of motor unit activation—the pattern encoding of the motor action potentials. Similarly, the frequency at which neural signals (rate coding) reach the muscles can be enhanced. These adaptations mean that muscles can be activated to produce much greater contractile forces through improved intramuscular coordination.[8]

These adaptations occur at a more global level; they are not restricted to individual motor units. Indeed, skilled performances are the result of sensory and proprioceptive or kinaesthetic feedback and the identified need to initiate responsive movements. Therefore, an important training adaptation is the ability to sense changes in the muscle fibre's length, tension and velocity of shortening to provoke corresponding signals to motor units that can produce corrective or responsive actions. The ability to organize motor action potentials to cause synchronization or coordinated sequencing of motor unit activations, or indeed larger muscle group actions, is a key training response.

# Bioenergetic System

All the work done within the body (thinking, moving, manipulating) requires energy. To improve the capacity of the athlete's motor system, training the availability of energy to fuel mechanical work is as important as developing the movement skills to perform the work with optimum efficiency. As the great sprint coach Loren Seagrave once said, 'Any idiot can make someone tired. The trick is to make them tired in the right way and without losing the quality of the technique' (personal communication).

Energy is created by breaking down a storage molecule. In sport, glycogen, the muscular storage of glucose, is usually broken down, but sometimes it can be fat. Breaking down these molecules involves a number of physical systems. For example, the respiratory system brings oxygen into the body; the vascular system transports the oxygen in the blood, which is pumped by the cardiac muscle (hence cardiovascular) and is used in the cell at the end stage of a series of metabolic reactions within a pathway to produce energy.

Rather than focus on each of these systems in turn, let's work on the premise that the function of these systems is to contribute collectively to the production of energy. Therefore, we will refer to them collectively as the bioenergetic system.

The bioenergetic system is responsible for producing the chemical energy that enables all work undertaken by the respective organs and systems within the body to occur. The primary factor that limits the rate at which physical work can be performed is the availability of the energy currency in the body, adenosine triphosphate (ATP), a molecule of adenosine that is chemically bonded with three phosphate molecules. These chemical bonds store energy that is released to enable work to be performed when the chemical bonds are broken.

Because little ATP is stored in the body cells (typically this supply is exhausted after 1 to 3 seconds of exercise), the athlete needs to train to produce ATP at an appropriate rate to enable the production of energy to support the imposed demand of the sporting activity. The availability of ATP limits the athlete's movement capabilities, so the coach needs to understand a little about how these energy-delivering mechanisms work with different intensities of activity.

Three energy systems are responsible for producing ATP from the body's stores of chemical energy:

**Phosphagen**. This system is sometimes referred to as the phosphocreatine or creatine phosphate system. It usually can produce energy for intense periods of exercise up to 10 seconds long by breaking down creatine phosphate stores in the body to produce ATP. After these stores are exhausted, the body uses glycolysis as the predominant means to create ATP.

**Fast glycolysis**. This system is sometimes referred to as anaerobic (without oxygen) glycolysis (the splitting of glycogen).

**Aerobic metabolism**. Slow glycolysis is a series of metabolic reactions that produce ATP in the presence of oxygen.

These three energy systems are not independent of each other. Indeed, they are integrated, and in any activity, a combination of these systems supplies energy. How they combine and which energy supply mechanism predominates in any given activity depends on the intensity of the exercise. The more intense the exercise is (i.e., the closer it is to maximum intensity at any given time), the greater the contribution that fast glycolysis will have. In this way, sports such as rugby league (figure 2.9) can be differentiated from sports such as soccer, which has many short bursts of high-intensity sprints interspersed with long periods of relatively low-intensity running and walking. The difference in the activity profiles between the sports needs to be reflected in the relative conditioning of the athletes. When demand for ATP begins to exceed supply, fatigue will quickly occur to prevent the body from reaching a point of systemic failure.

Glycolysis involves breaking down the muscular and liver stores of glycogen into a substance called pyruvate. This conversion requires 12 enzymatic reactions in total and produces a net gain of three molecules of ATP plus hydrogen, which is used at a later stage to produce more ATP in the presence of oxygen. The combined actions of the ATP–PCr (phosphagen) and glycolytic systems allow muscles to generate force when the demand for energy exceeds the rate at which energy can be supplied aerobically. In this way, these two energy systems are the major energy contributors during the early minutes of high-intensity exercise.

The fate of the pyruvate molecule depends on the intensity of the work being performed. The rate-limiting factor is the ability of the cardiorespiratory system to supply oxygen to the working muscles. In low-intensity exercise, in which the demand for oxygen can be met by the supply, oxygen-dependent (slow) glycolysis allows pyruvate to be transported into an organelle within the muscle cell known as a mitochondrion.

In the mitochondria, a series of chemical reactions occurs, which ultimately produces up to 36 molecules of ATP (thus, the potential total production of ATP from one molecule of glycogen is 39 molecules). The by-products of the reactions that occur to produce this ATP are water and carbon dioxide, which are removed from the muscle cells by the blood and exhaled through the lungs. This process (known as oxidative phosphorylation) can occur for as long as the athlete is able to deliver glycogen and oxygen to the working muscles.

When the intensity of exercise exceeds that at which the oxygen supply is sufficient, then oxygen-independent (fast) glycolysis becomes largely responsible for creating ATP. The net production of ATP is the same (two or three molecules), but the fate of the pyruvate

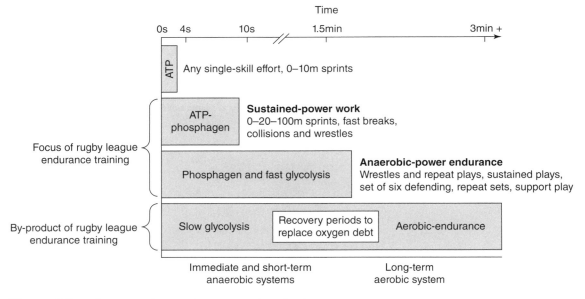

**Figure 2.9**   Bioenergetic requirements of rugby league.

molecule changes. Instead of being transported into the mitochondria, pyruvate is reduced to lactate in the muscle cell.

During medium-intensity exercise, lactate is formed. Lactate has two uses. When sufficient oxygen is available (for example, after intense work when the athlete is replacing the oxygen debt by breathing hard), lactate is transformed back into pyruvate, transported into the mitochondria and converted into 36 molecules of ATP. Alternatively, it is removed from the muscle cell, taken by blood to the liver and converted back into glucose for use as an energy store at a later stage. Thus, it can be seen that lactate, rather than being a toxin (as many coaches think it is), is actually a useful fuel source for the body, particularly in slow-twitch muscle fibres, which have a high number of mitochondria in them.

High-intensity anaerobic work, which forms the major components of the majority of game-based sports and all sports in which performances last less than 3 minutes, cannot be sustained for long periods. High-intensity anaerobic work

can produce immediately available energy for up to 2 minutes in fit players, but a significant fatigue component limits how long the player can keep working anaerobically. This occurs because the build-up of lactate in the muscle cell is accompanied by an increase in hydrogen ions (H+). High concentrations of these positively charged particles make the muscle cell more acidic. Higher levels of acidity interfere with the muscle contraction mechanisms and the efficiency of the enzymes involved in ATP production, thereby causing fatigue. The body has evolved this protective mechanism to limit the amount of work that a human can do before reaching exhaustion. For a review on the training adaptations to the bioenergetic system, see Kenny, Wilmore and Costill.[2]

Figure 2.10 summarizes the training adaptations possible within the biomotor systems. The importance of the neuromuscular and musculoskeletal systems in enabling the production of skilled movement has been discussed throughout this chapter. By understanding the basic principles for developing the components

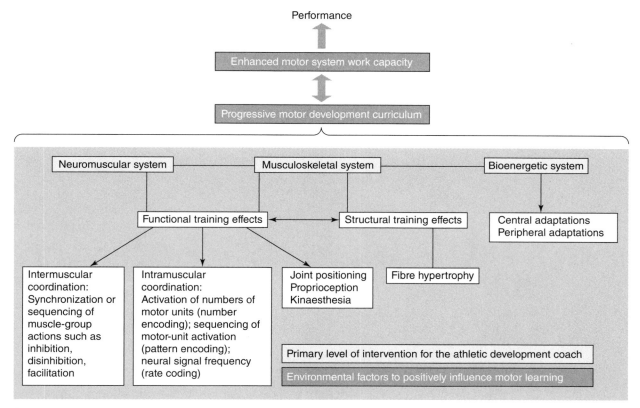

**Figure 2.10**    The athletic development coach can manipulate biomotor systems to enhance performance.

of the motor system, the athletic development coach can manipulate the type and volume loading of training to achieve the desired training outcome. This knowledge serves as a foundation for the specific skill development processes outlined in the subsequent chapters, which present a systematic set of functional guidelines that will support decision making about how best to develop these qualities.

## Summary

This chapter has built on the understanding that physical competence is a prerequisite to sporting achievement and that specialist movement skills are underpinned by foundational (or fundamental) movement skills. Indeed, the first role of anyone charged with the physical development of an athlete is to develop posturally correct movements, and through this to develop muscular actions in a functional and progressive manner. Understanding of the workings of the respective components of the biomotor system leads to training programmes that focus on comprehensive adaptations to all aspects of the motor system in a means that will transfer positively to performance.

# CHAPTER 3

# Patterns of Motor System Development

The objective of any athlete development programme is to optimize the potential for an athlete's performance at a predetermined time. This performance may be a target competition (Olympic Games, national championships, individual challenge) or, in team sport, it may relate to the maintenance of specific performance capacity throughout a season during which the team is required to perform weekly, or more often, over many months. This reality of sport requires the programme to use precise training interventions that develop specific motor system qualities at certain times to arrive at the target competition in the best physical state of preparedness.

Bompa and Haff[1] explain that a key part of this planning process is to understand that not all components of the motor system can be prioritized for development at the same time. For example, strength development is a required precursor to power development, and power is a necessary foundational quality for speed development. So to get faster, an athlete must first get stronger in the appropriate manner for the sport.[2] Similarly, to develop aerobic power, the athlete must perform some type of aerobic capacity training to enable the left ventricle of the heart to adapt to produce increased cardiac output. Aerobic training, however, will not provide a foundation for anaerobic capacity, although extensive anaerobic work may provide a basis for the development of certain aerobic capacity improvements as the athlete recovers from high-intensity efforts in a recovery interval.

The physiological qualities that underpin strength and power and longer-duration endurance are divergent; indeed, the training adaptations for each can be contradictory. Therefore, the key to effective programme planning is to determine what biomotor qualities will be emphasized at which point in the programme, a concept known as emphasis loading, and to ensure that the correct sequence is used to establish prerequisite qualities. This process isn't limited to elite-level performance or childhood development; practitioners working with all ages, experiences and performance levels need to understand it.

Planning is also important in programmes for developmental athletes, in which the objective is to deliver the appropriate biomotor abilities in the correct sequence to promote long-term development. Such a programme physically prepares athletes for the transitions they make throughout a progressive sporting career (for example, from youth to first-grade level, from high school to college, or from inactivity to recreational sport). Success requires knowledge of the developmental trainability of children's physiology and anatomy to the point of adulthood, when all physiological systems become fully trainable and adaptive to specific training stimuli,[2] as long as the prerequisite physical training has been undertaken to enable the athlete to be ready for such training experiences.

## Developing Youth Athletes

Young athletes are a unique population, and the practice and competitive schedules they are exposed to should reflect and support the wide-ranging physiological and psychosocial changes that occur during youth. Note that all aspects of fitness—strength, speed, endurance, mobility and combinations and derivatives of these—can be developed in children at every stage. As indicated in figure 3.1, however, the components of the motor system do not develop at a uniform rate. Knowledge of how the motor system develops enables a focus on two important determinants for an athlete development programme.

First, knowledge of how the motor system develops provides a guideline for the physiological constraints on programme delivery in terms of the methodology and volume or intensity. Second, it provides a framework for identifying how training programmes should be devised to support and reinforce the optimal development of the motor system. The concept of sensitive periods of development guides coaching practice.[3] Because many of the components of movement skills rely on the athlete's ability to produce multidirectional forces rapidly (a function of strength, speed and postural control), it is no surprise that neuromuscular and musculoskeletal system development is central to the athlete development model. Therefore, functional strength and power and motor skill competency are the major priorities for a practitioner working with young athletes.[4]

This concept becomes especially important in the context of movement skills. Indeed, most sports requiring exceptionally high levels of endurance as a performance priority, such as rowing, distance cycling and distance running (typically referred to as the engine sports), have relatively low skill requirements. As will be illustrated, endurance may be fully developed in adulthood, and many athletes have transferred into engine sports at elite levels after being successful athletes in other sporting contexts. They can do this because they have the ability to apply high levels of force at critical periods to enhance their movement economy (see chapters 8 and 10). Therefore, endurance isn't typically considered a targeted priority

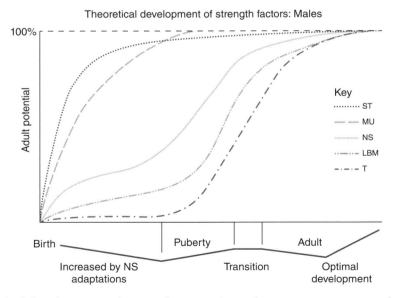

**Figure 3.1**   Theoretical development of strength output in males as a consequence of physio-mechanical development of the male motor system.

T = Alterations in testosterone levels due to maturation; LBM = Alterations in lean body mass due to maturation; NS = Nervous system maturation; MU = Motor unit maturation; ST = Maximum strength levels

Reprinted, by permission, from K. Pierce, C. Brewer, M. Ramsey, R. Bird, W.A. Sands, M.E. Stone, and M.H. Stone, 2008, "Opinion paper and literature review: Youth resistance training," *UKSCA's Professional Strength and Conditioning Journal* July: 9-22.

for the athlete development programme. That said, for reasons of general health and injury prevention, alongside the consideration that athletes typically shouldn't specialize too early if their choices of activity aren't to be narrowed too early, endurance shouldn't be ignored either; it should be a feature, if not priority, of most programmes. Therefore, the chapter presents considerations that the practitioner should bear in mind when looking at endurance activities.

## Motor System Development for All Athletes

Understanding the principles of athlete development is important even for practitioners who are not working with children. In its simplest form, athlete development relates the structure and nature of training to any athlete's developmental pathway so that people are doing the right things at the right time for long-term, not necessarily immediate, development. Ultimately, most coaches' aims are athlete centred, based on taking an individual and educational approach and based on a desire to make a long-term difference to their athletes. Therefore, when working with adults, practitioners need to understand the experiences they have had to date so that these can be built on. Likewise, coaches should understand the experiences they haven't had so that they can be remediated for or introduced into a progressive practice regime.

The ability to do this requires the practitioner to understand how the motor system develops and what training or practice experiences can positively enhance this development. Having this knowledge enables the practitioner who is working with an athlete of any age to base training decisions on the athlete's training age.

With this in mind, the developmental patterns of the neuromuscular, musculoskeletal and bioenergetic systems are discussed in line with a model of childhood (0 to 6 years of age), late childhood (6 to 9), early adolescence (9 to 12), adolescence (12 to 16) and late adolescence (16 to 18). These terms are presented purely in terms of biological (physical) development; these descriptors (i.e., when is someone an adult?) may not be fully applicable to social developmental contexts. Recall the points made in chapter 1 that although certain activities are suited to a child's biological stage of development, the athlete's training age determines whether he or she is ready to undertake such activity, especially with regard to high-volume work.

## Childhood

Although childhood isn't a time that requires large volumes of formalized coaching and practice, children need to have the opportunity to develop mature movement patterns in foundation movement skills such as running and jumping (figure 3.2). During this stage, the provision of informal learning opportunities in the home and school environments is essential. This activity should be aimed at developing rudimentary movement, early fundamental movement skills and a love and enjoyment of physical activity.[5]

During this time, the relationship between the psychomotor and physical aspects of development is inescapable. The major factor for the child to develop is confidence and a can-try aptitude. Encourage young children to explore a range of environments and to attempt novel tasks that challenge their development. This activity should include many basic skills that often link and combine (run, jump, climb), as well as skills that can be explored bilaterally (manipulate with two hands, manipulate with either hand).

The key is to keep the children 100 per cent engaged and 100 per cent active 100 per cent of the time! This practice helps to develop the phosphagen system and aerobic bioenergetic energy pathways. During this phase of development, the major emphasis should be on activities to develop the locomotive, stability and manipulative abilities. By age 5 or 6, the child should be able to integrate all the subcomponents of these skills into a gross movement pattern that, if successfully and consistently executed (a function of the opportunity to

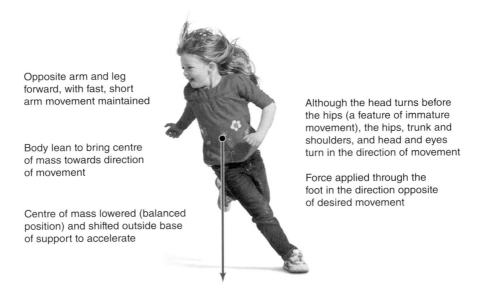

Opposite arm and leg forward, with fast, short arm movement maintained

Body lean to bring centre of mass towards direction of movement

Centre of mass lowered (balanced position) and shifted outside base of support to accelerate

Although the head turns before the hips (a feature of immature movement), the hips, trunk and shoulders, and head and eyes turn in the direction of movement

Force applied through the foot in the direction opposite of desired movement

**Figure 3.2**    Playground games enable a 5-year-old to demonstrate key aspects of running and change-of-direction skills.

play and practice), will provide a platform for the development of stable performances of transitional skills that link the individual skills. During this time, the focus should be on getting the child to execute skills with an emphasis on distance rather than accuracy; how far can the child kick or throw the ball is much more useful than aiming to hit a target. This focus will aid the development of the motor system and provide the underpinning for increases in motor unit trainability and strength development in later childhood.

## Late Childhood

This phase focuses on the provision of positive learning environments that develop a broad range of fundamental skills in a playful context. These key fundamental skills build basic competence and confidence and play an important part in contributing to participation in sport and developing more advanced skills in later years. Indeed, in many models of skill development, this foundation stage has been categorized as the phase of fundamental movement skills.[6]

During the years of age 6 to age 9, locomotive, stability and manipulation (object control) skills should be practised and mastered before sport-specific skills are introduced.

The development of these skills, using a positive, fun and largely games-based approach, will contribute significantly to future athletic achievements. Participation in a wide range of sports and physical activities should be encouraged. This emphasis on motor development will produce athletes who have better trainability for long-term sport-specific development. Indeed the evidence clearly suggests that U.S. colleges are more likely to recruit athletes who played multiple sports compared to those who specialized in one sport. The importance of this multisport education has been underutilized in many cultures.

Most sports are late-specialization sports. Elite performances are the consequence of many non-specialist skills (running, jumping, agility skills, throwing, catching, kicking) coming together with specialist sport applications (kicking a soccer ball versus punting a football, hitting a baseball versus striking a racquetball) to produce a sport-specific performance. The development of nonspecialist skills explains why many elite athletes in one sport have been pre-elite performers in another. Likewise, many good athletes can play recreational golf well because their sporting experiences have taught them coordination, timing and control.

In contrast, consider athletes who specialize early. These athletes develop highly repetitive motor actions that often lead to muscle imbalances and a linked predisposition to injuries. They have little ability to transfer their skills across different sporting contexts because they have little experience of the aspects of motor learning that enable this transfer. Another issue is athlete burnout; a person who has been subjected to many years of highly repetitive training in narrow practices and competitions may become demotivated to take part in that sport any more. A multisport experience that progressively narrows through adolescence is the recommended practice to develop highly transferable and athletic motor skills.

Early in the developmental years, the balance mechanism of the inner ear gradually matures. As kinaesthetic awareness improves, children have the opportunity to improve and refine the basic motor patterns relating to speed, agility, balance and coordination. This process can be supported by a programme that utilizes specific activities and games that emphasize coordination and kinaesthetic senses. Gymnastic and other body-control-based activities are useful for this purpose (figure 3.3).

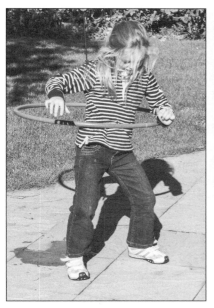
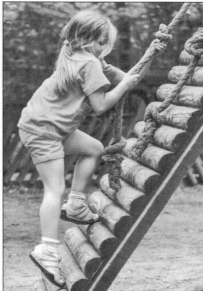
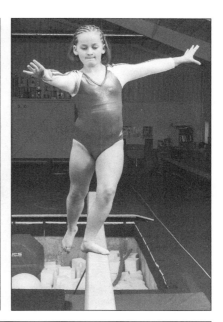
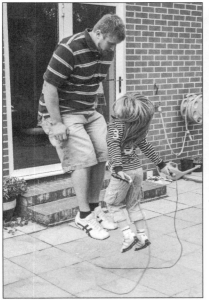
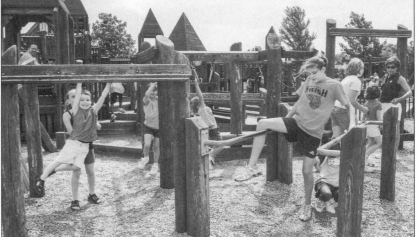

© Human Kinetics/Brenda Williams

**Figure 3.3**  Formalized practice and deliberate play activities that involve agility, balance and coordination tasks encourage the refinement of basic motor patterns.

Similarly, the larger muscle groups (for example, the quadriceps and hamstrings, the gluteus maximus) and consequently the larger motor units not involved in fine actions are more developed than smaller muscle groups (for example, the supraspinatus, infraspinatus, teres minor and teres major, which support the shoulder girdle). The development of the muscles responsible for fine control also explains why vision control isn't fully developed; the ability to activate motor units in the muscles that control positioning the eyeball is typically developed by the age of 10. Therefore, the child will be more skilful in gross movements that involve the large musculature.

Actions that involve precise and coordinated actions encourage the interaction of the smaller muscle groups and motor units, but these typically produce reduced success in comparison with less skilful movements. The ability to activate motor units maximally is a critical determinant of success in sport performance in later life, and this ability is developmental. Therefore, maximal activation of motor units needs to be encouraged by emphasizing explosive and speed-based activities. Speed and agility should be programmed (developed) independently of coordination-based tasks until temporal awareness (usually referred to as eye–hand or eye–foot coordination) becomes more stable. This goal is achieved through object-handling and obstacle-dependent activities such as striking, catching, clambering or hurdling.

The athletic activities related to running, jumping and throwing are a major emphasis in terms of developing both the motor skills and the neuromuscular system. Explosive, high-speed activities that last for 1 to 5 seconds are ideal for children of this age. Significant evidence shows that children benefit immensely from reactive plyometric and high-speed activities (e.g., figure 3.4), which rely on the neural aspects of the neuromuscular system.[7]

Similarly, a wide range of multiplanar activities encourages strength development through neuromuscular (motor unit) recruitment. Activities such as medicine ball throws, bodyweight exercises, pushing and pulling tasks, swinging, climbing, grappling, dynamic balance and weight transfer tasks also provide positive stressors to the development of bone and connective tissue. Total-body movements performed through a full range of movement also encourage postural management, flexibility

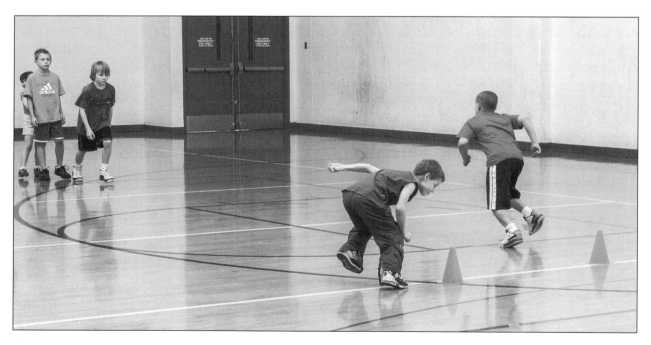

**Figure 3.4**   Agility courses and relay activities provide fun and basic movement skills for children whilst enhancing neural system development.

and mobility. Again, the practitioner should emphasize performing few repetitions to avoid excessive, repetitive stresses to the long bones, where the epiphysis is continuing to calcify.

These activities also link well with the psychological development of children at this age. They cannot sit and listen for long periods; they want to move and participate in activities. Their attention span is short, so continual variation is required. Indeed, physical education teachers have long used the analogy of age plus 3 minutes as a guide for the attention span of children. Therefore, activities need to be short and varied, and they should be delivered in an organized and effective manner using brief and easy-to-follow instructions.

During this time children are also developing their procedural and affective knowledge base. The motor cortex is developing programmes that form the basis of skill acquisition and skill execution. Therefore, the balance between repetition of an action (to ingrain the motor programme) and variation in the task (to enable the child to adapt the basic skill model to a novel task) is essential. All these concepts are further explored in chapter 7 which looks at planning learning curriculums.

During childhood, the proportions of the body segments change in relative terms. The head grows to twice its original size; the trunk grows up to three times, the arms up to four times and the legs up to five times their original proportions.[8] This transformation has implications for children in terms of coordination. As they grow and develop, the arms and feet are not where they were relative to the head. In these late childhood years, boys and girls have few structural or physiological differences between them, so they should be encouraged to participate in activities together. The major areas of skeletal growth are the limbs, a pattern that continues through to puberty. Therefore, spatial awareness and kinaesthetic sense can be developed as limb length increases through multiple sporting activities in three dimensions (planes of movement).

Children's bones are continuing to calcify at this age, and the ends of the bones are still largely composed of cartilage. Therefore, the skeleton is highly susceptible to injuries induced through excessive stresses or heavy pressure. The ligaments that support the joints are becoming denser and therefore stronger throughout these years. Activities that promote neural recruitment are important, but a slow progression should be used to allow time for adaptation to hopping, skipping (including for height and distance), strength exercises that involve moving the child's own body weight and explosive medicine ball exercises. The number of repetitions should be kept relatively low.

Children are naturally flexible, and their joints relatively mobile. Therefore, a focus on developing flexibility in children is unnecessary unless hypermobility is required (for example, for gymnastics). Recognize that where there is a range of motion around a joint without the specific strength to support that joint, the joint is potentially compromised in a dynamic action. By promoting a spectrum of full-range movements under muscular control, the practitioner encourages the child to maximize flexibility and mobility and develop strength. Indeed, mobility cannot be developed independently of neuromuscular activation and will not come simply with passive stretching. As the child matures and the musculoskeletal system grows, the challenge is to maintain the flexibility naturally present in childhood. In adolescents, strength movements through a full range should be continued, and specific activities that encourage stretching under active muscular control (such as Pilates or yoga) should be incorporated to maximize the range of movement around specific joints.

The specific technical requirements of these exercises are introduced later in the book, including suggestions for adapting the exercises to suit athletes of different stages. But key aspects of running and jumping mechanics, such as active ground contact with dorsiflexed toe, dorsiflexed toe during flight phase (see chapter 8) and a countermovement in jumps for height and distance (see chapter 9), can be encouraged by coaches through fun and games-based activities. Movement mechanics can be developed and expressed through agility games that incorporate movement in the sagittal and transverse planes.

Children are less fuel efficient than adults.[9] This deficit is exacerbated by the child's relative biomechanical inefficiencies because the length of the child's limbs are not completely in kinetic balance with the muscles. Indeed, children have only approximately 28 per cent of their body mass composed of muscle in comparison with 35 to 40 per cent (or more) in adolescents and young adults.[10] The child's small stature (limb length and ability to express forces through the musculoskeletal system) leads to a biomechanical disadvantage in terms of movement efficiency in tasks that older children or adults would find less demanding. This disparity leads to an increased oxygen requirement for a given workload compared with a working adult.

Games and games-based practices should encourage short-duration, high-intensity, high-speed efforts of approximately 5 to 7 seconds followed by self-determined periods of rest and recovery. These activities develop the bioenergetic system within the endurance capacity of young, active participants. Getting children active is of paramount importance for health, but high-speed, high-velocity and chaotic change-of-direction activities are ideal for promoting athletic development in children at this stage. In children in activities such as swimming or rowing, in which technique is endurance dependent, higher volumes of work can be developed through higher repetitions of shorter technical practices as opposed to high-volume, endurance-specific activities.

**Table 3.1**   Multiactivity Week for an 8-Year-Old

| Day | Activity |
| --- | --- |
| Monday | Physical education (60 min.), swimming (45 min.) |
| Tuesday | Gymnastics (60 min.) |
| Wednesday | |
| Thursday | Physical education (60 min.), basketball (60 min.) |
| Friday | Soccer (60 min.) |
| Saturday | Track and field (60 min.) |
| Sunday | Football (60 min.) |

Table 3.1 shows the sample weekly programme of an active 8-year-old who is not yet identifiable as a performer in any specific sport but whose parents are encouraging the development of foundation movement and sport skills.

If the coaching programme within each sport is well devised, the emphasis within each sport-specific session will be on developing foundation movement skills, usually delivered within the context of the specific sport being coached. Table 3.2 provides an example of a practice session that illustrates this intention within the context of a track and field environment, but this approach might be applicable to any of the sports identified in table 3.1.

Undertaking year-round activity of this nature will enable the child to have a well-rounded movement skills vocabulary that will provide the foundation for building sport-specific skills as the child progresses through his or her sporting career.

# Early Adolescence

Some sports have been identified as early specialization sports; to achieve success in these sports, the athlete typically needs to specialize during early adolescence. These sports require highly specialized skill ranges, such as tennis and swimming, or rely on special strength and hypermobility, such as gymnastics. Specialization at this stage does not necessarily mean exclusivity; the child should be encouraged to participate in a range of formal and informal sport opportunities outside his or her focused practices.

With the exception of those who are progressing towards a focus in an early specialization sports, the focus of a child aged 9 to 12 should be on sampling a range of sports, developing basic sport skills and further building competence and confidence. In particular, transitional movement challenges (linking skills) and environmental-specific challenges (within sport-specific situational contexts across multiple sport experience) are the key programme drivers. These activities should incorporate stimulus detection and recognition so that the child can build on foundation

**Table 3.2**   Sample Multiple Skills Practice Session for an 8-Year-Old

| Time (min.) | Activity |
|---|---|
| 0 to 10 | Follow the leader: Children work with a partner. The leader moves in various ways, and the other child imitates the movement. |
| 10 to 20 | Turn the cones over: Divide the group into two teams. Place 16 to 30 cones on the ground with half turned upside down. On the 'Go' command, team 1 has 3 minutes to turn over as many cones as possible. Team 2 has to reverse the cones. The winning team is the one that turns over the most cones. Progress to relays. |
| 20 to 30 | Agility course: Lay out a course that encourages children to run, jump, climb, hurdle, go under, and perform other movements related to as many objects as practically possible within 1 minute. This activity can be developed into games such as off-ground tag. |
| 30 to 40 | Skill and movement activities<br><br>Speed bounce: Double-foot lateral jumps over a 10- to 20-centimetre foam hurdle (height depends on competency). How many bounces can be done in 20 seconds?<br><br>Multiple-throw challenge: From a standing start, the child has to perform four basic medicine ball throws (chest pass, overhead throw, rotation throw left, rotation throw right). After the ball is thrown, the distance is measured. The child then sprints, retrieves the thrown ball and returns to the starting line. A stopwatch starts as the child starts to sprint and stops when the child returns to the throw line. A break occurs between throws. The distance thrown in metres for each throw is added up and combined with the total sprint time for all efforts to give a score for the athlete in this task. |
| 40 to 50 | Game time activity relay: Teams of three children work in a relay (or alternating-turns) format. Working over a set distance, the team races to cover the distance by hopping, sprinting and passing a baton, or skipping over a rope. Activities can be changed as required. |

movement qualities and begin to determine when and where skills should be executed.

During this stage, programme design should reflect biological age more than chronological age, because individual differences will start to become apparent. Indeed, differences also will emerge between the sexes; at this biological stage, girls generally are about a year ahead of boys in terms of physical development. Skeletal growth, predominantly from the limbs, is typically slow and steady; a typical increase in height is 3 to 5 centimetres annually.

The larger muscles are still better developed than smaller muscles. Coaches need to be aware of movement compensations in which large-muscle groups responsible for powerful movements begin to perform the roles that smaller, postural muscles might undertake in controlling joint stability. Appropriate joint positioning in all running, jumping, throwing and striking activities as well as any derivative movement patterns will correct or help prevent compensations. Indeed, the incorporation of dynamic warm-ups based on movement games enables an appropriate focus for activities that

encourage dynamic balance and good muscle sequencing through correct joint positioning. The coach must view the warm-up as a time for positive coaching experiences rather than preparation for the session that follows it. Examples of movement-specific warm-ups can be found in chapter 11.

The process of myelination along the axons of the neurons is finished towards the end of this stage, which might be referred to as one of neural proliferation. As identified in chapter 1, myelination is the developmental process in which the person's ability to activate motor units voluntarily exhibits potential for adaptation in response to a range of strength, speed and power stimuli. Therefore, a continued emphasis on explosive speed activities in a multidimensional context should form the basis of the athlete's physical conditioning.

High-intensity running, jumping, hopping and skipping activities for 4 or 5 seconds are ideal and build on the skills learned in the fundamental stages. With the improved transmission of motor action potentials, reaction times improve with appropriate reaction (simple stimulus–response) practices built into the acceleration and agility practices. This improved transmission of neural signals also means that eye–hand and eye–foot coordination is well established by the biological age of 12.

Appropriate practices lead to demonstrable improvements in strength during this time. Indeed, the relative gains in strength before puberty can be greater than those achieved during adolescence.[11] These gains are primarily because of improved neural stimulation of the motor unit as opposed to any morphological changes at muscle fibre level. Any activity that provides a positive stressor to the musculoskeletal system will improve strength and connective tissue structure, as well as encourage appropriate postural management.

Suggested activities include gymnastic and strength balances (for example, press-ups or handstands), climbing activities (ropes, wall bars or chin-ups) and progressive plyometrics (see chapter 9). Double-footed jumping, leaping (taking off from one or both feet and then landing on either the other foot or both feet), basic bounding (repetitive transfer of weight from one foot to the other in an exaggerated running action), and basic three-step explosion techniques (chapter 8) are all well suited to be introduced during these ages. Technical guidance for each of these activities is offered in more detail later in the book.

Medicine balls can be used either for ballistic (explosive power) exercises such as maximal overhead throws and chest passes or as a resistance-training modality, providing an external load for exercises such as squats and multidirectional lunges. The principle of using a low number of repetitions to avoid damaging the epiphysis of the bones (which are still calcifying) applies to these activities.

Note that the potential damage to the bone does not necessarily result from the intensity of the activity but from the repetitive stress that a large volume of work can inflict. Indeed, bone growth is encouraged by mechanical loading. The tissues respond to pressure, so resistance is a good thing to incorporate into the programme for skeletal and neuromuscular development. Grappling, wrestling, pushing and pulling tasks require minimal equipment and involve groups of children in interactive activity that is maximally intensive, short duration and fully involving.

The coach should continue to emphasize correct movement mechanics in all activities. Besides developing postural control and strength, gymnastic and dynamic body management activities also teach children some of the key principles of movement biomechanics. (Examples of gymnastic and dynamic body management activities, such as animal walks and strength balances, can be found in chapter 10.) The specific detail underpinning these principles is discussed more in chapters 4 and 5. In summary, several key principles underpin movement mechanics:

1. When resisting or transferring forces, straight is strongest.
2. Force generation develops from large-muscle groups to small-muscle groups.
3. Slow movements progress to fast movements as inertia is overcome.
4. Off-centred forces cause rotation.
5. The athlete needs to control rotation around a secondary axis to produce linear movement.
6. Short levers move faster than long ones.
7. For every action, there is an equal and opposite reaction.

These principles are evident in all the movement sequences introduced through the progressions in subsequent chapters. The athlete does not need to know these principles, but he or she must be coached to be able to demonstrate them in the movements produced, especially when presented with a novel task.

For example, if asked to perform a fast and repetitive spinning motion, a child will bend the arms to increase speed of movement. The child does this not because he or she understands that by reducing the lever arm of the limb he or she will move faster (principle 6), but simply because experiential knowledge has taught the child that this action helps produce a more rapid movement.

Because during this stage of neuromuscular system development the motor system is so open to learning, these ages often have been called the skill-hungry years. This stage is an excellent time to introduce the skills of complex weight-training techniques into the programme as a supplement to the speed, agility and plyometric activities that form the central themes within the programme. The full-range movements of the squatting action (including lunge patterns and single-leg variations) and pulling motions associated with lifting from the floor to overhead, and their various derivative movement patterns, become important strength-training modalities in any performance training programme (chapter 10). Therefore, learning the techniques at this stage, as a precursor to later strength development programmes, is an important step in the athlete development process.

The emphasis should always be on developing technique and skill and learning the coordinated movement sequences, but as these become more developed, progressively heavier loads can be incorporated into practices. Indeed, such activities challenge the athlete to move explosively through a full range of movement, promoting strength and mobility.

Children need to learn that being strong through a full range of movement allows them to access greater ranges of skill and maintain the connective tissue length that can prevent injury. These activities also develop the child's ability to control posture through the full kinetic chain rather than in isolated portions of the body or in isolated joint actions. This principle is a foundation on which movement skill development practices build throughout this text.

The popularity and use of resistance training, including training for sport, appears to be increasing among children and adolescents. This development is positive, despite anecdotal reports and conjecture regarding potential injury to the epiphyseal plates in the bones (the growth plates). Indeed, current scientific data indicate that when children are properly supervised, resistance training can enhance performance, reduce injury potential and enhance health aspects of children of all ages, including those in early adolescence.[12]

Children enter elementary school with what can be seen as a base of high energy and low endurance. Although the cardiovascular system is still developing, the child's continued biomechanical disadvantage also leads to increased oxygen requirements for a given workload. This circumstance is further exacerbated by the peripheral circulatory system, whereby oxygen is less able to be extracted from the blood at the working muscles.

One of the major means of thermal regulation in the human body is for the blood to transfer heat energy to the skin where it evaporates. But because the total skin surface area of children is small and their blood volume is low (compared with adults), their mechanisms for heat dissipation are limited. Before puberty, children cannot produce ATP anaerobically because of the absence of key enzymes (anaerobic adaptations following puberty are discussed later in the chapter). Anaerobic energy production creates an acidic environment within muscle cells, which is a fatigue mechanism, slowing the chemical reactions that cause muscle contractions and creating a burning sensation in the muscle. An important physiological function of fatigue is to prevent muscle damage through excessive effort.

Without this fatiguing system, children can easily be pushed in team or individual coaching situations to the point at which they are overheated, dehydrated and distressed. Because children cannot easily dissipate heat, overexertion is an important issue that needs to be kept in mind when considering high-intensity activity, prolonged activity or training activity, especially in hot environments.

# Adolescence

Adolescence is arguably the most important phase of athletic preparation. During these years, programmes can really make an athlete in terms of enabling him or her to reach full physical potential. Athletes who miss the opportunities afforded by this phase of developmentally appropriate training may find it difficult to achieve their full capabilities, because the opportunity for individualized development has potentially been compromised (or at least not optimized). The reason that so many athletes plateaus during the later stages of their careers is thought to result primarily from an overemphasis on competition at the expense of training or practice during this important period in their athletic development.[3]

These ages transcend the onset of puberty, so this phase can be seen as having both prepubertal and postpubertal considerations. Puberty refers to the somatic (anthropometrical) and physiological changes that occur in young people as reproduction organs change from an infantile state to an adult state. Puberty is often confused with adolescence; adolescence is largely regarded as the period of psychological and social transition between childhood and adulthood, which largely overlaps the period of puberty, but with less well-defined boundaries.

Puberty is initiated through hormonal signals from the hypothalamus in the brain to the gonads (the ovaries in females, the testes in males). These signals stimulate a sustained release of a variety of hormones (testosterone in males, estradiol in females) in large concentrations that stimulate the growth, function and transformation of the musculoskeletal, neuromuscular and bioenergetic systems, which can significantly influence performance improvements in the child. Anthropometrical changes between males and females now also become evident, as body shapes and proportions change in response to the evolutionary (reproductive) function of males and females.

Puberty is associated with the onset of peak height velocity (PHV), commonly known as the adolescent growth spurt, which provides the coach with a reference point for making informed decisions about the nature of the activities that a child is undertaking. During this time, children may grow up to 15 centimetres in a 2-year period (figure 3.5). The growth increase commonly starts at any age between 10 and 12 in girls and between 12 and 14 in boys, although in both it may start earlier or later. Indeed, around the chronological ages of 12 to 15, a programme may have a group of players who are biologically 11 to 18 years old. A 3-year variation typically occurs within a year group, so a coach of a U14 soccer team may have players who are biologically 11 to 17 years old (figure 3.6), although they may have similar training ages.

The biomechanical differences between individual skeletal sizes at these stages contribute to differences in the energy cost of work, efficiency during exercise and effectiveness in performance. This circumstance creates two problems related to how young performers are coached and how we seek to identify athletic talent within children.

Those who enter the growth spurt early often do extremely well in age-group sport and become used to success without training hard or focusing on skill mastery in their practice. In their later teens, however, when their slower-growing peers catch up and skill

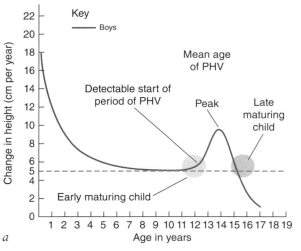

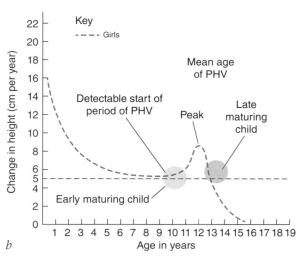

**Figure 3.5** Typical rates of growth in *(a)* males and *(b)* females.

Adapted from P. Rieser and L.E. Underwood, 2002, *Growing children: A parent's guide*, 5th ed. (SanFrancisco: Genentech).

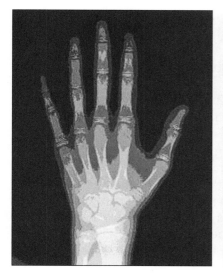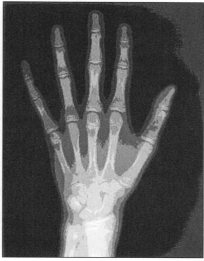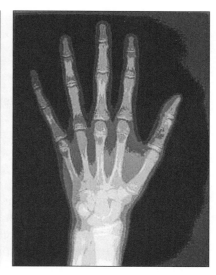

**Figure 3.6** X-rays from children of the same chronological age show markedly different biological ages, as shown by the bone density and growth plates of these children.

Courtesy of Viswanath B. Unnithan and John Iga.

development and game understanding become more important, the early maturers are not accustomed to being beaten and often drop out of the sport.

Likewise, many of the children who experience their growth spurt later than their peers do (and who ultimately may have the potential to be equally skilled physically) may feel hopelessly overpowered from the start and believe that they are simply no good at sport.

Thus, both ends of this normal distribution need to be accounted for through programmes that focus appropriately on skill mastery and a more individualized, or differentiated, approach to coaching children. Research into the relative age effect within sport has recognized this point. Early developers, or those born in the first half of a year group for a sport, tend to be advanced as talented performers compared with their relatively younger peers born later in the respective year. This circumstance has been thought to narrow the talent pool in a sport artificially, because later-maturing children often become discouraged about further participation and may ultimately never achieve the potential they may have had if they had gone through the full spectrum of the physical development process.

The coach who is able to work closely with the child's parents may be able to identify when a child is approaching, entering and leaving PHV. This stage can be determined by having adults make accurate and consistent measures of a child's height at monthly (before PHV onset) and weekly or fortnightly (after PHV onset) intervals. As the pattern of skeletal growth begins to change with the onset of puberty—the principal region of growth is now the trunk instead of the limbs—seated rather than standing height is often a more appropriate reference point for coaches and parents to use to monitor the increase in height.

During PHV, the child's body is using energy to grow. Therefore, coaches should consider reducing the training volume load on the child during these periods and instead focus on skill-based tasks that encourage the neuromuscular system to adapt to changes in spatial patterning caused by the changing proportions of the body.

This change in body shape may have stronger implications for the coach working with female athletes. Widened hips may mean a more steeply angled femur (thigh bone), resulting in changes to running and landing techniques (for example, heels kicking outwards when running, knees rotating inwards when landing; see figure 3.7). As we will see in chapter 5, these changes can potentially cause a number of injury problems. As figure

3.7 illustrates, this valgus position has a force vector (a concept explained in chapter 4) that tends to cause medial rotation.

The changing hip position also tends to cause asynchronous firing patterns between the quadriceps and hamstrings. The result is that the predominant angle of muscular force tends to be outwards. This asynchronous firing pattern not only contributes to knee instability on impact but also can affect the lateral tracking of the patella, often causing problems to the medial and anterior cruciate ligaments and the patella itself.

For example, chondromalacia patella is an abnormal softening of the cartilage under the kneecap that can be alleviated by stretching and strengthening the quadriceps and hamstrings, especially on the medial (inside) portion. Coaches need to invest time in developing and reinforcing correct landing mechanics in

running, hopping and jumping actions through puberty and beyond both to promote movement efficiency and to reduce injury. The later chapters of this book are largely devoted to this concept.

The widening of the hips and lengthening of the trunk lead to changes in the child's centre of mass. In females, the centre of mass tends to lower as hip width increases, which means that females become relatively more balanced and stable. In males, the centre of mass tends to rise, which means that they tend to become relatively less stable. Lowering the centre of mass is beneficial for some activities, such as those requiring balance and stability. To accelerate in any direction, however, an athlete has to place the centre of mass outside the base of support. The coach needs to work with the child to develop strategies to do this effectively as body proportions change.

Reductions in training volume load during periods of rapid growth are not recommended simply because of the need for energy conservation. Muscular and external loading (pulling forces) on the bones stimulate bone growth and increase bone mineral density. Repetitive force loading at this time, however, can injure musculotendinous structures where the muscle connects to the bones. Complete fusion of tendons to their respective apophyseal locations (a projection on the outside of the bone) occurs at various ages between 12 and 20 years old for different sites, potentially leading to a number of traction injuries.

These conditions include Osgood-Schlatter's disease at the tibial tuberosity (12 to 16 years old) in young soccer players, runners and jumpers, and Sever's disease at the calcaneum of the heel (10 to 13 years old) in young swimmers, runners and jumpers. The iliac crest at the top of the hipbone is especially vulnerable to apophysitis (inflammation of the bony projection on the bone surface) between 14 and 17 years old, especially in activities that twist the trunk, such as throwing, pitching, grappling and hurdling. Similar apophysites may occur

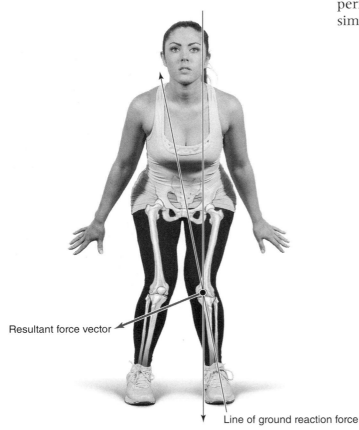

Resultant force vector

Line of ground reaction force

**Figure 3.7**  The increase Q angle at the hips means that practitioners need to reinforce landing mechanics in postpubertal females.

in the shoulder and arm in young pitchers, swimmers and throwers. Such traction stresses, associated with crescendo pain (i.e., pain above a certain threshold of activity), occur particularly through high-repetition training.[13]

After the completion of PHV, the myotendinous structures are more developed and less vulnerable. At this stage, androgenic hormones (principally testosterone) are also at their highest levels. This stage provides an ideal opportunity to maximize strength and speed–strength gains. The correlation between maximal strength (the ability to produce maximal force) and power production is well documented.

With the onset of puberty, the hormonal profile of the child changes significantly. Change occurs in the strength, speed and endurance capabilities of the child. Given that the long-term power-producing potential of an athlete depends heavily on his or her long-term force-producing capabilities, the athlete should be given the best chance to develop this characteristic through exposure to resistance and high-force training.

This approach is especially important given the high concentrations of anabolic hormones in the adolescent athlete. This characteristic means that the neurological and morphological training benefits of strength training, plyometric and speed-based activities can be optimized.

Such training methods promote bone development and enhance protein synthesis, contributing to muscle hypertrophy (increase in muscle fibre size) and, to a lesser extent following the earlier years of growth, hyperplasia (increase in the number of cells or muscle fibres). These changes increase muscle cross-sectional area, which is closely correlated with the ability of the muscle to produce force. Increased muscle cross-sectional area is a positive training adaptation, regardless of the sport that a person is training for. By puberty, a child typically is beginning to focus on a specific sport. Not all sports require large muscles, but as explained in chapter 4, all sports require the body to be able to exert and withstand forces. This ability is primarily a function of the recruitment of motor units through the central nervous system, but when a motor unit has been stimulated, an increased contractile mechanism in which more protein filaments can bind together enhances the force-producing capabilities of the muscle. Therefore, an increase in the muscle cross-sectional area benefits all athletes, although not all athletes need to be bodybuilders!

Understanding the difference in muscle cross-sectional area required by different sports is important, because it is directly related to the athlete's training regimen. High-volume, submaximal resistance training (typical bodybuilding exercises or weight-training circuits of more than 10 repetitions) tends to result in more increases in the volume of noncontractile proteins and fluid components of the sarcoplasm of the muscle. This substance is the plasma volume that surrounds the contractile elements of the muscle fibre. Because this has no direct influence on the contractile proteins, it has little effect on the force-producing capabilities of the muscle and therefore is of little direct benefit to sport performers.

Conversely, near-maximal-force resistance training (Olympic-style weightlifting; low-repetition, high-load resistance training; plyometrics) results in sarcomere hypertrophy. The sarcomere is the functional contractile unit of the muscle (explored in depth in chapter 4), and an increase in the size, number and arrangement of the sarcomeres is possible with the appropriate training. With high-speed training, sarcomeres can be added in series (i.e., end to end), which improves the velocity of the muscle contraction. High-force resistance training has been shown to increase myofibril density by adding sarcomeres in parallel. The density of the contractile structures increases, expanding the number of connections between the contractile proteins and enhancing the ability of the muscle to produce greater forces. World triple-jump record holder (18.3 m) Jonathon Edwards personified an athlete with little muscle bulk but high-density muscles with high cross-sectional area within his leg muscles. He cleaned 2.23 times his body weight at 68 kilograms (the clean technique is reviewed in chapter 10).

A progressive and balanced approach to the incorporation of such activities into the programme allows the connective tissue strength to develop at the same time as the muscle architecture. An inappropriate emphasis on increasing muscle volume can lead to connective tissue injuries when the athlete is performing in the sporting context. Because training is done to enhance sport performance, this approach would be a negative (rather than positive) transfer of training effect.

Strength gains are achievable at any age, because the neural components of the contractile mechanism respond positively to strength stimuli. The hormonal changes brought by puberty, however, enable athletes to maximize strength gains caused by changes in muscle structure. Appropriate high-force and high-velocity modalities should be incorporated into the training programme to maximize these morphological benefits during puberty.

Increased strength means increased ability to apply forces. This force production must be associated with two key elements to ensure successful transfer of training benefits to the ability to move well within sport. First, training to produce maximal force should be appropriately combined with training to produce force quickly so that the athlete is able to execute sport-specific movements (see chapters 4 and 10). Second, the athlete must always be challenged to use mechanically efficient postures to reduce short- and long-term injury potential.

Because athletes are able to exert more force into the ground and their legs are getting longer, running stride typically increases in length. As a result, athletes speed up, even with little or no technical input into a speed or agility programme. But the athletic development professional wants to maximize the potential for this developing power production. Appropriate integration of technical practices for multiplanar movement with physical development work will ensure that the athlete is able optimize speed and agility potential because of the programme rather than accept speed improvements that might occur despite the programme.

The focus of speed work at this time should be related to the technical and force-producing aspects of ground contact in linear running. As chapter 8 details, acceleration and maximal velocity running speeds depend on the athlete being able to exert sufficient impulses (chapter 4) within short ground contact time frames. The athlete must have optimal technique to make efficient use of the plastic properties of the Achilles tendon at the ankle joint and elastic properties of the stretch-reflex mechanism in the neuromuscular system. This technique will be developed through the increasingly complex and intense plyometrics that should be a focus of the power-training programme, as well as technical practices channelled towards enhancing ground contact mechanics that transfer the benefits of the physio-mechanical properties to skilled execution.

Chaotic changes of direction also rely on physio-mechanical properties of the stretch-reflex mechanism. The ability to apply and use highly reactive forces to change direction efficiently and powerfully in a sport context is an essential skill for a high-level sport performer. Change-of-direction techniques are important, but as explained earlier, these techniques ideally will have been learned during the skill-hungry years that precede adolescence. The focus during adolescence should be on the reactive and decision-making components and explosive application of forces through executing the techniques that make up agility skills (chapter 8).

Puberty also marks an important physiological change for the bioenergetic system. Testosterone stimulates development of the anaerobic system and promotes the capacity of the aerobic system. The higher levels of serum testosterone increase the production of the oxygen-carrying red blood cells. Therefore, aerobic training could be given primacy with the onset of PHV to coincide with this increase in testosterone. Aerobic training, however, should not be used in preference to, or at the expense of, strength, skill or speed development, especially in athletes who are not going to specialize in sports or events that require high aerobic capacity (distance running, rowing, distance cycling, middle- and long-distance swimming). Although many propose that team sports and intermittent, high-intensity sports such as boxing and tennis require a large aerobic capacity, these sports last 90 minutes or longer, so that is not really the case (figure 3.8).

Success in invasion and combat sports depends on the ability to perform at the highest intensity and sustain powerful performances for long durations. Athletes in these sports require training that promotes the recruitment of Type IIa and IIx motor units and the development of high anaerobic power and capacity within these fibres and the central and peripheral aspects of the cardiovascular networks. The priority for developmental training at this time should be maximizing the development of the neuromuscular and musculoskeletal systems so that the athlete becomes as strong and fast as possible. This training will provide the athlete the best basis for transfer to higher levels of performance later in his or her career.

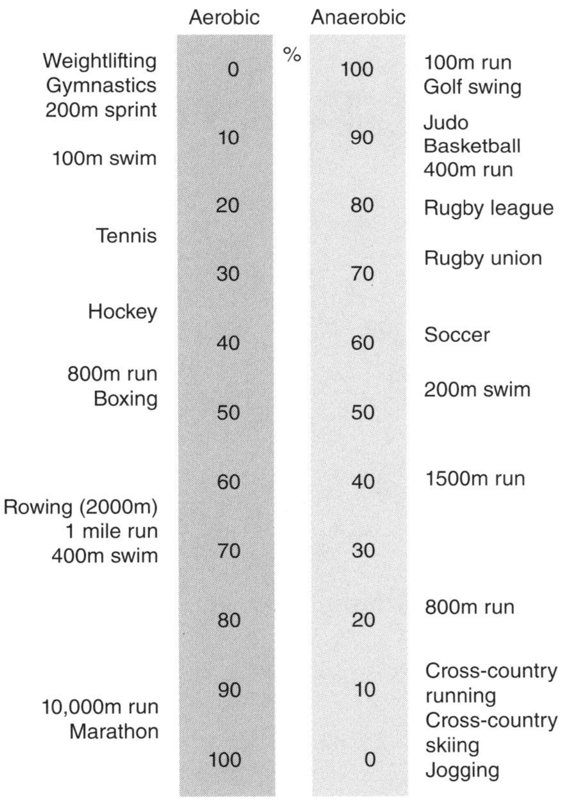

| Aerobic | % | Anaerobic | |
|---|---|---|---|
| Weightlifting Gymnastics 200m sprint | 0 | 100 | 100m run Golf swing |
| 100m swim | 10 | 90 | Judo Basketball 400m run |
| | 20 | 80 | Rugby league |
| Tennis | 30 | 70 | Rugby union |
| Hockey | | | |
| 800m run Boxing | 40 | 60 | Soccer |
| | 50 | 50 | 200m swim |
| | 60 | 40 | 1500m run |
| Rowing (2000m) 1 mile run 400m swim | 70 | 30 | |
| | 80 | 20 | 800m run |
| | 90 | 10 | Cross-country running Cross-country skiing Jogging |
| 10,000m run Marathon | 100 | 0 | |

**Figure 3.8**  The bioenergetic contribution to performance in various sports.

The training focus should be fitness preparation for activities that support the neuromuscular system. From a health perspective, the bioenergetic system should not be ignored, but sufficient sport-specific practices that involve high-intensity, low-volume work typically promote sufficient endurance in a complimentary manner to the primacy of motor system development, ensuring that the athlete is able to meet the endurance needs of the activity.

As figure 3.8 illustrates, the importance of high-level aerobic fitness is overestimated for many sports. Most team or invasion sports require an athlete to perform at high intensity (high speed, high strength) and recover quickly. An athlete who is able to work for a long time but not with enough intensity (not fast enough, agile enough or powerful enough) will not be able to transition to higher levels of performance.

As figure 3.9 demonstrates, elite-level intermittent sports, such as rugby league, require players to be able to run in excess of 7 kilometres in 80 minutes. Players are also required to reach top speeds in excess of 8 metres per second, be involved in more than 60 collisions (making or being tackled) and recover quickly enough to be able to perform another high-intensity effort. Figure 3.9*a* shows that heart rates are above 160 beats per minute for 61.5 per cent of the game (typically exceeding the anaerobic threshold); figure 3.9*b* shows heart rate against speed efforts. This figure illustrates that the key capacity in a player is to be able to recover quickly from high-intensity efforts so that he or she can become involved in the game again as tactics require.

Although athletes typically should not yet be identified as specialists in sport or event disciplines, this often happens early in adolescence. Certainly, preferences will begin to narrow the choices. But all the energy-supply mechanisms in the athlete should be fully developed. Whatever the sport, the athlete will require speed, agility and power. Short-interval training (for example, 10 seconds of high-intensity intermittent running at 100 to 120 per cent of maximal aerobic speed) will develop the anaerobic alactic and aerobic systems in

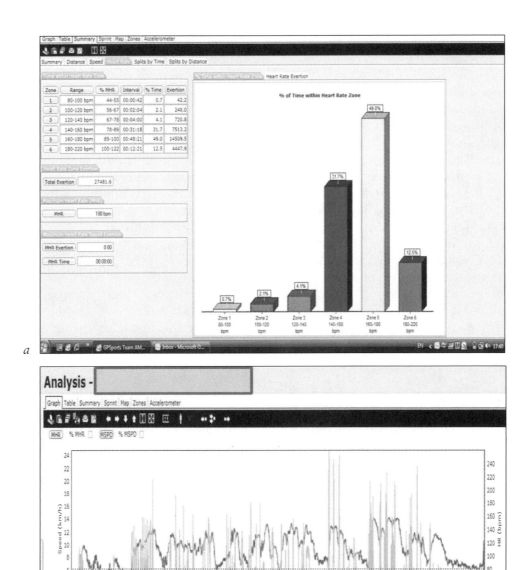

**Figure 3.9** Activity analysis using GPS in elite rugby league demonstrates the importance of repeat high-intensity efforts to team performance.

terms of maximal oxygen uptake and maximal aerobic speed before PHV.[14]

After puberty, the ability to tolerate and use the anaerobic and lactate systems becomes more developed because of the increase in PFK, an enzyme that regulates the conversion of glucose into ATP, enabling anaerobic metabolic pathways to operate. Anaerobic energy production results in the accumulation of lactate in the blood and an acidic environment within muscle cells. This acidic environment acts as a fatigue mechanism that the adolescent needs to be trained to tolerate so that he or she can perform the intense activity that characterizes many sport performances. Appropriate training includes high-intensity and longer-duration interval methods as well as conditioning games and sport-specific practices. This type of training permits differentiation between those who are moving towards specialization in multisprint sports and those who will be participating in prolonged endurance events. Note that short-interval intermittent training also has been linked to other aspects of fitness, such as lower-limb explosive strength,[14] thought to be primarily caused by neurological rather than morphological adaptations.

Let's consider three endurance-training sessions for 16-year-old athletes who have different sporting ambitions.

### Speed Endurance Session for a Track Athlete Moving Towards Sprint Specialization

Dynamic warm-up and mobilization drills that progress into technique drills

Technique drills largely incorporated into a simple low-intensity training unit that leads into a speed–endurance session:

- 2 × 150 metres at or greater than 90 per cent; walk back between repetitions
- 5-minute recovery
- 3 × 120 metres at or greater than 90 per cent; walk back between repetitions
- 5-minute recovery
- 4 × 90 metres at or greater than 90 per cent; walk back between repetitions

Cool-down

### Running Anaerobic Lactic Capacity Session for a Track Athlete Moving Towards Endurance Group Specialization

Dynamic warm-up and mobilization drills that progress into technique drills

Technique drills largely incorporated into a simple low-intensity training unit that leads into an anaerobic lactate capacity session:

- 3 × 3 × 300 metres at 85 per cent of 300-metre time trial
- 3-minute recovery between repetitions and 8-minute recovery between sets

Cool-down

### Running Anaerobic Lactic Capacity Session for a Soccer Player

Dynamic warm-up incorporating mobilization drills and movement skill drills

Progress into 4 × 3 × 100 metres at or greater than 85 per cent max velocity, 30-second recovery between repetitions (jog between repetitions), 4-minute recovery between sets

5 × 200 metres in 30 seconds; easy walk back between repetitions

Cool-down

Note that using small-sided games to develop endurance applies to this age group, especially in a soccer player for whom endurance and game play are emphasized within the same session. Specific examples of this type of work can be found in the case study in chapter 11. The practitioner needs to balance the benefits of using this approach with the realization that skill levels and player choices can limit the intensity of such sessions. Without intensity, anaerobic endurance will be hard to develop. Running or other equally valid endurance training modalities such as grappling, rowing or cycling can be simplified so that the session achieves the desired intensity and bioenergetic outcomes.

Because of the great individual variation among adolescent athletes, the coach needs to build both capacity and skill (movement- or sport-specific) through individual development programmes. Training should be based on maturation as well as training age; early, average and late maturers need different timing relative to the training emphasis.

The concept of individualized programmes requires a radical change in mind-set from many current coaching practices. At present, many of these decisions are based on chronological age (age groups), not training age and individual maturation. No form of individual skill is universally valid for everybody. This concept is known as differentiation, which has been a central theme of education programmes for many years. Differentiation learning methods provide athletes (pupils) different avenues to acquiring the session content, whether in how they process information, construct solutions or make sense of ideas. In a practical context, differentiation means structuring practices or providing prescriptions or equipment so that all students within a practice can learn effectively, regardless of ability or physical stature. This concept is further explained, and examples are provided, in chapter 7.

The important thing is for the coach to identify each player's technical qualities and the ways in which those skills may be developed further. Technically gifted young players are able to learn skills faster than ordinary players can. The athletic development specialist must ensure that a training session works on all the interdependent motor faculties of the players, such as speed and strength together or speed and agility. The physiological effects of the training are bound to complement each other and do not in any way cancel each other out. Additionally, individual skills depend on perceptual, and maybe intellectual, abilities. Motivation for individual skill training depends on how complex or simple and how real or artificial the training is.

During competitions athletes perform to win and do their best, but the major focus of practice is on learning to express the movements, sport-specific skills and tactics in a competitive (fun!) arena, as opposed to focusing on the competition outcome (win or loss). Training and competition ratios need to be optimized; too much competition wastes valuable training time, but not enough competition inhibits enjoyment.

Skill and physical development must have a priority over competitive results. Athletes following this philosophy and undertaking this type of preparation will be better prepared for competition in both the short and long term than those who focus solely on winning.

# Late Adolescence

Shortly after puberty, the athlete will have reached physiological maturity. Females will have reached skeletal maturity, although this may not occur in males until they are 21 or 22 years old. The training emphasis now shifts towards individualized skill and physical development to improve sport-specific competition performance as opposed to longer-term development needs. At this stage the athlete learns to optimize and maximize biomotor abilities to facilitate peak competitive performance within a sport-specific programme.

The focus on physical training now depends on two distinct but not mutually exclusive factors. The first is to determine the physical performance variables that determine success within a given sport:

- What force-producing capacities are required: high force, high strength–speed, high speed–strength?
- What locomotive capacities are required: linear maximum velocity, multidirectional, chaotic and agility-based?
- What endurance capacities are required: anaerobic alactic power, anaerobic lactic power, anaerobic lactic capacity, aerobic power, aerobic capacity?
- What mobility capacities are required: postural hypermobility, joint-specific hypermobility, full movement range?

Answering these questions will enable the practitioner to determine the training parameters or objectives for a programme, typically a sport-specific programme at this point in the athlete's career. In this context, some training priorities are complementary and some objectives are divergent in terms of the physiological consequences.[15] See figure 3.10.

The next question is arguably the most important follow-up to the previous questions: How should the individual athlete be trained to achieve the desired performance priorities? Answering this question requires understanding the athlete's training age and experiences and anatomical strengths and weakness in relation to achieving the desired outcomes. For example, little can be done to influence the athlete's height or limb length. What does the athletic development professional need to do to maximize the athlete's strength, power, speed, agility and so on based on the athlete's anatomy? Some anatomical limitations are transient, but some are the consequences of poor postural control or movement skills. Chapters 5 and 6 identify why these might occur, how they can be developed and how they can be remediated within a programme.

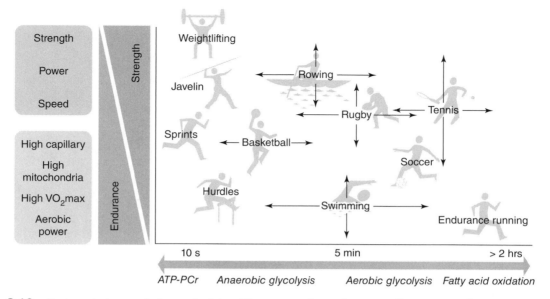

**Figure 3.10** Determining training priorities: The strength–endurance divergence of priorities.

Adapted, by permission, from D. French, 2014, "Programming and adaptation implications for concurrent training: Optimising divergent physiology in strength/power sports." Presented at UKSCA's 10th Annual Conference, July 2014.

Training age is the most important consideration. Many sport-specific practitioners quickly identify the performance determinants of a sport and channel training towards these elements. But the progression towards specific and complex movements will lead to poor performance and increased risk of injury if the athlete doesn't have sufficient background in the progressive development of generalized motor skills. Regardless of the athlete's age, the practitioner should be guided by the athlete's competency and preparedness to execute a task rather than what the sport-specific demands would dictate. The competency-based approach to development is explained further in chapter 7, and it forms the basis of the movement-specific skills discussed in chapters 8 through 10. Differentiating an athlete's programme based on training age and movement skill competencies is an essential characteristic for the athletic development professional.

Note that these principles do not apply only to young athletes. To perform in a certain sport, athletes should meet prerequisite training volumes and have experiences and capacities. To approach a training programme without these prerequisites will ultimately limit the athlete's performance and significantly increase the risk of injury.

For this reason, those working with adults also need to understand and engage in the developmental process. Robust structures need strong foundations, and athletes are no different. An athlete development specialist needs to understand an athlete's training and prerequisite physical development and be able to identify the experiences that the athlete may need to undertake to be successful in his or her chosen activity. A needs analysis can identify strengths and deficiencies to be addressed. Any subsequent programme objectives will be based on this process. What are the needs of the individual athlete based on his or her training age, experiences and injury history? What are the athletic challenges posed by the sport for which he or she is preparing?

The practitioner who understands how the body develops and which activities can best promote optimal development will know how to differentiate and appropriately structure specific training interventions with any athlete.

Regardless of the sport, the required movement skills and physio-mechanical capacities that enable the effective execution of these skills should be part of any training prescription at a sport-specific level. These are summarized in figure 3.11. The guidelines and technical details for prescribing and progressing all

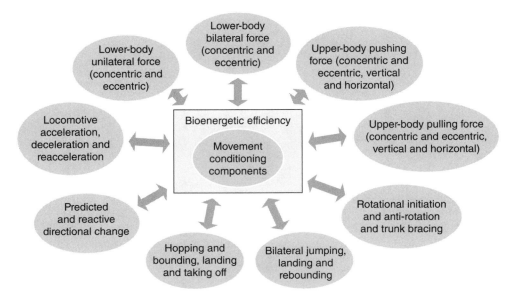

**Figure 3.11**   Generic movement skill programme components.

aspects of each of the specific programme elements form the basis for chapters 8 through 11.

The successful athletic development professional has the ability to construct curriculums or progressions based on knowledge of the physiological development of a young athlete and understanding that certain physical characteristics are prerequisite to others. An applied example of this knowledge is presented in table 3.3, in which growth and development considerations have been summarized and aligned to a progressive curriculum for soccer players. The table presents the specific programme elements of movement skills and physical conditioning, identified from the training components in figure 1.4.

## Summary

Athletic development programme progressions need to be developmentally appropriate, regardless of the athlete's age. The athlete's level is predominantly determined by his or her biological stage of development; the athlete's preparedness for a specific activity is determined by his or her training age.

Practitioners equipped with the necessary knowledge and skills to structure and monitor training programmes to match the anatomical and physiological development processes of the child will be able to maximize the potential of their athletes. This chapter has explored in depth some of the key aspects of motor system development and the way in which they should influence coaching practice. In young athletes, the development of the neuromuscular system is a primary objective. Specific emphasis should be placed on developing strength, power and speed through mechanically efficient postures that optimize the athlete's potential for effective movement skill performance at any stage of his or her career.

**Table 3.3** Soccer Conditioning Curriculum That Aligns Growth and Development Considerations to Movement Skill and Physical Conditioning

| Learning to move | Learning the skills | Learning the game | Playing the game, developing performance |
|---|---|---|---|
| Late childhood | Late childhood to early puberty | Early puberty to late puberty | Late puberty to early adulthood |
| **GROWTH AND DEVELOPMENT CONSIDERATIONS** | | | |
| Emphasis on development of fundamental movement skills and generalized physical literacy (multidirectional movement and handling, catching, throwing, evasion and posture, support skills)<br><br>Stability, object control and locomotion<br><br>Central nervous system development to promote primary speed development (reactive agility and quickness) | The skill-hungry years: emphasis on overall sport skill and soccer-specific skill development (multidirectional movement and throwing, catching, kicking [directive passing and long distance], evasion and support skills)<br><br>Earlier maturation of girls compared with boys<br><br>Major focus on strength and speed: technique and motor skill development | Early in the stage, brain and neural control mechanisms disregard nerve connections that are not used. Therefore, use varied and challenging movement, strength and speed training opportunities at all times before puberty. 'Use it or lose it' phenomenon.<br><br>Neural system training through plyometrics and speed and agility work remains a priority.<br><br>Opportunities to maximize availability of hormones to develop morphological and neurological aspects of strength. Females at end of PHV and again at the onset of menarche (puberty).<br><br>Males 12 to 18 months after PHV.<br><br>Onset of growth spurt (PHV). Typically girls 11 to 13 years old, boys 13 to 16 years old. Differentiation in coaching practices to avoid relative age effect precluding late maturers from development opportunities.<br><br>Anaerobic system development following PHV. Opportunity to develop alactic (short time and distance, long recovery) capacity.<br><br>Increased capacity for aerobic system training (as appropriate) following the onset of PHV through intermittent, high-intensity and games-based activities. | Training process is based on individualized programmes within team schedule; physiological optimization; maximizing power (strength–speed and speed–strength); acceleration, chaotic and multidirectional speed; top-end speed (position specific); technique; flexibility.<br><br>Need to ensure that postural integrity is maintained as strength and musculature increase.<br><br>Maturation is finished for females.<br><br>Skeletal maturation in males typically is complete by 21 years of age. |

*(continued)*

55

**Table 3.3** *continued*

| Learning to move | Learning the skills | Learning the game | Playing the game, developing performance |
|---|---|---|---|
| Late childhood | Late childhood to early puberty | Early puberty to late puberty | Late puberty to early adulthood |
| **MOVEMENT SKILLS PROGRESSIONS** | | | |
| Stability, object control and locomotion skills emphasis<br><br>Games-based approach to agility and body-weight exercises<br><br>General movement, manipulation and stability skills; static into movement situations<br><br>Development of coordination, body management and awareness (kinaesthetic sense) through multiskill activities<br><br>Use of traditional PE and playground activities within a soccer environment | Learning (understanding movement) through action in games<br><br>Gymnastic and body management (incorporating dynamic balance) activities to develop appropriate neuromuscular recruitment patterns<br><br>Mechanics, posture and body awareness emphasized through running, jumping, throwing and other skills and linked into games-based practices<br><br>Grappling, rotation, ground to feet and athletic development activities through appropriately qualified and experienced individuals<br><br>Neural development through jumping and other plyometric skills<br><br>Agility training based on closed, confined movements that apply agility mechanics, with increasing decision-making involvement throughout the stage | Challenge the posture by changing base of support, speed of execution, planes of motion, length of lever, position of centre of mass and so on.<br><br>Focus on pelvic and shoulder girdles and knee tracking in female players.<br><br>Coordination and technique drills should be used to develop coordination as body proportions change.<br><br>Functional (running, jumping, pushing, lifting, rotational movement, resisted movement) postural integrity training introduced and progressed so that it eventually is fully integrated into the player's training.<br><br>Total-body movements develop posture and functional strength and power for soccer. High-force and velocity-dependent activities. are the focus of the programme.<br><br>The major developments in terms of physical gains are targeted at the neuromuscular system (fast delivery of sound technique through high-intensity, low-volume, low-fatigue programmes).<br><br>Small-muscle groups are becoming more developed. Programmes emphasize control in these muscles (putting the joints in the right position).<br><br>Reactive change of direction and forceful application of change-of-direction mechanics increase in importance as neuromuscular system develops. | Every session has a warm-up (speed, agility, balance, coordination) that prepares the neuromuscular system for training and playing.<br><br>Functional posture integrity and muscular recruitment exercises are fully integrated into player's individualized training.<br><br>Strength technique is transferred into technical work (strength training, warm-up, gymnastic activity, grappling activity). Posture is always in a position to exert and withstand forces.<br><br>Ensure that all muscle groups are recruited in appropriate sequences through performance analysis and dynamic screening process with communication between players, physiologists, strength and conditioning coaches (review after every session and game).<br><br>Individual programmes are used to ensure that proprioception, balance and coordination are maximized.<br><br>Use tactical-based, stimulus-identification response practices.<br><br>Use agility training based on open and reactive movements<br><br>Refinement of footwork patterns and skills are linked to decision making, position and game-based activities. |

| Learning to move | Learning the skills | Learning the game | Playing the game, developing performance |
|---|---|---|---|
| Late childhood | Late childhood to early puberty | Early puberty to late puberty | Late puberty to early adulthood |
| **PHYSICAL CONDITIONING PROGRESSIONS** | | | |
| 'Make it fun, kids will run' | Major focus is on strength and speed: technique and motor skill development. | Use diagnostics to analyse strengths and weaknesses in all physical performance factors. Key principle is to do better individual monitoring as players move on to more regular contact with performance programme delivery | Training process is based on maximizing power (strength–speed and speed–strength); maximizing acceleration, chaotic and multidirectional speed; optimizing anaerobic capacity and power, with aerobic system benefits as a consequence; improving flexibility. |

Development means that practice should encourage multiple activities of 0 to 10 metres and 0 to 5 seconds with recovery after each.

Running mechanics: Use linear, lateral and multidirectional movement games.

Use fun, games-based and individual challenge approach to developing strength and power through faster, higher, stronger (e.g., jumping, throwing, kicking, grappling, climbing, pulling) games.

Use few repetitions to avoid excessive or repetitive stresses.

Introduce endurance and develop it through small-sided games and general play.

Develop understanding of range of movement in skill development.

Monitor children to ensure they receive and progress in a variety of movement skills.

---

Development means that practice should encourage activities of 0 to 20 metres (0 to 5 seconds).

Basic movement mechanics are reinforced for running, jumping, throwing.

Running and jumping mechanics (one and two feet).

Acceleration: linear, lateral and multidirectional movement.

Introduce movement mechanics in warm-up and game play.

Develop strength and improve body mechanics using medicine balls, hopping and body-weight exercises, pushing, pulling, swinging, climbing, wrestling games and tug-of-war activities.

Use a games-based and individual challenge approach to developing endurance. Training is not formalized and is continually developed through games-based activities and small-sided games and play

In early maturing and older age groups, introduce planned repetitive short-duration high-intensity interval activities (up to 10 seconds). These can be games-based, wrestling-based or skills-based activities as well as running and other activities.

Introduce habit of warming up and cooling down through fun and dynamic activities.

Recognize the importance of range of movement in skill development and injury prevention.

Use a competency approach to monitoring individual process outcomes: how not to, how high, how far, how fast.

---

Use appropriate balance between quality of work and quantity of work depending on session objectives.

Optimize movement mechanics and emphasize intensity of reactions and movements: reactions and decision making, acceleration, deceleration, direction change, reacceleration, position-specific top-end speed development.

Increase intensity (as strength base develops) of plyometric jumping skills. Emphasize high-force and rapid foot contact activities.

Individualize weightlifting programmes under qualified supervision. Focus on multijoint, multimuscle activities through full posture and kinetic chain. This activity emphasizes neural and structural development and coordination at periods of major growth and development.

Introduce principle of progressive overload at an individual level led by monitored training records.

Endurance training is based on short intervals (5- to 15- second efforts with 1- to 3-minute active recoveries). Activities can be game based or relay based. Introduce endurance training from the start of this phase.

After PHV, introduce intermediate and longer, more intense game-based intervals. Conditioning can be done through small-sided conditioning games for those who are appropriately developed.

Emphasize and develop flexibility (important in maturing person because skeleton grows rapidly) through dynamic exercise and static stretching sessions.

Dynamic, athletic warm-up and a comprehensive and total-body cool-down are essential components of athletic development.

Prescribe individual stretching sessions away from the training environment.

---

Emphasize postural integrity as strength and musculature increases.

Integrate individual and position-specific programmes into annual and weekly training programmes.

Use advanced training methods for strength, power and endurance.

Use musculoskeletal screening, athlete-monitoring technologies and diagnostic tools to analyse strengths, weaknesses and physical performance factors in training and games.

Increasing intensity of intervals is important for speed–endurance. Work-to-rest ratios are important.

Emphasize flexibility.

Optimize individual training routines in accordance with individual needs and team training and playing demands.

# CHAPTER 4

# Efficiently Controlling Forces: Mechanical Functions of Movement

Well-executed movement patterns form the solutions to the problems of any sporting situation. A core principle of this book is that motor (movement) control pertains to the patterning of muscle activation, that is, the timing of when muscles are active and when they are not. Efficient movement requires coordination of muscle action such that stability is ensured (chapter 5) and effective load, or force, transfer is achieved. This chapter explains why skilful movement patterns in sport require the athlete to get into a position from which he or she can continually and consistently exert and withstand forces. After reading chapters 4 and 5, you will understand the science of force management that underpins practical techniques (chapter 8 through 10) and know how to apply the principles of science to progress an athlete's movement control capacities (as exemplified in chapter 11).

The character of the force developed in the athlete's body depends on the interaction between the alignment of the joints and the environment. Chapter 5 focuses on the correct organization of the posture by the neuromuscular system. Many of the remaining chapters apply these principles to developing the motor patterns of skilful movements that use the kinetic chain in the most effective and efficient manner in sport. This chapter focuses on the importance of forces in determining the observable outcome of a sporting movement.

## The Three Laws of Motion

Biomechanics is the study of the internal and external forces acting on the body and the observable effects of these forces in performance. The mechanics of movement are governed by the three basic laws of motion identified by Isaac Newton in his *Philosophiæ Naturalis Principia Mathematica*, published in 1687. The practitioner who understands the principles of biomechanics and their application will provide athletes the best opportunity to reach their potential. Similarly, injuries in sport tend to have a mechanical cause.[1] Therefore, understanding how the body works in sport reduces the probability that an athlete will experience an injury within a programme.

### Law of Inertia

The first law is that of inertia, which is also called the laziness law. An object at rest and an object in motion are two examples of the same thing: An object will continue in its state of rest or uniform motion (i.e., constant speed and direction) unless acted on by an external force. For example, a ball thrown in the vacuum of space would continue to move at the same speed and in the same direction ad infinitum. On earth, the ball would slow and eventually stop because of the forces of gravity and the external resistance (friction) of the air that the ball moves through.

This law explains the parabolic flight path of a punted soccer ball, a driven golf ball and a thrown javelin. It also explains why a swimmer who dives into a pool will slow down after entering the water; the momentum of his or her body will be slowed by the frictional drag of the water.

## Law of Acceleration

The second law is the law of acceleration. A change in uniform motion or rest occurs because of an externally applied force. It can also be said that the change in motion (i.e., momentum) is proportional to the force acting on the object, is inversely proportional to the mass of the object and acts in the direction of the forces. This law gives rise to the classical formula of force equals mass times acceleration (F = MA). Simply put, the more mass an object has, the more force will be required to move it (relative to an object of less mass), the more force will be required to accelerate it (i.e., get it to change speed) and, once it is moving (i.e., it has some momentum), the more force will be required to decelerate or stop it.

Alternatively, given the fact that the mass of an object rarely changes in sport, the faster an object must accelerate or decelerate (i.e., change speed of movement), the greater the force-producing capabilities the athlete must have. An ideal example of this is the tennis serve; the ball has a constant mass that is the same for both players. But analysis of the world rankings and indeed individual games quickly demonstrates that some players are able to apply more force to accelerate the ball more rapidly from the racket head when serving, thus enabling them to achieve a greater serving speed.

In sport, force is plural because more than one force may be acting on the body. The body (whether the athlete's body or an object such as a ball) is subject to gravity at all times (a constant force of 9.81 metres per second times mass of the athlete or object), frictional forces (from the ground or the air), forces applied through the momentum of external objects (for example, from an implement or an opponent in a collision) and internal forces (those exerted by muscles pulling on bones). The resultant force is the vector sum of all the forces acting on the body at once. As shown in figure 4.1, a vector is quantifiable as having direction as well as magnitude (size), which determine both the direction of the resultant action and the distance of the resultant action.

In figure 4.1*a*, the vector force applied through the planted leg is predominantly horizontal (to accelerate the centre of mass forward) with a large vertical component as the centre of mass is propelled forward with a takeoff angle of approximately 20-22 degrees for optimum travel distance in the long jump. Figure 4.1*b* shows a basketball player attempting a lay-up. As the player approaches the backboard, he or she needs to have enough speed to gain momentum. The force vector applied in the final stride transfers the momentum generated through running into the vertical jump (i.e., the body movement must be transferred upwards instead of forwards). As the take-off foot plants, the vertical body angle, flat-foot push and sharp lift of the jumping leg give the body the right angle to the basket. The magnitude of the force applied to the floor determines the height of the jump; the magnitude of force applied to the ball at the top of the jump determines how high up the backboard the ball makes contact.

Similar factors can be applied to the reasoning behind club selection and shot execution in golf. The vector force applied through the ball is a function of the angle of the club head as it strikes the ball. This angle is determined by the club selected (drivers have a flatter club head for more horizontal force; smaller irons and wedges have a greater angled face for more vertical force). Similarly, as this chapter explains in more detail, drivers have a longer shaft length and a greater lever arm, which serves as a speed multiplier (so that the club head

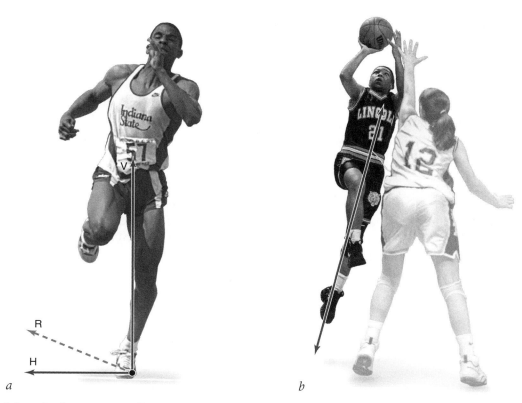

*a*                                                                                     *b*

**Figure 4.1**   The force vector illustrated in two sporting contexts: *(a)* long jump; *(b)* basketball lay-up.

contacts with more momentum, imparting more impulse into the ball), whereas smaller irons have a shorter lever arm for greater control, which results in a slower swing and less club head speed (less impulse into the ball). This all influences the magnitude of the force applied to the ball. The swing angle also influences the final vector. Longer, flatter swings for drives contribute greater horizontal force; shorter, chopping swings contribute greater vertical components to the force through the ball.

In the case of sport, athletes generally are trying to change momentum (the product of mass times velocity). This notion applies to tackling in American football, as the player attempts to stop the forward momentum of the opponent, as well as hitting a golf shot or performing a basketball lay-up. Impulse is applied to the object (body, ball, floor and so on). Impulse is defined as the integration of the forces acting on the body with respect to the time in which they are acting. Many physics texts explain that a small force applied

for a long time can produce the same change in momentum as a large force applied briefly because the product of the force and the period through which it is applied are important. The impulse is equal to the change of momentum, known as the impulse–momentum relationship.

In sport, however, athletes typically do not have long periods in which to apply forces. They need to apply impulse in very short periods. For example, the ground contact time in sprinting is 0.08 to 0.12 seconds, depending on the ability of the athlete. Peak forces may take a well-trained athlete 0.6 to 0.8 seconds to achieve. But after the athlete is no longer in contact with the floor or an object (for example, a tennis ball on a racket), no forces can be applied to it to cause a change in momentum. Even in relatively unexplosive actions (for example, cycling or rowing), performance usually depends on the performer generating forces quickly and therefore producing a critical impulse output. Consequently, the prime concern for the athletic development professional is to coach the athlete to produce large impulses—large forces in minimum time—to cause large changes in momentum in short periods.

By changing momentum, the athlete is accelerating or decelerating, depending on the context. The ability to accelerate is generally accepted as the critical factor in whether a person will succeed in most sports.[2] In short, the greater the force that the athlete is able to exert at critical times (for example, in the support phase of running, the take-off phase of jumping or the ball contact time when hitting a baseball), the greater the acceleration the athlete can achieve and the faster, higher or farther the result. In a movement context, an athlete can be deemed to be accelerating when a change in direction occurs without an increase in velocity because acceleration is a vector quantity; it has magnitude and direction. This concept is important in understanding high-speed running and change-of-direction mechanics (chapter 8).

In sport, power athletes are identified as successful, but what does it mean to be powerful? Power is a measure of work that can be derived from dividing the energy expenditure to perform a task by the time taken to achieve the task:

$$power = energy / time$$

The energy requirement for that work can be determined by multiplying the force required by the distance moved in the direction of the force applied:

$$power = (force \times distance) / time$$

Velocity is calculated by dividing the displacement of an object (the distance between a starting point and the finish point) by the time taken to achieve that distance:

$$velocity = displacement (distance) / time$$

Following this thinking process, by substitution the logical conclusion is the following:

$$power = force \times velocity$$

The relationship between force and velocity needs careful consideration in the context of long-term training plans. The relationship typically can be explained by considering a force–velocity curve. Although the force–velocity curve has been derived from studies looking at activation of a single muscle fibre,[3] the same curvilinear relationship applies for total-body movements. As figure 4.2 demonstrates, at any given time, power can be expressed as the product of force times velocity; altering the input of either variable changes the nature of the power produced. But the gradient of the force–velocity curve is constant. To shift the power line to the right (to make the performer more powerful), the coach must improve both the force-producing capacity and the velocity-producing capacity of the athlete.

Some sports require higher maximum force-producing capabilities; for example, a bobsled athlete has to move a large external resistance, and an offensive lineman in American football has to block a rushing player. Other sports depend more on velocity-specific actions; for example, in tennis, power is the product of racket-head speed. Regardless of the nature of the sport, time within the programme must be spent increasing the athlete's maximum strength proportionally to the velocity component of the programme. That suggestion doesn't necessarily mean that the same amount of time must be spent developing each objective for every athlete. Some athletes may need more maximum strength, others more velocity, but some time must be spent

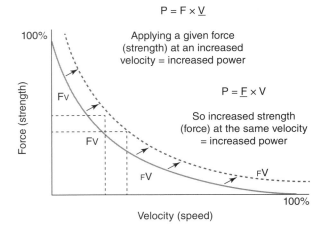

**Figure 4.2** Intention of training is to increase the athlete's power application.

developing each section of the curve if the curve is to be moved, thereby increasing the athlete's power-producing capabilities.

The objective at any particular stage in the athlete's coaching programme determines the range of methods that a coach might adopt. To improve the force-producing component of the curve, multimuscle, high-mass loadings in exercises such as squats, deadlifts, and pulling and pushing movements (see chapter 10) might be employed. To develop the velocity-producing components of the curve, the practitioner should choose activities that require higher speeds but produce lower force, such as plyometric exercises, detailed in chapter 9.

The practical implication is that a basic objective of an athlete's training is to improve the power of a movement or management of forces during a movement (figure 4.3). This insight applies to all biomotor qualities; even bioenergetic capabilities will be enhanced with more efficient movement (the same work can be done for less energy cost, or more work can be done for the same energy cost). This point relates to the concept of mechanical efficiency, which is explored through high-speed running in chapter 8.

Increasing power output in sport means improving the rate of force development (RFD), the ability to generate greater impulse during short periods and over short distances in which forces can be applied in skilled movements. Therefore, explosive force application is the basis of strength training for sport. The functional strength of an athlete can be expressed only in terms of forceful execution of a skill (i.e., the period in which the force can be applied) or the acceleration or velocity capabilities of an object (or body). This idea is shown in figure 4.4, whereby impulse (the product of force and contact time) is represented by the area highlighted under each force–velocity curve. The force–velocity curve can be increased by enhancing the RFD (the time it takes for the force to be manifested).

The differential between the maximal force that can be developed by an athlete and the useful force that can be developed (i.e., the force that can be expressed within the requisite contact time for a movement) is known as the explosive strength deficit (ESD) (figure 4.5). If the time available for force development is limited (for example, ground contact time in a long jump), then athlete A is able to produce more force (i.e., is stronger). But with no time constraint (as in a maximal strength lift), athlete B is stronger (i.e., can produce more force).

Producing powerful accelerations (high rates of force development, enabling high impulses)

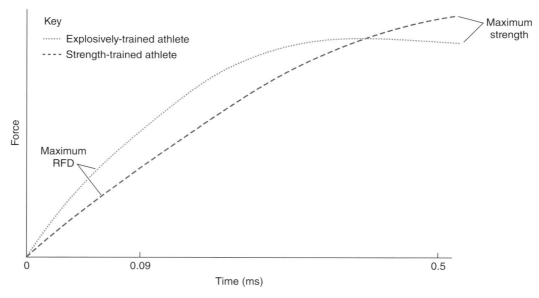

**Figure 4.3** Force-producing characteristics as a result of training history.

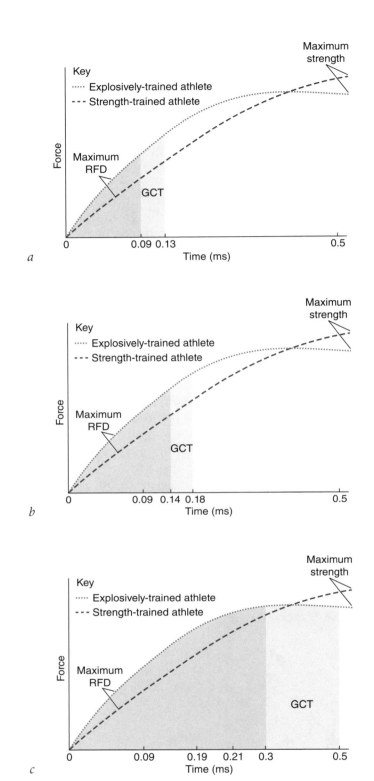

**Figure 4.4** Impulse requirements in explosive performance contexts: *(a)* sprinting; *(b)* vertical jumping; *(c)* rugby scrum.

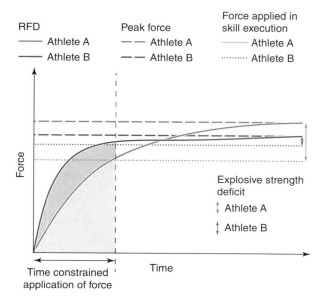

**Figure 4.5** Explosive strength deficit.

is the goal of any functional athletic development programme. Training programmes that disregard this basic understanding of physics may be fundamentally compromised.[4] The objective of the athletic development programme is to progress, in simplistic terms, from generating large forces to generating large forces quickly and expressing these forces in the right periods and in the right directions. The impulse and timing relationship is a central tenant of motor control in relation to movement skills. This relationship has implications for the mode and method of training that the coach puts together in terms of developing characteristics of force and velocity within athletes.

## Law of Action and Reaction

Newton's third law is commonly called action–reaction, as in 'For every action in movement there is an equal and opposite reaction.' In other words, for every force exerted on an object there is an equal, opposite and simultaneous force. When you apply a force to an object, you don't have to wait around for the reactive force; it happens simultaneously.

For example, to generate acceleration in running, the athlete pushes his or her foot into the ground; the ground reaction force is equal and simultaneous. Newton's first two laws explain the need to apply large forces in minimal periods for acceleration; the greater the force applied in the necessary ground contact period, the greater the acceleration. Newton's third law indicates the importance of technique in a movement, because technique determines the direction of the resultant force and therefore the success of the skill attempt.

The importance of this law can be seen through analysis of the required pattern for forces generated during linear running, from the acceleration phase through a transition phase and into high-speed (maximum velocity) running mechanics. During this time, the magnitude of the impulse needs to send the athlete back into flight (i.e., working against gravity to achieve an unsupported phase of a stride cycle, with neither foot in contact with the floor) for sufficient time to reposition the limbs (this aspect is put into context by the technical models presented in chapter 8) and to overcome horizontal forces (e.g., wind resistance and friction forces from the ground).

During the acceleration phase of running, the athlete tries to keep the centre of mass in front of the base of support by generating forces into the ground; the reactive force from the ground pushes the body forwards. The posterior chain muscles (gluteals, hamstrings) extend the hips, the quadriceps extend the knees, and the gastrocsoleus muscles extend the ankles to push fully into the ground. The reactive force from the ground accelerates the centre of mass forward along the line of direction of the ground reaction force.

This action drives the athlete into a fully extended (trunk, hip, knee, ankle) position illustrated in figure 4.6. The other leg moves into the triple-flexed position in preparation for the next ground contact with the shins at the same angle so that the pushing force will be in the same direction. The effect of this movement, and the actions of the arms, is explored later in this chapter with the consideration of rotational forces.

In acceleration, the athlete has a longer contact time relative to maximum velocity running, so there is more time to reach peak force. Large components of this force can be

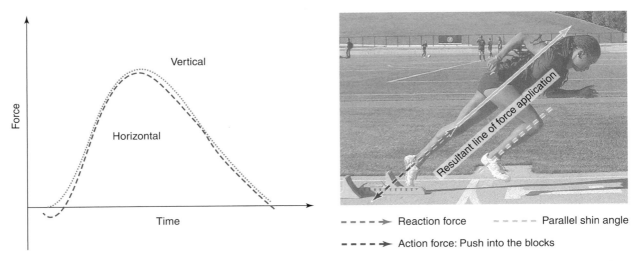

**Figure 4.6** The shin angle in sprinting acceleration determines the line of action in reactive force. When the shin angles are correct, the shin of the unsupported leg is prepared to drive into the floor at the same angle as the driving leg.

distributed to generating a significant horizontal force (the reaction force in figure 4.6). The centre of mass will accelerate forwards with each step so that the athlete's body gains momentum, which is important in track acceleration and in other sport contexts.

During acceleration, vertical forces will be smaller than they are in top-speed running because of the decreased falling pattern of the centre of mass and a much shorter flight phase. Imagine an athlete performing a wall sprint, an acceleration technique drill explained in chapter 8. The aim of this drill is to complete a driving action with the legs so that the shins of both legs are at the same angle when one leg is fully flexed and the other leg is fully extended. When the shins are at different angles, the vertical component of the resultant ground reaction forces is greater than the horizontal component. This less-than-optimal positioning causes the athlete to march up the wall during the wall sprint drill (i.e., the feet move closer with each successive action to the increased vertical forces). In a running action, the athlete would adopt a position that is too upright too early in the action, decreasing horizontal momentum and deviating from the optimal technique.

As the athlete's velocity increases, he or she transitions into maximum velocity. At this phase, the athlete's centre of mass has a lot of horizontal momentum propelling the body forwards. At maximum velocity, the body position is much more upright and the ground reaction forces are predominantly vertical (figure 4.7). The athlete has very short ground contact times (less than 0.08 seconds in an elite sprinter), and all force production is used to overcome the downward force of gravity. The athlete can therefore keep the centre of mass high and maximize stride length, the distance between the centre of mass at the point of touchdown on one foot to the position of the centre of mass at the point of touchdown on the other foot.

Faster sprinters do this by applying higher peak forces during a shorter contact period (i.e., the same total impulse is generated but in a shorter time). The front leg does not reach, and the ankle joint does not push off in this phase, because the centre of mass needs to be above the foot at ground contact. Trying to perform either of these actions results in overstriding, which slows the horizontal velocity of the centre of mass because the foot contacts too far forwards. Stride length is therefore effectively determined by the athlete's ability to generate vertical impulse (practical application of Newton's second and third laws) and the athlete's limb length.

For example, when he broke the world 100-metre record (9.58 seconds) Usain Bolt

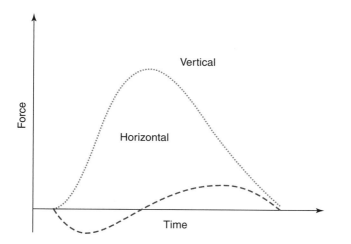

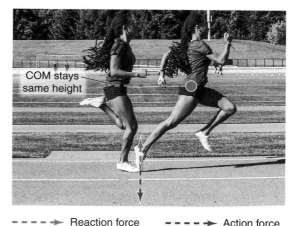

**Figure 4.7** Vertical force generation dominates in maximal velocity running.

was able to maximize his ground contact time without increasing it beyond a critical period to generate sufficient vertical ground reaction forces to propel his centre of mass forward with an average stride length of 2.47 metres per step. (At 93 kilograms and 1.96 metres tall, Bolt is both heavy and tall for a sprinter.) This average stride length masks the effective maximal stride length; in the 41 steps that he took in the race, those taken during the acceleration phases were smaller (1.43 metres for 0 to 10 metres; 2.38 metres for 10 to 20 metres) than at the later stages of the race (2.94 metres for 80 to 90 metres). Throughout the race Bolt had an average step frequency (cadence) of 4.23 steps per second.[5] His maximum stride length of 2.94 metres is a product of his long legs and his ability to generate high vertical impulses in ground contact.

# Coaching Multidirectional Movement

Newton's third law is also essential in understanding the coaching of multidirectional movement. The direction of body movement is determined by the angle of the force that is directed into the ground. To accelerate rapidly to one side from a two-footed stance, an athlete needs to be able to push through the inside of one foot and the outside of the other foot; this

ability is one of the most important skills an athlete can learn.

For example, in figure 4.8a, the goalkeeper has to push through the inside of the left foot and outside of the right foot to accelerate towards the right to make the save. This skill is even more complex when an athlete has to change direction forcefully and rapidly from a single-foot plant when moving at speed. Indeed, one of the hardest movement skills to master is the inside foot cut, or lateral push through the outside of the foot (figure 4.8b).

## Relation of Centre of Mass to Stability and Mobility

The centre of mass has been referred to several times. The terms centre of mass and centre of gravity often are used interchangeably in sport to represent the unique point in an object or system (in this case, the human body) that can be used to describe the body's response to external forces and torques. Although a solid object has a fixed centre of mass that cannot be altered, the human body is a shape that is not only complicated but also continuously altering as it changes positions.

As the position of the limbs relative to the trunk changes (and the mass of any implements or load that is being carried is considered), the position of the centre of mass changes as well. As figure 4.9a shows, in a standing human the centre of mass typically is at the level of the

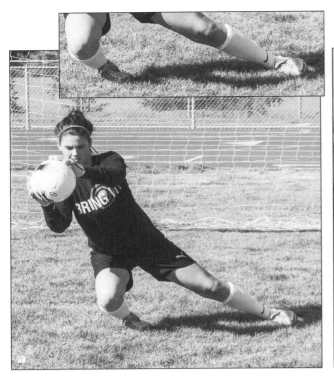

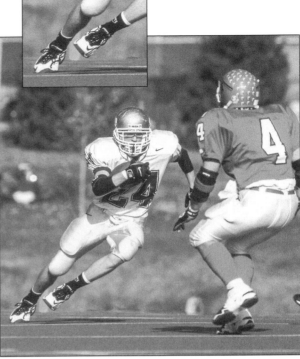

**Figure 4.8**  Applying force into the ground through different parts of the foot: *(a)* double-foot stance; *(b)* single-foot plant.

upper third of the sacrum, slightly towards the front of the body. But as the positioning of the trunk changes relative to the positioning of the limbs, the centre of mass changes. Coaches and athletes can use this reality to manipulate the selection and execution of techniques to achieve a given skill challenge.

For example, a tall athlete who has relatively long femurs or a long spine may struggle to achieve a mechanically efficient squat position (detailed in chapters 6 and 10), but placing the bar overhead instead of behind the neck raises the centre of mass relative to the hip (figure 4.9*b*). This technique enables the athlete to maintain a much more upright trunk position.

The centre of mass can also move outside the body to achieve a technical advantage. The best-known example of this is the Fosbury flop high-jump technique (figure 4.9*c*). Gravity influences every segment of the body, but in terms of total-body movement, gravity acts through the centre of mass. Vertical jump

height is therefore determined by how high the athlete can raise the centre of mass. After take-off, height cannot be achieved by exerting more force.

In the flop technique, the athlete's body is supine; the body is 90 degrees to the bar, and the head and shoulders cross the bar before the trunk and legs do, giving the flop its characteristic 'backwards over the bar' appearance. While in flight the athlete can progressively arch the shoulders, back and legs in a rolling motion, keeping as much of the body below the bar as possible. As figure 4.9*c* illustrates, this technique positions the centre of mass outside the body and indeed at a point below the bar, allowing the body to travel higher over the bar. The athlete who executes this technique well may clear the bar while the body's centre of mass remains as much as 20 centimetres below it.

The centre of mass of an object, whether a human body, a discus, or a kicked ball, follows a parabolic curve flight trajectory following

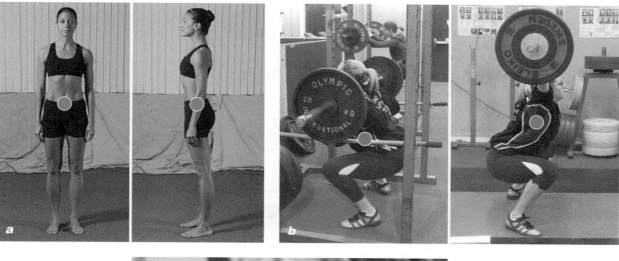

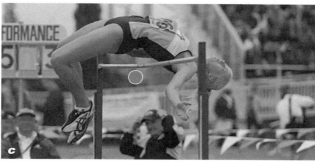

**Figure 4.9** Position of the centre of mass changes with body position: *(a)* normal standing; *(b)* different bar positions in a squat exercise; *(c)* Fosbury flop high-jump technique.

release or take-off. Gravity acts on the object, forcing it towards the floor, because air resistance slows the speed of the object. The larger the object is, the more influential air resistance will be. How far the object travels is primarily influenced by the magnitude of the force imparted into the object (the product of force and velocity) and the angle of take-off or release, which determines the direction of the force.

In some athletic endeavours, such as throwing, the height of the centre of mass at release is also an important consideration. For that reason, elite throwers typically are tall; a tall height at release means that the thrown object has farther to fall to the ground, extending its parabolic flight path.

When the athlete is in contact with the ground, the position of his or her centre of mass determines how stable the body is at any time. Indeed, as long as the centre of mass falls within the base of support, an object will retain its equilibrium. Ergo, the more stable the body (or any object) is, the harder it is to accelerate the body. In performance, therefore, athletes need to be able to adjust their base of support (relative to their centre of mass) according to whether they need to be anchored and stable (figure 4.10a) or mobile and able to change direction rapidly (figure 4.10b).

Although the size of the base of support (figure 4.11) is a primary influence on the stability of the body, a number of biomechanical principles come into play (table 4.1). Note that these principles apply to making an athlete not only more stable but also more unstable. Stability makes movement easier to achieve; an inverse relationship operates between stability and mobility when referring to the movement of the body as a whole.

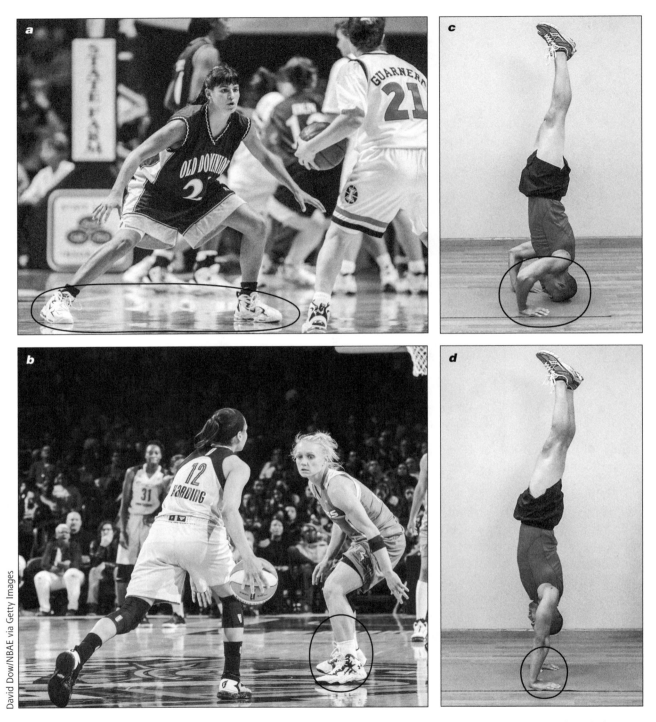

David Dow/NBAE via Getty Images

**Figure 4.10** Altering the base of support influences the stability of the movement: *(a* and *b)* defensive positions of stability and mobility; *(c* and *d)* vertical strength balances.

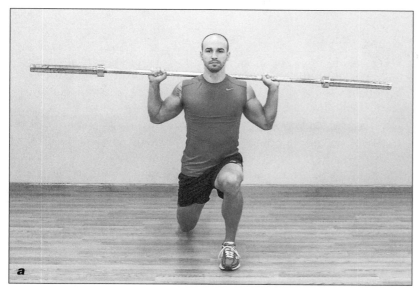

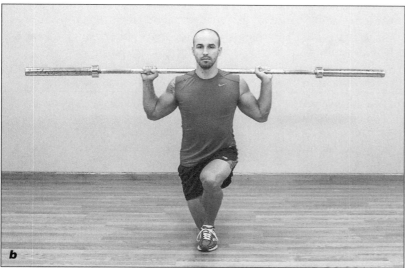

**Figure 4.11** The wider base of support in *(a)* a lunge requires less neuromuscular control for transverse and front plane motion than required in *(b)* the in-line lunge.

## External Forces

Additional forces influence the movement of an athlete or an implement that the athlete controls. The coach must plan for these forces or at least be aware of their influence on the athlete's movement. At all times, a number of forces are acting simultaneously on the athlete's body. These forces must be controlled and managed for efficient and effective movement.

As discussed in chapter 5, the crucial consideration for efficient movement is dynamically placing the posture where it is always optimally aligned to resist the force of gravity. An inability to control the posture causes additional stresses to act on the musculoskeletal system, increasing the mechanical load on the body and therefore increasing the workload. Coaches can use their knowledge of the effects and influence of gravity. If the centre of mass is outside the base of support, the centre of mass will accelerate towards the ground as determined by gravity.

Drills such as up tall and fall (chapter 8) put the athlete into a position where, after the support position is removed, the athlete must control and go with the acceleration (i.e., the coach is using gravity to teach the body). In this situation, both the coach and the athlete get immediate feedback if the athlete loses control of his or her body position when the support is removed. If the correct straight body alignment is not maintained, the athlete stumbles forward. Alternatively, if the first step taken is too large, the centre of mass is brought back inside the base of support and the body stops rather than accelerates. Maintaining the optimum posture and taking small steps allows gravity to cause the body to accelerate forward; the athlete uses this movement to increase stride frequency and enhance the horizontal translation of the centre of mass.

Friction is the force resisting the relative motion of solid surfaces, fluid layers or material elements sliding against each other. In human motion, friction typically relates to the front-to-back and side-to-side motion of the foot in contact with the ground and the movement of the body or thrown implements through

**Table 4.1** Principles of Stability

| Principle | Examples |
|---|---|
| The lower the centre of gravity is, the greater the level of stability is. | When landing from a jump, an athlete flexes at the knees to absorb the force and lowers the centre of mass to increase stability and aid balance. |
| | An athlete moving into a collision (e.g., a rugby or American football tackle) bends from the hips to increase stability on impact. |
| Greater support is achieved if the base of support is widened in the direction of the line of force. | Boxers stand with a wide staggered stance so that they can transfer weight in the line of force from the back foot to the front foot as they throw a punch. |
| | The in-line lunge uses a narrow base of support in the sagittal plane; therefore, it is more unstable than a normal lunge in which the feet are hip-width apart. |
| | To decelerate a fall when pushed forwards, an athlete automatically takes a big step forwards to bring the centre of mass back into the middle of the base of support in the direction of travel and prevent a fall. |
| For maximum stability, the line of gravity intersects (crosses) the base of support at a point that allows the greatest range of motion within the area of the base of support in the direction of forces causing the motion. | In the ready position (see chapter 8), a tennis player centres the line of gravity so that he or she can shift the centre of mass in any direction without loss of balance as the opponent returns the ball. |
| | At the 'Take the strain' command, a tug-of-war player leans backwards in anticipation of the forward pull of the opponents. |
| | To achieve optimum acceleration in a sprint, the athlete must move the centre of mass in front of the base of support to become unstable. |
| The more mass an object has, the more stable it will be. | This principle relates to Newton's second law. The greater the mass of an object is, the more gravity influences it and the more force is required to move it. |
| | In contact sports in which the ability to create effective collisions and withstand impacts is a performance requirement, heavier, more solid athletes are more likely to maintain equilibrium than those with lighter mass. For that reason, defensive linemen in American football typically weigh more than 280 pounds (127 kg). |
| The greater the friction is between the surface and the body parts in contact with it, the more stable the body will be. | A strength balance (see chapter 10) with three points of contact with the floor will be more stable than one with only two points. |
| | Training shoes with flat rubber soles have increased friction, aiding stability in static transition positions between quicker or more explosive movements in court sports such as basketball and badminton. |
| The most stable position of a standing human body (vertical alignment) is one in which the centre of mass is positioned centrally over the base of support or a position that enables the balancing of off-centred forces that would cause rotations. | In the overhead squat with a load on the bar, the trunk should be upright and the weight should be directly above the middle of the foot. If the weight is in front of or behind this position, the mass of the bar will cause it to fall forwards or backwards. |
| | A handstand can be maintained only when the trunk is positioned fully upright. |

the air or water. Generally, friction is a much bigger consideration in equipment design and selection (for example, what footwear to wear on a given playing surface) than in human movement. Typically, friction is considered important only for the development of movement skills when practitioners seek to minimize braking or frictional drag forces in an athlete running at maximal velocity. Fluid resistance may be influential in specific environments in which movement cannot be considered without reference to sport-specific technique such as in swimming and cycling.

In collision sports, the impact from external objects—typically the opponent—cannot be ignored. The latest technology, including accelerometers integrated into GPS units in playing garments, makes it increasingly easy to measure the intensity of impact and the cumulative load stresses from collisions. Indeed, international rugby league impacts have been recorded at levels in excess of 16 times body weight during tackles. The important consideration for such impacts is that the athlete needs to be posturally strong enough (explored in chapter 5) to resist the forces generated by the opponent's momentum into the collision. From a safety perspective, youth coaches should be aware that collisions with the ground following a tackle can be in excess of the force of the impact, because the fall is accelerated by gravity and the opponent often lands on the tackled player.

## Internal Forces

Skilful movement results from the forceful application of correct technique at the correct time. Besides controlling external forces, the athlete needs to be able to create and control internal forces through the action of the muscles and the myotendinous structures (figure 4.12), as explained by the sliding filament theory of muscular contraction.[6] Practitioners need to understand this mechanism of muscular contraction to conceptualize how muscles work to exert forces. As identified in chapter 2, motor units within the muscles contract in response to a stimulus from the motor nerve; these motor units are either contracted or they aren't (the all-or-nothing principle).

The more motor units that are activated, the greater the force that is generated along the length of the muscle, creating a pull on the bones to which the muscles are attached. If this pull is greater than the mass of the bone (the example in figure 4.13 is the lower arm, with the hand holding a weight), then the bone will move. The role of the athletic development professional is to help the athlete develop the skill of sequencing the timing of the motor action potentials within the requisite number

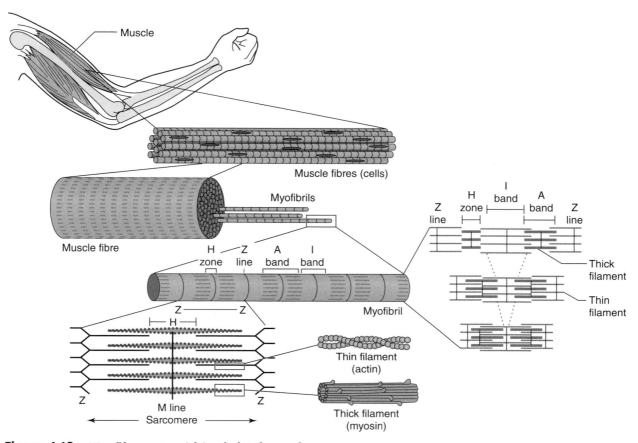

**Figure 4.12**  Myofilaments within skeletal muscle.

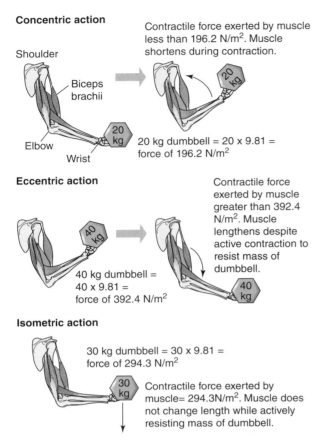

**Concentric action**

Shoulder

Biceps brachii

Elbow

Wrist

Contractile force exerted by muscle less than 196.2 N/m². Muscle shortens during contraction.

20 kg dumbbell = 20 x 9.81 = force of 196.2 N/m²

**Eccentric action**

Contractile force exerted by muscle greater than 392.4 N/m². Muscle lengthens despite active contraction to resist mass of dumbbell.

40 kg dumbbell = 40 x 9.81 = force of 392.4 N/m²

**Isometric action**

30 kg dumbbell = 30 x 9.81 = force of 294.3 N/m²

Contractile force exerted by muscle= 294.3N/m². Muscle does not change length while actively resisting mass of dumbbell.

**Figure 4.13**    Muscle actions: concentric, eccentric and isometric.

of motor units to ensure successful coactivation of the muscles and thereby achieve the desired action. The physical qualities associated with timing and coordination cannot be separated from the decision-making aspects in analysing the effectiveness of a technique in an applied context.

Not all muscle force is caused by shortening the muscles. Indeed, many of the most important muscular actions within sport are brought about by lengthening the muscle under tension. These eccentric muscle actions (not contractions, because the muscle length doesn't contract or shorten) are essential in controlling movements and all deceleration actions and in producing high-force, high-velocity actions through the stretch-shortening or plyometric actions described in chapter 2.

As illustrated in figure 4.13, eccentric actions can be caused only by an opposing force, because a muscle cannot actively lengthen

through conscious control. In figure 4.13, the opposing force of gravity acting on the dumbbell is greater than can be resisted by the biceps brachii and other assistance muscles responsible for elbow flexion. The load is still being resisted by the architecture of the muscle at a myofibril level (i.e., it is still actively trying to contract), but the muscle cannot generate enough internal force to oppose the action of gravity. Besides ensuring that the muscle is working hard, this type of eccentric loading causes greater damage to muscle tissues. This damage occurs because the heads of the myosin filament are actively pulled off the actin filament before reattaching further along the protein strand. (In a concentric contraction, these would attach and reattach to cause the muscle to shorten progressively.) This process continues until the load is no longer being lowered (i.e., the arm is fully extended). The rip and reattach process causes damage, inflammation and swelling to the protein filaments, experienced as delayed onset muscle soreness (DOMS). This soreness is the aching stiffness often felt after strenuous exercise, often (incorrectly) attributed to lactic acid in the muscles.

Coaches should be aware that eccentric actions do not occur only when an external mass greater than the muscle's maximal concentric capabilities forces a muscle to lengthen. Indeed, being able to perform strong eccentric actions is as vital as being able to control the movements required in sport. Consider this first in a training context. In the fundamental movement pattern known as the squat, the athlete lowers the body until the hip is below the knee before returning to standing. Typically, this exercise is performed with an external load on the back, but the single-leg squat (figure 4.14) is a variation (small base of support, body mass through a single limb) that doesn't necessarily require an external mass to overload the musculature.

The squat is an important movement pattern in both assessing (chapter 6) and progressing (chapter 10) the athlete's functional strength and control. As with any resistance exercise, lowering and raising actions are involved in this movement. Rising (returning to standing) is achieved through the concentric contraction

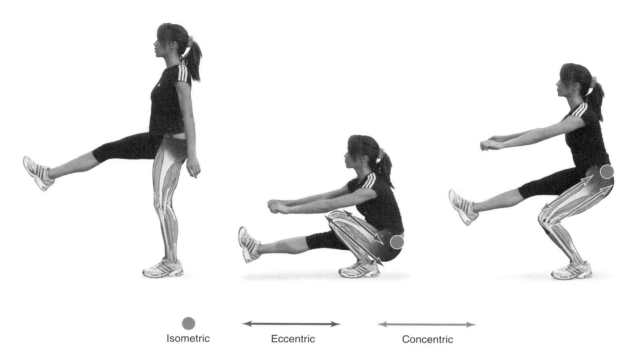

Isometric          Eccentric          Concentric

**Figure 4.14**    Muscle actions: single-leg squat.

of the hip and knee extensors, which contract to exert a force into the ground (action),
resulting in a reaction force that overcomes
gravity. During the lowering (descent) phase,
the flexion movements in the hip and knee are
assisted by gravity, which means they need to
be resisted (or controlled) by the muscles that
contract to cause hip extension. These muscles
work eccentrically, that is, they are lengthened
under tension, even though this action is not
maximal. Note also that during this movement,
the gluteus medius contracts isometrically to
maintain the level pelvic position.

Eccentric control function is extremely
important in controlling dynamic movement
in sport. Indeed, any athlete who must decelerate and change direction needs to be strong
eccentrically in the muscles that oppose the
joint action. For example, in figure 4.15,
the right leg of the tennis player is acting to
brake (decelerate) forward momentum. This
action involves eccentric contraction of the
quadriceps, hamstrings, gluteus maximus and
gastrocsoleus (calf) muscles to establish a low,
flexed position in the hip and knee and prevent
momentum from carrying the athlete's trunk
forward and over the planted foot.

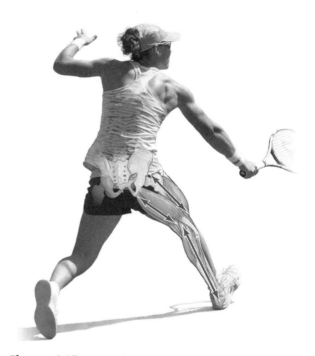

**Figure 4.15**    Deceleration.

Similar muscle mechanics are required
in any deceleration position. If an athlete is
moving from an acceleration position and is
required to stop or slow, these muscles need
to work eccentrically to enable this action to

occur. Deceleration requires a great deal of strength to prevent the muscles from being damaged too much as they resist the forces exerted on them.

Eccentric actions are used in various ways to achieve different training objectives. Submaximal loads can be lifted or lowered slowly. This approach may be extremely useful from a rehabilitation training perspective, such as when a muscle has atrophied after disuse following injury or when the goal is to increase connective tissue strength, such as in managing a tendinopathy. Slow lowering increases the time during which the tissues are under tension, which is thought to stimulate fibre hypertrophy.

Training slowly, however, has a negative effect on the athlete's neuromuscular system because training with slow movements leads to slowed movement speeds. From a functional perspective (see chapter 10), the development of eccentric strength may be better achieved by using resisting supramaximal loads or undertaking plyometric actions (chapter 9), depending on the overall balance of the athlete's training programme.

The stretch reflex also requires high eccentric strength to store elastic energy and transfer it into a forceful reflex contraction. The majority of effective movement patterns across sport require the athlete to create and use the stretch-reflex mechanism and the stored elastic energy benefits to move efficiently. This concept can be illustrated in reactive jumping actions. In preparation, the ankle dorsiflexes (toes are pulled towards the knees) to prestretch the gastrocsoleus muscles and place them under tension. This action also creates tension within the Achilles tendon, which will be maintained because the ankle remains dorsiflexed. This tension and the accompanying storing of potential energy are responsible for much of the ankle stiffness that is a feature of the reactive jump, as detailed in chapter 9.

As the athlete makes active flat-foot contact with the floor, gravity exerts a large vertical force through the ankle, knee and hip joints, which is resisted by the simultaneous actions of the hip (gluteus maximus, hamstrings), knee (quadriceps) and ankle extensors (gastrocsoleus complex) working rapidly and eccentrically to maintain stiffness in these joints. Gravity exerts a force equivalent to many times body weight (magnitude depends on the height or distance jumped).

The vertical force of gravity lengthens the muscles resisting the force, which in turn activates the muscle spindle fibres to initiate a strong reflex contraction in the opposite direction. The greater the athlete's eccentric strength is, the more rapidly this response occurs. Simultaneously, or indeed maybe even quicker than the neuromuscular response, the Achilles tendon recoils; the tendon is non-elastic, already stretched and under tension because of ankle dorsiflexion. In an athlete who is not eccentrically strong, the golgi tendon organ also activates, effectively inhibiting the eccentric muscle action as a protective mechanism, meaning that the forceful reflex action will not occur.

In chapter 9, specialist strength-training methods known as plyometrics are detailed. Plyometrics develops reactive strength in the neuromuscular system, strengthens and maximizes the nonelastic recoil potential of the tendon, maximizes the response of the muscle spindle fibres and aids in the inhibition of the golgi tendon organs to maximize the elastic properties of the muscle tissue.

The final muscle action in the neuromuscular system is an isometric action. Isometric contractions occur when a muscular force is exerted but no resulting change occurs in muscle length (i.e., the force generated by the muscle is equal to the opposing mass resisting it); therefore, no change occurs in the joint angle of the attached muscles. Relatively few performances in sport require the performer to hold a static position. The classic example is in gymnastics, shown in skills such as the crucifix on the rings or a handstand on a beam.

Although static hold positions are rare in sport, the coach should not underestimate the importance of isometric muscle actions, because these are key in the maintenance of posture. The importance of maintaining posture for the sport performer is explored in detail in chapter 5. The importance of isometric muscle actions in sporting movements can be illustrated through the analysis of the pelvis in running (see figure 4.16). As shown in chapter 8, the pelvis must not have an anterior or posterior tilt in the running action or any form of lateral deviation (i.e., a side-to-side sway). Either of these errors can result from ground reaction forces caused as the legs drive forward, lack of hip mobility as the thigh is lifted towards a horizontal position to accommodate leg swing or rotations in the trunk because of arm-driving action. Rotations caused by ground reaction should be balanced by the opposing arm action, and hips should be mobile enough to enable the leg lift. But if the pelvis is to act as a stable platform through which forces can be transferred, the trunk must be maintained in a stable upright position. The arrangement of the ribs, spine and pelvis must be maintained by the isometric actions of the trunk (external oblique, rectus abdominis), pelvic muscles

Pelvic rotations – causal factors

Arm action + core stability

Hip flexibility + posture

Ground reaction forces

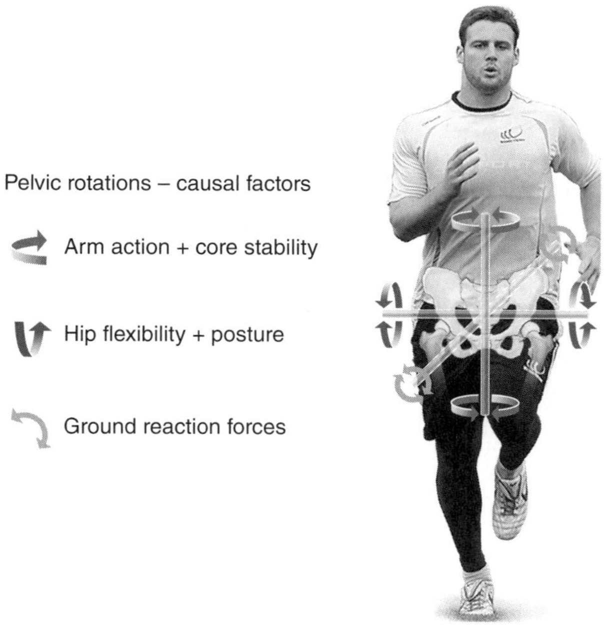

**Figure 4.16** The isometric actions of the trunk stabilizers maintain spinal–pelvic alignment when challenged by ground reaction and rotational forces through the pelvis in running.

(transversus abdominis, multifidus) and hip (predominantly gluteus medius).

Athletic development practitioners may hear about other types of muscle actions such as isotonics (constant tension throughout the movement range) or isokinetics (constant velocity of muscle shortening). These terms are often used to describe various types of machine-based exercise protocols. If these actions can be achieved only with machines and contractions of this nature do not occur naturally in sport, why would coaches want to incorporate them into routines?

# Muscle Structure and Force Production

As figure 4.17 illustrates, the shape and size of muscle fibres vary. Generally, thicker muscles that have a larger cross-sectional area (for example, pectoralis major) produce greater forces. Conversely, longer muscles (for example, rectus femoris) can develop higher velocities of shortening. The orientation of fibres within these muscles alters as a function of both purpose and training exposure.

As with external forces, the internal forces generated by the muscles are vectors; they have a magnitude and a direction. The line of action of the muscles' force is determined by the orientation of the fibres[6] and the location of the myotendinous junctions. As we will see in chapter 5, an important goal is to balance the force vectors throughout the kinetic chain between the muscles of the anterior and posterior to maintain stability within the joints and equilibrium across the posture.

A good illustration of this can be seen in the rotator cuff (figure 4.18 and table 4.2), the muscle group that stabilizes the shoulder joint by holding the head of the humerus into the shallow glenoid fossa of the scapula. The line of action of the muscle during contraction indicates the direction of force that will be generated. From this, the function of the muscle can be determined.

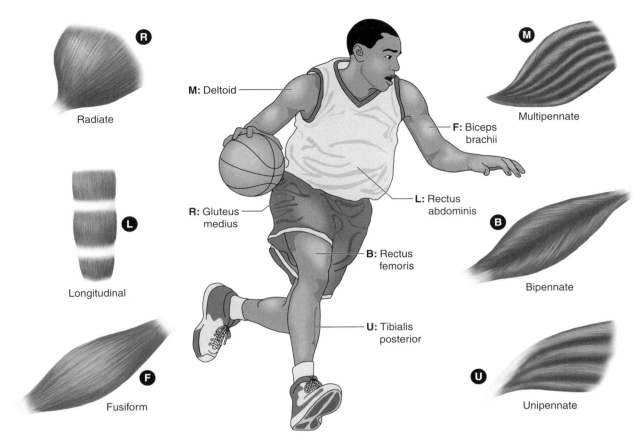

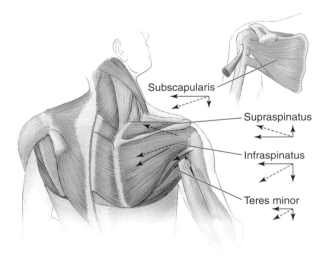

**Figure 4.17** Different muscle shapes have different force-producing capabilities.

**Figure 4.18** Lines of action of force in the rotator cuff.

Consider the slightly different function and line of muscular action in the supraspinatus compared with other muscles in the rotator cuff. The combined rotator cuff actions enable a stable shoulder position from which other muscles can produce forceful movements of the arm (for example, a tennis serve or a baseball pitch). Excessive tightness in one of these muscles limits the range of movement in opposition to the line of force in the muscle. Weakness in a muscle means limited force produced in the direction of muscle action. A weakness in the rotator cuff muscles may mean that the athlete is unable to stabilize the shoulder joint when the arm is brought sideways across the body as in an overarm throwing action or during overhead movements such as a tennis serve.

Forces cause movement. In general, the total force influencing the movement of an athlete at any one time is a sum of several forces produced by external (reaction force, impact force, air resistance and so on) and internal (muscular) forces. A basic understanding of angular movement is critical in understanding human movement in sport because nearly all human

**Table 4.2**    Rotator Cuff Muscles and Their Functions

| Muscle | Function |
|---|---|
| Supraspinatus | Abducts (pulls towards the body) and laterally rotates the shoulder while stabilizing the head of the humerus in the glenoid fossa |
| Subscapularis | Laterally rotates the shoulder while stabilizing the head of the humerus in the glenoid fossa |
| Infraspinatus | Laterally rotates the shoulder while stabilizing the head of the humerus in the glenoid fossa |
| Teres minor | Laterally rotates the shoulder and stabilizes the head of the humerus in the glenoid fossa during movement of the glenohumeral joint |

movement involves the rotation of body segments about a joint axis. For example, the forearm rotates about the elbow in the flexion–extension movement. Figure 4.19 illustrates how rotational movements of the thigh, lower leg and foot cause translation (straight-line movement) of the body in sprinting.

# Rotational Forces

Rotational movements, or torques, are caused by off-centred forces, forces that do not pass through the axis of rotation. Forces that do not pass through an axis of rotation but instead are balanced on either side of it will not cause a rotation; they are in equilibrium. Children easily understand this idea. They realize that a heavier person will cause one end of a seesaw to dip. The concept of torques in relation to body movements is explored in more detail in the discussion of the posture and lever systems in chapter 5. Indeed, the concepts of forces, levers and movements are not easily separated. But a chapter on forces cannot be

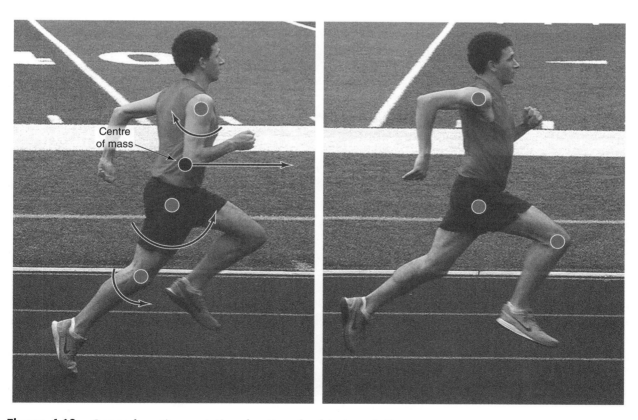

**Figure 4.19**    General motion: rotational actions lead to translation.

complete without explanation of how the laws of mechanical motion apply to angular or rotational movements.

At first glance, the principles of angular and linear motion appear similar, and one can almost be directly substituted for the other. For example, the law of inertia states, 'A rotating body will continue in a state of uniform angular motion unless acted upon by an external torque.' Inertia is the resistance of a body to a change to its velocity; in linear movement, this relates to the mass of the object. In angular motion, the equivalent to mass is the moment of inertia, which represents the resistance of an object (or body) to a change to its angular motion. The moment of inertia depends not only on the mass of the body but also on the distribution of its mass relative to the axis of rotation. In a moving body, which might have many axes of rotation and therefore a complex distribution of mass, the moment of inertia can be altered by changing the position of the body. For example, a platform diver performing a somersault is rotating about a transverse axis. He or she can rotate more quickly by making the tuck movement tighter and bringing the head into the knees. The tighter the tuck is, the closer the distribution of mass is to the axis of rotation. Therefore, the moment of inertia is reduced, and a faster rotation is achieved.

Consider also the swing phase of sprinting during which the athlete brings the heel as close to the buttocks as possible. This action reduces the moment of inertia of the leg relative to the rotational axis (the hip joint), meaning that the recovery of the leg is much quicker. The ability of an athlete to perform this well contributes to higher sprint speeds. The athlete must have sufficient hip mobility to achieve the desired action.

An external torque produces an angular acceleration or deceleration of a body that is proportional to the torque in the direction of the torque and inversely proportional to the moment of inertia (Newton's second law). Similar to the concept of momentum in linear moment, this principle gives rise to the concept of angular momentum, an indication of the quantity of angular motion in an object.

Angular momentum remains constant within a system unless an external force is applied. When gravity is the only external force applied to the object (for example, in projectile motion after take-off), angular momentum remains constant during flight until landing, when ground reaction forces rapidly decelerate the momentum. Because angular momentum remains constant, sport performers know that, following take-off, the moment of inertia of an object can be altered to increase the angular velocity of an object because of the principle of conservation of angular momentum.

Gymnastics provides an example to illustrate this concept. As a gymnast performs a vault, his or her angular momentum is constant following take-off. But as the gymnast tucks into the somersault, the angular velocity increases as the moment of inertia decreases and the distribution of mass around the rotational axis changes. As the gymnast exits the tuck position and the body opens out, the moment of inertia increases and angular velocity decreases as the athlete prepares to land. In track and field, sound hammer-throwing technique uses this principle. The mass of the hammer is constant. After momentum is generated in the initial swing, the athlete rotates with a straight arm to conserve angular momentum. The mass of the hammer does not change, so by maximizing the lever in the arms, the moment of inertia is maximized.

The law of action–reaction is also crucial to the athlete who is seeking to control total-body movement in any sporting situation. Newton's third law states, 'For every torque exerted on a body by another, there is an equal and opposite torque exerted by the former body on the latter.' This law applies not only to the collision of two bodies but also to the movement of one body part in relation to another. For example, a long jumper who brings his or her legs forward in preparation for landing in the pit sets up a lower-body torque. The equal and opposite reaction can be seen in the trunk, which leans forward, and in the arms, which come forward.

Although this example pertains to a specific sporting skill, a more general example that athletic development coaches need to think about concerns running movement skills. As the leg drives forward from toe-off, the ground reaction force drives the thigh forwards and upwards, and the rotational axis is through the hip joint. This powerful movement creates angular momentum within the lower body that needs to be countered to prevent a torque that would detract from the translation (forward movement) of the centre of mass. The backwards-driving action of the arms (rotational axis through the shoulder) sets up the counter-rotational movement through the upper body equal and opposite that of the lower body. Therefore, running with the correct arm action typically produces faster leg movement than running without the use of the arms.

# Summary

This chapter introduced some complicated, yet fundamental, elements of physics. At first glance, these topics may seem inconsequential. But a basic grasp of the ways that forces influence movement and the forceful expression of technique is essential for the athletic development coach. Indeed, skilled movement is the result of the athlete's ability to manage external and internal forces through well-coordinated neuromuscular actions and effective musculoskeletal positions.

Generally, coaches do not need to have detailed knowledge of anatomy, but an appreciation of muscular structure and the way that muscles produce force is important. This knowledge enables a practitioner to prepare athletes to be strong and powerful enough to reproduce the challenging and rapid forces necessary for running, jumping and evading opponents. This knowledge also helps coaches contextualize and evaluate the relative contribution that the practical techniques presented in chapters 8 through 10 will make to their overall athletic development programmes. Similarly, coaches should understand that skeletal muscles have a line of force determined by the alignment of their attachments to the skeleton. Coaches can then focus on joint positioning in skill execution, enabling functionally correct muscular actions to underpin movement patterns. This knowledge is important to help train athletes to maintain the dynamic postural control essential for the execution of movement skills. This topic is the focus of the next chapter.

# CHAPTER 5

# Importance of Posture in Athletic Movement

The goal of an athletic development programme is to enhance the athlete's movement efficiency and symmetry so that he or she is better able to implement sport-specific movement (technique) mechanics and thus enhance performance. As identified in the previous chapters, the concept of movement efficiency is related to the body's ability to produce and control forces. An athlete must be able to control the positioning of the body segments relative to each other and intentionally and habitually assume the best positions (or postures) for enabling the neuromuscular and skeletal systems to function and achieve the performance requirements.

This chapter explores this concept in detail. The practitioner is introduced to the various considerations that define an effective body position and the positions that enable the optimal functioning of the various muscle groups. This should arguably be the first goal of a functional training progression within an athlete development programme.

## Planes of Motion

The previous chapter showed that the human body is subject to multiplanar forces whatever position it adopts. Practitioners must understand that movement occurs (and needs to be controlled) in three dimensions. Although this statement may seem obvious, and indeed common sense, training to prepare athletes in

this way is not always common practice. For example, performing linear sprints may help a soccer player become faster, but if he or she hasn't mastered the mechanics of lateral movement or isn't strong enough in the muscles that produce and control forces in the transverse and frontal planes (figure 5.1), the resulting movement pattern will be inefficient and may cause injuries.

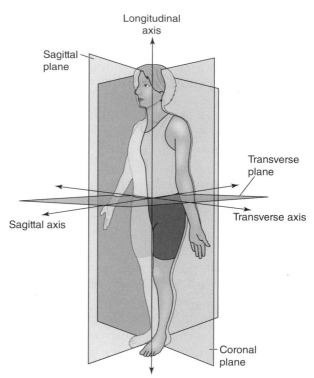

**Figure 5.1**  The three planes of motion and axes of rotation.

Even more simply, think about the use of resistance-training machines that control the movement of the weight (or the athlete) throughout the motion in a single plane. This training neither replicates the everyday demands of movement nor educates the athlete to control his or her body position in three planes of motion throughout a movement pattern. This principle is one of the keys to using functional training to develop athletic movement skills, a concept explored in detail in chapter 10.

To understand movement better, a universal system of describing motion has been devised. This approach has a basis in three planes of motion that exist at right angles to each other and that transect at the centre of mass (figure 5.1). Movement of a body part, or the whole body, is described as being in, or parallel with, a specific plane. The distinction is important, because movement in a plane requires the plane of movement to pass through the centre of mass; the majority of body section movements, however, will not do this.

For example, consider an athlete who is sprinting (figure 5.2). The movements in the upper and lower leg are in the sagittal plane as the athlete sprints, but they are parallel with the movement of the sagittal plane, which runs through the centre of mass. Individual joint and total-body movement in linear sprinting movements are in the sagittal plane. The arm (flexion and extension of the shoulder), thigh (flexion and extension of the hip) and lower leg (flexion and extension of the knee) movements are all in the sagittal plane with rotation through a transverse joint axis. Note that in describing the motion of the entire body, the axis of rotation would be an external one, about the point where the toe contacts the ground.

When a gymnast performs a crucifix on the rings (figure 5.3), the shoulders abduct in the frontal plane about a sagittal (anteroposterior) axis. The difficulty of the movement is increased by simultaneously extending the hips and knees in the sagittal plane.

Figure 5.4 shows that the total-body movement of the tennis player is forward, in the sagittal plane, as the forehand is struck. The

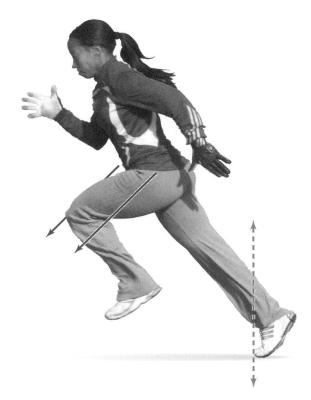

**Figure 5.2**  Movement in the sagittal plane about a transverse axis: the sprinter.

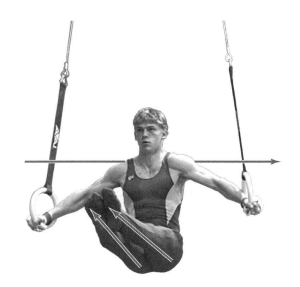

**Figure 5.3**  Movement in the frontal plane about a sagittal or transverse axis: the gymnast.

shoulders and trunk, however, are moving in the transverse plane. The shoulder horizontally adducts in the transverse plane about a longitudinal axis. In the same movement, the trunk rotates internally in the transverse plane about a sagittal (anteroposterior) axis.

Movement in a particular plane will also be about a specific axis of rotation, which will be perpendicular (at a 90-degree angle) to the plane of motion. These axes of rotation can be internal (through joint centres), through the centre of gravity or external to the body. Practitioners must understand and be able to describe these different movement patterns and movements of the various body parts during sporting movements. When coaching or analysing movement in any form (for example, through video evaluation), the most accurate view of any particular plane of motion is best obtained perpendicular to the plane of motion; for example, movement in the sagittal plane is best viewed from the side.

True motion within sport usually occurs in three planes simultaneously (figure 5.5). In a baseball pitch, the throwing arm simultaneously extends and flexes in the sagittal plane and abducts and adducts in the frontal plane. As the player throws, he also laterally flexes the trunk (leans to the side) in the frontal plane. The trunk internally rotates from an externally rotated position in the transverse plane as the ball is thrown. The hip and knee flex and extend in the sagittal plane.

The coach and the development programme need to prepare the athlete for simultaneous movement in all three planes. Indeed, one of the principles of advancement or progression in exercise difficulty is to increase the planes of motion that an athlete is required to move through (figure 5.6).

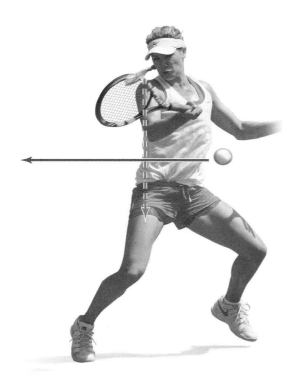

**Figure 5.4** Movement in the transverse plane about a longitudinal axis: the tennis player.

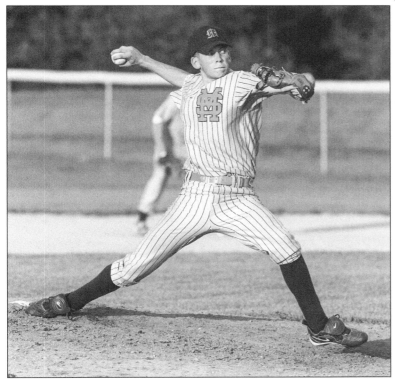

**Figure 5.5** Most sporting movements occur in all three planes simultaneously: the baseball pitcher.

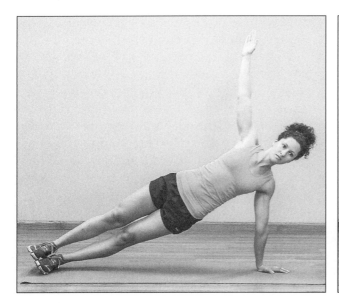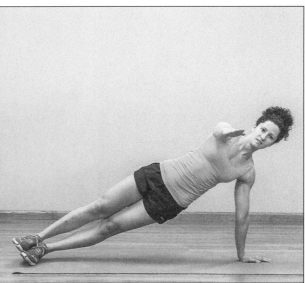

**Figure 5.6** Increasing the number of planes of motion that need to be controlled significantly increases the difficulty of the side plank exercise.

In multidirectional sports such as soccer or basketball, this concept is crucial, because to perform a cutting action, the player needs to be strong and stable in the muscles that exert forces through the hip joint. In the lateral (frontal plane) motion, hip motion is related to adduction using the gluteus medius, sartorius, pectineus, adductor magnus, gracilis, adductor brevis and adductor longus muscles. To control hip and trunk rotation in the transverse plane, the gluteus medius, internal and external obliques and transversus abdominis need to be contracted. To extend the hips forcefully in the sagittal plane, the gluteus maximus, biceps femoris, semimembranosus and semitendinosus contract to produce the rapid and forceful movements that characterize chaotic invasion games.

Athletic development practitioners don't need to learn the muscle groups responsible for each action, but they do need to understand that during high-force, high-speed movements in sport, the athlete needs to be able to coordinate a number of simultaneous muscular actions in a number of planes of motion to produce an effective action. The athlete's ability to recruit muscles and produce multiplanar forces through multiple muscle groups around a joint (remembering that multiple other joints are involved in the action) needs to be factored into the progression of skilled movements that are introduced in chapters 8 through 10. Effective movement coaching requires a different approach to exercise progression from the more traditional faster, more weight approach often prescribed by coaches.

Modern technology allows the contribution of forces in each plane to the overall movement to be measured in real time. This measurement can be achieved through a force platform built into the floor over which the athlete runs or from which the athlete jumps or lifts. In team sports, where such controlled actions do not exist, multiplanar forces can be measured using accelerometers located within GPS tracking units that the athletes wear during training or games (if the rules of the sport allow). Such information can prove vital when attempting to understand performance demand, injury occurrence and factors such as the influence of different surfaces (for example, grass versus artificial turf) on performance and athletic preparation.

The importance of controlling three-dimensional forces in such a performance context can be seen in figure 5.7. The athlete (in the example, a rugby league player) has to work all the muscles in the kinetic chain to

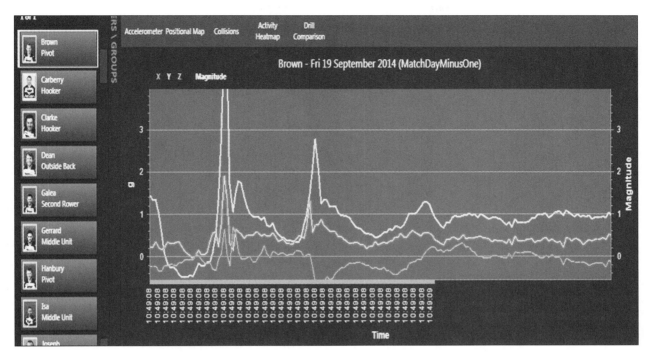

**Figure 5.7** Vertical (gravity and ground reaction), lateral (side-to-side) and anterior–posterior (front-to-back) forces in a rugby league player performing a series of cutting actions as measured by a GPS unit.

resist the forces of gravity (the predominant cause of the vertical forces), as well as side-to-side and front-to-back accelerations and decelerations when performing a double-cut action to exploit available space. The more control the athlete is able to achieve, the more efficient the actions will be and conversely the less demanding the performance requirements are.

Indeed, one way in which the athletic development professional can analyse movement economy needs (in terms of enhancing quality and durability) in an athlete in a movement context within sport is to look at the lateral and anterior–posterior forces that the athlete is subjected to within a performance. The more mechanically efficient the player is, the better he or she will be able to resist external forces and produce internal forces with less energy cost and the lower the chance will be of incurring an injury because of either chronic (repetitive) exposure to high forces or acute exposure to excessive and unanticipated forces.

# Effective Posture

The opening chapter explained that the musculoskeletal system is capable of responding to challenges in any situation. The aim of an athlete development programme is to implement a series of educational measures (training equals learning) that influence the motor system components of the body to use mechanical solutions to respond positively to the environmental stressors to which it is subjected. Meeting this goal requires sound postural mechanics—a coordinated integration of joint positioning, muscle alignment, muscle recruitment and force production. Traditionally, coaches have focused on *what* athletes are doing in their athletic development drills; developing sound postural mechanics requires a focus on *how* athletes are performing movements and techniques.

In 1947 the posture committee of the American Academy of Orthopaedic Surgeons[1] produced the following definition of good posture, and this description has provided an operational definition for coaches and therapists alike for many years:

> Posture is usually defined as the relative arrangement of the parts of the body. Good posture is that state of muscular and skeletal balance that protects the supporting structures of the body against injury or progressive deformity, irrespective of the attitude (erect, lying, squatting or stooping) in which the muscles are working or resting. Under such conditions, the muscles will function most efficiently and the thoracic and abdominal organs are in their optimum positions. Poor posture is the faulty relationship of the various parts of the body, which produces increased strain on the supporting structures and less efficient balance of the body over its base of support.[1]

This definition demonstrates the real importance of emphasizing postural integrity, the correct positioning of the joints relative to each other in a dynamic context. First, postural integrity is the basis for efficient movement, because the joint positions optimize the biomechanical efficiency of the musculoskeletal system. The human body is basically a combination of structures designed to withstand compression (bone, cartilage) and pulling (tendons, muscles, ligaments) forces. Chapter 2 illustrated that joint positioning determines muscle function. This chapter explains this concept in detail, highlighting the importance of length, tension and velocity relationships in muscular actions and illustrating to practitioners why it is important to emphasize correct joint positioning (technique) throughout all aspects of movement training.

Correct joint alignment also improves stability and balance by minimizing compressive forces and optimizing the base of support as well as maximizing the efficiency of the neuromuscular system. Correct joint alignment maintains balance in the muscles around joints and enhances inter- and intramuscular coordination and the proprioception elements of the motor system.

Second, allowing an athlete to adopt poor postural positions will predispose him or her to injuries within the musculoskeletal system. This factor is functionally related to the performance-enhancing aspects of posture. Poor positioning increases the stress on the ligaments that provide stability to the joints, increases the tension on the myotendinous connections between muscles and bones and, by creating shear forces within the joints, increases the risk of joint injury. These injuries might be chronic (long term) or more acute (because of a single incidence). Practitioners who emphasize correct joint positioning and movement mechanics will be rewarded with athletes who are biomechanically effective and less predisposed to injuries, making them available to practice and perform more often. Indeed, the basis for rehabilitation from injury is a progressive re-education through proprioceptive control and strengthening of mechanically correct postures or positioning around a single joint. Therefore, this principle should be used in everyday training to decrease the probability of injury.

An athlete's generic movement competency relates to his or her ability to adapt the most effective and efficient postural positions during movement and do this reasonably quickly. In this context, posture doesn't differ much from the concept of mobility. Sport-specific movement patterns—that is, the postural positions specifically related to the techniques and movement requirements of the sport—are built onto generic movement competencies and facilitate the optimal transfer of forces into the sport-specific context. Although many general movements—such as running, jumping and turning—are required in most sports, some examples of the specific movement demands for various sports are identified in chapter 11.

Postural control—the ability to get into a functionally stable position within a given range of motion—is essential in a movement context. Therefore, as chapter 6 explains, static assessment of a person's posture will never provide a complete assessment. The standing position, however, is a good point from which to begin to explore the concept. In addition, beginning the assessment of an athlete's posture from the standing position is relatively easy. The only tool needed is a weighted piece of string—a plumb line—that can be hung down next to the standing athlete (figure 5.8).

Viewed from the rear, the athlete should display symmetry in the left and right sides of the body, and the shoulders and hips should be level. The weight should be evenly distributed through both feet, and no muscular effort should be needed to maintain this equilibrium. Athletes may stand with their toes pointing slightly outwards (figure 5.8*a*), but the degree of turn in the toes should be equal for both feet.

Viewed from the side, a straight line should run between the ear lobe (with the head facing forward), the spine, hip, knees and ankles (figure 5.8*b*). This imaginary line is used to differentiate between the muscles of the anterior and posterior kinetic chain (figure 5.9). In sport, the anterior muscles often are referred to as mirror muscles, the muscles that the athlete sees every day and usually is most aware of. Consequently, these muscles often become the focus of strength training, which can lead to

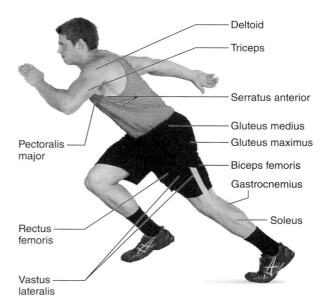

**Figure 5.9**   The anterior and posterior kinetic chain.

postural problems. A good motivational technique is to remind athletes often that it is what is behind them that makes them powerful and pushes them forwards.

Imagining the posture as a chain is useful. It is easy to see that if a chain were suspended from the ceiling, altering the position of a section of links in the chain would alter the orientation of those above and below this section. This idea is well illustrated in the spine. To resist the forces of gravity, evolution has determined that the spine should have a series of curves in the cervical (neck), thoracic (upper back) and lumbar (lower back) regions. One of the essential things to realize is that when the lumbar curve is neutral, ideally, the vertical plumb line will come down through the midline of the shoulder with the scapula lying flat against the upper back. But a change in the position of the scapula, head, neck or lumbar spine will produce compensatory movements in the other spinal curves, which lead to a number of maladapted postural positions.

In an active population, these positions tend to be caused by poor habits when standing, sitting or moving. They generally originate from misuse of the musculoskeletal

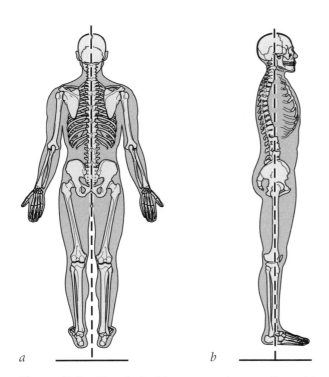

**Figure 5.8**   The desirable posture in standing: *(a)* back view; *(b)* side view.

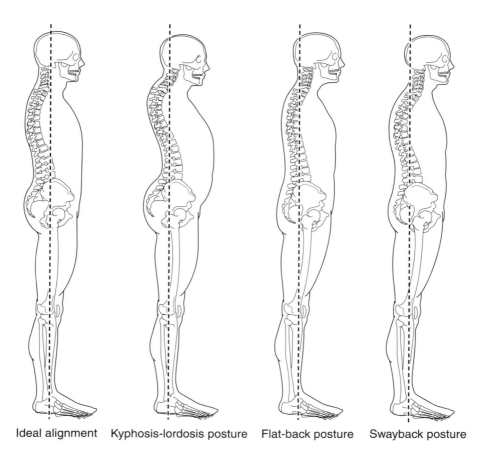

Ideal alignment   Kyphosis-lordosis posture   Flat-back posture   Swayback posture

**Figure 5.10**   Ideal posture compared to kyphosis–lordosis, flat-back, and swayback postures.

system (as opposed to resulting from a structural defect in skeletal design). As figure 5.10 and table 5.1 illustrate, maladaptive postures affect the functioning of the muscles around the trunk and the hip as well as other muscles throughout the kinetic chain. A poor posture not only influences the athlete's ability to move effectively (i.e., engage the muscles to produce optimal forces at the right time) but also may predispose the joint structures to injury from shear and compression forces.

## It's About the Posture, Not the Core

The neuromuscular and musculoskeletal systems are complex. Those working with athletes needs to appreciate, if not fully understand, this complexity. Rather than learning about and focusing on isolated muscle groups, a more effective strategy for a practitioner is to ensure correct positioning of the shoulder girdle, lumbar spine, pelvis, hip, knee and ankle through all the athlete's movements. Correct positioning enables the athlete to recruit the appropriate muscles to generate and absorb forces more strongly and efficiently.

One of the underpinning philosophies of this book is that, simply speaking, coaches should train the athlete's movement rather than focus on specific muscles. The premise is that by positioning joints correctly throughout a movement, muscles will perform the correct actions. In reality, exercises are more effective when they mirror athletic movements, a cornerstone principle of the movement skills component of the model for programme development. The functional neuromuscular activation patterns required can vary according to the demands of the task and the joint positioning undertaken to execute it.

**Table 5.1**  Maladaptive Standing Postures

|  | **Swayback posture** | **Flat-back posture** | **Kyphosis–lordosis posture** |
|---|---|---|---|
| **Description** | Pelvis tilts posteriorly, extending the hips and flattening the normal lumbar curve. The thoracic spine has increased flexion throughout (kyphosis), and the cervical spine (neck) is typically extended. This posture gives the upper trunk the backward-leaning look and puts the head in a slightly forwards position | Pelvis tilts posteriorly, extending the hips and reducing the curvature in the lumbar spine. The lower thoracic spine is similarly flattened, but the upper thoracic spine has increased flexion (narrowing of the internal angle). This posture puts the cervical spine in an extended position with the head forwards. | Pelvis is tilted anteriorly. Flexion occurs in the hip joint, which increases the forwards arching in the lumbar spine (lordosis) and the flexion in the thoracic spine (kyphosis). The cervical spine becomes hyperextended. |
| **Spinal erectors** | Lumbar spine muscles become very strong, whereas the upper spine extensors lengthen and become very weak. | Spinal erectors often lengthen, although they do not necessarily weaken in movements that increase the lumbar curve. | Neck extensors shorten and become strong; neck flexors are weak. Lower back muscles may shorten or become tight, but not always. |
| **Abdominals** | Abdominal muscles lengthen and weaken, especially the external obliques. | Abdominal muscles often become disproportionally strong, increasing the flexion in the lumbar spine. | Abdominal muscles may elongate and weaken, depending on the extent of thoracic kyphosis. |
| **Hip extensors** | Hamstrings become tight and disproportionally strong. | Hamstrings become tight and disproportionally strong. | Hamstrings lengthen. |
| **Hip flexors** | Iliacus and psaos (iliopsoas) lengthen and become weak relative to the hip extensors. | Iliacus and psaos (iliopsoas) lengthen and become weak relative to the hip extensors. | Hip flexors become tight and disproportionally strong relative to the hip extensors. |

A stabilization exercise is any exercise that repeats movement patterns that maintain the balanced, dynamic positioning of the centre of mass in a way that does not produce excessive (abnormal) loading of the spine or other joints.[2] Stability is important, because an athlete who is unbalanced and has to work hard to maintain posture cannot achieve optimal force production or rapid rates of force development. For example, when in neutral position, the position of the pelvis and its relationship with the lumbar spine are extremely important in the maintenance of good posture. This neutral pelvic position is hard to define anatomically, but in this position the lumbar spine has a natural curve. When an anterior pelvic tilt (a tipping forward of the top of the pelvis) is observed, lordosis (an exaggerated curve in the lumbar spine) is evident (figure 5.10). Lordosis typically elongates the muscles

to the rear of the pelvis (the hip extensors) and shortens or tightens the muscles at the front of the pelvis (the hip flexors, such as the iliopsoas). Understanding the cause-and-effect relationship here is important; poor positioning of the pelvis can cause the muscle to shorten. But an imbalance in training stimuli (i.e., an overemphasis on hip flexor work) can lead to overdeveloped muscles that pull the pelvis into anterior tilt. With a posterior tilt in the pelvis (rotation of the top of the pelvis towards the rear), the lumbar curve disappears as the spine flattens (figure 5.10).

The maintenance of the neutral pelvic position is important not simply in standing but also in most movements within sport. Neutral pelvic positioning is the optimal position from which muscular length–tension relationships function, and forces are generated by the muscles around the hip, trunk and groin.

Determining whether the athlete is managing to maintain the desired neutral alignment as he or she moves is difficult. But knowing that the pelvis position influences (and is influenced by) the trunk position enables the use of some basic anatomical landmarks to determine the extent to which the athlete is successful in maintaining neutral pelvic positioning when performing skills.

When the athlete is standing with good posture, the practitioner can identify the distance between the navel (belly button) and the xiphoid process at the base of the sternum (breastbone) (figure 5.11). An athlete who is able to keep the distance between the navel and the xiphoid process constant throughout any movement, based on the distance achieved when standing with good posture, has maintained the pelvis in neutral. With a posterior pelvic tilt, the distance between these landmarks decreases. With an anterior pelvic tilt, the distance between these landmarks increases.

Besides influencing muscle function, maintaining the position of the pelvis during movements is important for maintaining the health of the intervertebral discs in the lumbar spine,

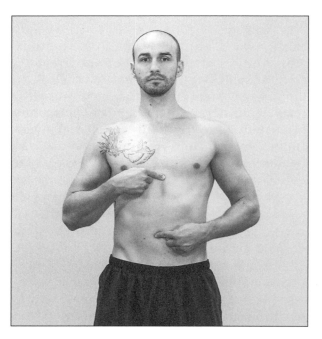

**Figure 5.11**   Identification of neutral pelvic positioning in good standing posture.

particularly in loaded squatting movements, as illustrated in figure 5.12. When squatting (or any similar movement), if the pelvis doesn't maintain alignment, the lumbar vertebrae positions will be adjusted as the pelvis tips. This adjustment commonly takes the form of a posterior pelvic tilt, which flattens out the lumbar spine. Posterior pelvic tilt has implications for muscle recruitment, and it has an effect on the intervertebral discs, especially when the spine is being loaded by a weight acting down through the axis of the spine.

In a normal squatting movement, the vertebrae remain level throughout the movement, and the compression forces of the load are evenly distributed through the cartilage disc that forms the intervertebral articulation. In the instance of a posterior pelvic tilt, however, the front side of the disc is squashed by the two adjacent vertebrae and the rear of the disc is stretched. As the athlete rises, this action is reversed. Repetitious loading patterns of this nature seriously threaten the integrity of the disc wall, increasing the risk that the disc will bulge, or herniate, an extremely debilitating condition.

Over the last 10 years, much of the focus of physical conditioning work within training has been on developing postural control based on the mythical core stability. The focus of this work has often been on the athlete's ability to control the pelvis position using isolated recruitment of muscles within the deep abdominal area of the trunk (figure 5.13 and table 5.2). Often, little thought is given to the athlete's overall postural integrity or to the fact that muscles such as multifidus or transversus abdominis (muscles deep within the abdomen that are the focus of classical core stability work) do not act in isolation, but are in fact phasic and sequential in their recruitment. They work effectively when they contract after certain muscles and before others. This activation pattern is an important part of any progression towards a functional sequence of actions.

Indeed, just because in healthy subjects the transversus abdominis activates before all other anterior muscles (muscles at the front of the body) in certain movements does not

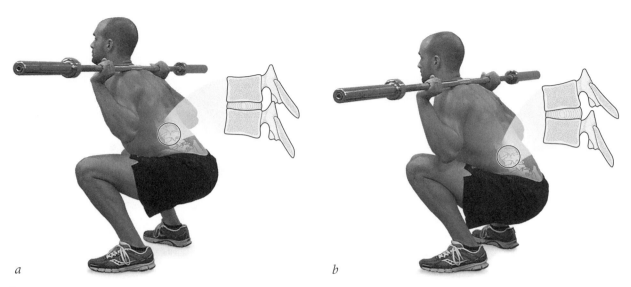

*a*                    *b*

**Figure 5.12** Disk compression and pelvic positioning during dynamic and axial loaded movements such as the squat: *(a)* correct squat; *(b)* incorrect squat.

mean that it is more important in any way. It just means that it is the first muscle that activates in a sequence of events. This debate has often arisen as practitioners have taken practices from rehabilitation contexts (where the ability of the neuromuscular system to recruit a muscle group is trained) and tried to place these into a conditioning or movement context.

Motor control is needed to maintain stability in all sporting movements, yet isolated muscle strength is rarely important in sport, and indeed training a muscle to work in an isolated manner may, in many cases, compromise stability and function.[3] Muscles typically need to co-act as part of a sequence, rather than act in isolation. The rehabilitator is concerned with isolation to teach motor recruitment; the athletic development coach needs to build on this and develop coordinated and skillful recruitment of groups of muscles to achieve stability and mobility. Therefore, coaches need to be thinking about developing postural control in the movement context.

The previous chapter focused on how muscle actions can generate force. That topic is important to understand in looking at the roles of muscles in supporting and mobilizing the spine, pelvis and hip during movement (table 5.2). Understanding the roles of these

muscles in stabilizing or moving the trunk enables the coach to be prescriptive in the type of training movements incorporated into the programme to develop the appropriate strength in these muscles. After all, these movements are important in developing the muscles. The postural muscles in the trunk (internal obliques, external obliques, transversus abdominis) isometrically act to increase intra-abdominal pressure into the abdominal region. This region has no skeletal infrastructure to aid in supporting the spine, so muscular effort is required to achieve it.

The importance of the postural muscles has led to the concept of bracing the posture.[4] When the athlete pulls the abdominal muscles tight ('bracing the trunk musculature') and inhales before performing a movement, the combination of tightened musculature and flattened diaphragm significantly increases the pressure within the abdomen. This intra-abdominal pressure provides necessary support to the spine during movement. Exhaling and relaxing the brace releases this intra-abdominal pressure, and if this is done when the spine is being loaded, the back becomes vulnerable.

Now that stability has been achieved in the pelvis and lumbar spine, the 'power muscles' can provide the powerful mobilization forces, as either prime movers or synergists (assisting),

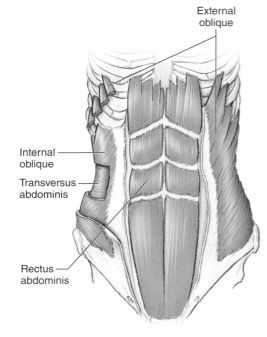

External oblique

Internal oblique

Transversus abdominis

Rectus abdominis

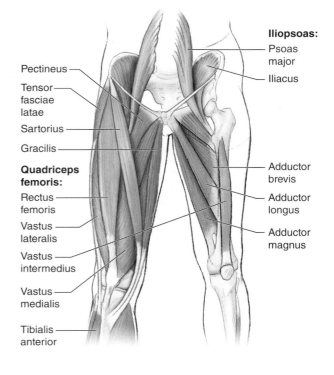

Iliopsoas:
Psoas major
Iliacus

Pectineus

Tensor fasciae latae

Sartorius

Gracilis

Quadriceps femoris:
Rectus femoris
Vastus lateralis
Vastus intermedius
Vastus medialis

Tibialis anterior

Adductor brevis
Adductor longus
Adductor magnus

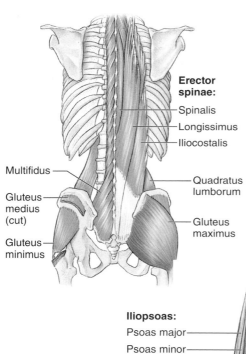

Erector spinae:
Spinalis
Longissimus
Iliocostalis

Multifidus

Gluteus medius (cut)

Gluteus minimus

Quadratus lumborum

Gluteus maximus

Iliopsoas:
Psoas major
Psoas minor
Iliacus

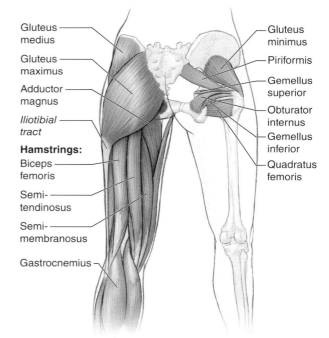

Gluteus medius
Gluteus maximus
Adductor magnus
Iliotibial tract
Hamstrings:
Biceps femoris
Semitendinosus
Semimembranosus
Gastrocnemius

Gluteus minimus
Piriformis
Gemellus superior
Obturator internus
Gemellus inferior
Quadratus femoris

**Figure 5.13** Posture and power muscles in the midsection.

**Table 5.2** Power and Postural Muscles in the Midsection

| Muscle | Major function |
|---|---|
| Transversus abdominis | Deepest of the three lateral abdominal muscles. Compresses the abdominal wall, aiding in the stabilization of the abdominal tissue and in the action of the other trunk muscles. Especially important in forced expiration (bracing). |
| Internal oblique | If activated bilaterally (on both sides of the trunk), this muscle flexes the vertebral column, tilting the pelvis anteriorly and bringing it closer to the trunk. If activated unilaterally, the muscle acts with the external oblique to flex the spine laterally and rotate the vertebral column. |
| External oblique | Acting bilaterally, this muscle flexes the lumbar spine, tilting the pelvis posteriorly. If activated unilaterally in conjunction with the internal oblique, this muscle causes side (lateral) flexion of the trunk. Also involved in the rotation of the vertebral column. |
| Multifidus | Extends the vertebral column and rotates it towards the opposite side. |
| Gluteus medius | Abducts the femur at the hip and medially rotates the thigh, thus assisting in stabilization of the knee in extension. In locomotion, co-acts with the gluteus minimus to maintain the level position of the pelvis so that the leg can swing forward, not across the body. May also assist in flexion and extension of the hip. |
| Gluteus minimus | Abducts the hip joint and medially rotates the thigh. It may also assist in hip flexion. |
| Rectus abdominis | Flexes the spine (i.e., bends the vertebral column forward). If the pelvis is fixed, the trunk moves forward; if the trunk is fixed, the pelvis moves towards the trunk. Also important in compressing the abdomen. |
| Erector spinae | Composed of three muscles: iliocostalis, longissimus and spinalis. They extend the lumbar and lower thoracic spine, assist in lateral flexion of the spine and rotate the spine for forceful inspiration. |
| Iliopsoas (psoas major and iliacus) | When the trunk or pelvis is fixed, it flexes the hip joint by bringing the femur (thigh bone) towards the trunk (e.g., swinging the leg forward in walking). Also assists in the lateral rotation and abduction of the hip joint. When the thigh is fixed, it flexes the trunk by bringing it towards the femur. Bilateral action in this situation increases lordosis in the lumbar spine; unilateral action assists in lateral flexion of the trunk to the same side. |
| Rectus femoris | Extends the knee as part of the quadriceps femoris group that also includes the vastus lateralis, vastus medialis and vastus intermedius. Rectus femoris flexes the hip joint by raising the femur towards the trunk. |
| Sartorius | Flexes, laterally rotates and abducts the thigh at the hip joint and aids in the flexion and medial rotation of the knee after flexion. This muscle swings the leg forward in the unsupported phases of running and walking. |
| Gluteus maximus | Typically used only in forceful extension and lateral rotation of the hip joint and stabilization of the knee joint in extension. |
| Biceps femoris | One of three muscles that make up the hamstring group. Flexes and laterally rotates the knee. The long head has a function in extending the hip. Assists in the lateral rotation of the hip. During locomotion, the hamstrings decelerate the forward swing phase of the thigh and prevent trunk flexion at the hip. |
| Semitendinosus and semimembranosus | With the biceps femoris, make up the hamstring group. Flex and medially rotate the knee, extend the thigh at the hip and assist in the medial rotation of the hip. |

through either flexion or extension of the trunk (rectus abdominis or erector spinae) or the hip (rectus femoris and iliopsoas or gluteus maximus and hamstrings, respectively). In sport contexts, these movements often are accompanied by rotational or lateral actions, so the associated muscular involvements become more complex. But the basic premise needs to remain—the postural muscles need to be able to co-act to provide a stable platform from which the power-producing muscles can mobilize joints and develop and express large forces.

Optimal movement performance relies on this stability and mobility. If either muscle group is producing compensatory movements, the athlete will be compromised and the musculature around the lumbar–pelvic area will have to compensate in some ways.

A common example can be seen in teenage athletes who are performing high-intensity running intervals. As fatigue sets in, the athlete may complain of pain in the lower back. Often this occurs because the athlete has compensated by using the rectus abdominis to maintain pelvic position. When the athlete reaches the point at which the rectus abdominis becomes involved in other actions (such assisting in breathing at high intensities) and can no longer maintain the pelvic position, the pelvis begins to tilt in an anterior–posterior movement. This tilt decreases movement efficiency and causes pain in the lumbar spine.

Other common movement compensations are seen around the hip; the athlete overuses the hip flexors and quadriceps to perform actions and consequently underuses the gluteal muscles. Often, imbalances and reduced mobility around the hip are the result. A chronic problem develops over time as the movement pattern becomes habit, and the muscle imbalance and loss of mobility worsen unless addressed. Although experience shows that the better the athlete's performance level is, the better he or she is at achieving movement compensations, this situation is not ideal and almost always leads to further complications down the line.

The correct movement mechanics are facilitated by the ability to produce forces through a full range of mobility from a stable platform. Incorrect mechanics lead to poor mobility, poor stability and inefficiency (increased energy cost for the same amount of work), all of which negatively affect the athlete's performance capabilities.

Injuries are also an important consideration in the alignment of joints as the athlete moves. As figure 5.8 shows, typically the hips are level during standing and the knees are in line with the toes. This positioning is also important during movement. As table 5.3 shows, the knee is a hinge joint; it is designed to flex and extend but not to rotate to any significant degree. Indeed, the ligament structures around the knee are specifically designed to allow movement only in the sagittal plane. Frontal plane movement is potentially damaging to the medial and lateral collateral ligaments, and transverse plane movement can cause damage to the anterior and posterior cruciate ligaments.

Because the knee is a complex articulation of the femur (thigh bone) and the tibia (major shin bone), any rotational or lateral movement that occurs here (without considering a direct blow from an external source) is largely the result of movement at either the hip joint (misalignment of the femur) or the ankle (misalignment of the tibia). This rotational or lateral movement can have catastrophic consequences for an athlete, because large forces that occur through an inappropriate plane can lead to shear forces, which can compromise some or all of the structures within the knee joint.

# Recognizing the Power of the Glutes

In saying that observation needs to focus on movements with respect to the alignment or positioning of the hip, knee and ankle, practitioners need to realize that, in motion, the coactivation of muscles is extremely important in positioning and stabilizing joints. In considering this, practitioners should understand the actions of one of the most important muscle groups within the athletic body, namely the gluteals (glutes). Coaches often ignore this muscle group, and evidence suggests that athletes underutilize it.

For example, in a single-leg landing, the gluteal muscles are extremely important in aligning the knee so that flexion occurs along the line of the foot. The simultaneous coactivation of the quadriceps and hamstrings stabilizes and braces the knee. The knee can then perform the powerful flexion and extension

**Table 5.3**  Movement in the Major Joints

| Joint | Articulation between bones | Classification | Degrees of movement | Movement capabilities |
|---|---|---|---|---|
| Shoulder: glenohumeral | Head of the humerus (upper arm) and the glenoid fossa of the scapula | Synovial ball and socket joint | 3 | Flexion and extension (sagittal plane); abduction and adduction (transverse plane and frontal plane). |
| Shoulder: sternoclavicular | Clavicle, sternum and first rib | Cartilaginous joint | 3 | Not directly influenced by muscle action, but all actions of the scapula cause action at this joint. |
| Shoulder: acromioclavicular | Acromion process on the scapula and the clavicle | Gliding synovial joint | 3 | Abduction (protraction); adduction (retraction); upward and downward rotation. |
| Spine | Vertebrae | Amphiarthrodial-cartilaginous | 3 | Flexion and extension (sagittal plane, frontal plane); left and right rotation; circumduction in some cervical vertebrae. |
| Elbow | Humerus of the upper arm and combined radius and ulnar from forearm | Synovial hinge joint | 1 | Flexion and extension (sagittal plane). |
| Wrist | Radius of forearm and carpus (complex of eight carpal bones in the hand) | Synovial ellipsoid joint | 5 | Flexion, extension, circumduction, abduction, adduction. |
| Hip | Head of the femur and the acetabulum of the pelvis | Synovial ball-and-socket joint | 3 | Flexion and extension (sagittal plane); abduction and adduction (transverse plane, frontal plane); medial and lateral rotation. |
| Knee | Femur of the thigh and tibia of the lower leg | Synovial hinge joint | 1 (2) | Flexion and extension; slight medial or lateral rotation about the axis of the lower leg when the knee is in a 90-degree flexed position. |
| Ankle | Tibia and fibula of the lower leg and the talus of foot | Synovial hinge joint | 1 | Plantarflexion and dorsiflexion (sagittal plane). |

actions that it is supposed to perform and resist lateral or rotational movements. Asynchronous firing of these muscle groups leaves the knee vulnerable to injury. As will be illustrated, the lack of coordination in this muscle firing sequence can be caused by an ineffectual motor programme (i.e., a coordination thing) or the faulty positioning or alignment of the hip and knee, meaning that the muscles cannot fire in sequence because of the relative positioning of their insertions across the respective joints.

# Joint Positioning and Muscle Function

Joints are articulations of the bones, and the positioning and actions of the joints play a key part in the movement, and the analysis of such, in the athlete. Joints are mainly classified structurally and functionally. Structural classification is determined by how the bones connect to each other, whereas functional classification is determined by the degree of movement between the articulating bones.[6]

Joint positioning throughout the posture is important, because it governs not only how forces are transferred through the body but also how the muscles function. The dynamic relationship of how joints are positioned determines the recruitment sequence of the muscular system. To demonstrate this concept to athletes, use this practical task (figure 5.14):

- Put your left hand on your right biceps brachii muscle so that the palm and fingers cover the belly of the muscle.
- As hard as you can, perform five biceps curls of the right arm with the palm of the right hand facing upwards (the wrist is supinated). The left hand will feel the biceps brachii muscle working.
- After five repetitions, turn over the wrist of the right hand so that the palm is facing down (the wrist is pronated). Keep the left hand in the same place.
- With the wrist pronated, perform five reverse biceps curls. The left hand will feel the action of the biceps brachii as the elbow joint flexes.
- Then ask the question, 'Did the muscle action feel the same in both exercises?'

The answer should be no. With the wrist supinated and the shoulder remaining in one fixed position, both the short and long heads of the biceps brachii act as the prime movers in elbow flexion, pulling the forearm towards the humerus. The brachialis also is a prime mover in this action. But with the wrist pronated and the radius crossing over the ulna at the radioulnar joint, the biceps brachii (in particular the short head) is less active, because of its attachment point to the radius. The role of the brachialis doesn't change because of its attachment to the ulna bone in the forearm, but with the wrist pronated, the brachioradialis has a more pronounced action in elbow flexion, particularly through the midrange of the movement.

This phenomenon of the influence of joint positioning on muscle function has been explored previously. This concept is emphasized in terms of practical technique in chapters 8 through 10, where the concept of 'form' (posture or technique) determining function (athletic outcome) is emphasized. Similarly, figure 5.10 illustrates the long-term influence of various postures on chronic muscle function. This highlights a key feature of teaching movement skills and techniques: Put the joints in the right position (adopt the best posture) and the muscle recruitment will take care of itself.

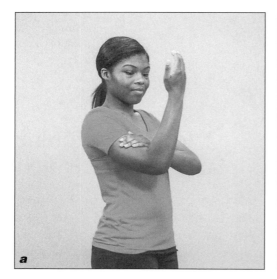 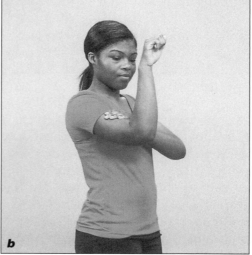

**Figure 5.14** Understanding the importance of joint positioning: *(a)* biceps curl (wrist supinated); *(b)* reverse biceps curl (wrist pronated).

Practitioners should strive to observe and provide feedback on the joint actions during any skilled performance to maximize movement efficiency in their athletes. How an athlete moves is arguably more important than how he or she performs (i.e., times, distances, and so on) in many situations. Indeed, I have often stood on a sideline and missed key game situations because I was focussed on how the athlete was moving rather than what was going on in the game. Such is the role of the athletic development professional.

# Muscle Recruitment and Length–Tension Relationships

In describing movement, athletic development professionals often refer to posture as the kinetic chain (the interconnections in the neuromuscular and connective tissue systems that link the head to the toes). As with any chain, a series of linkages form the connective structure, and, as with any series of attachments, the weak point in the chain limits the functional capacity of the structure. The point to which load is applied and the shape of the chain at that particular time determine the performance capacity of the chain. In moving, the articulations of the body change constantly, and the angles of the joints relative to each other change simultaneously and in combination.

Chapter 2 demonstrates how muscles cross joints and are attached to bones. If the positioning of the bone changes relative to another bone as the articulation (joint) is moved, then the distance between where the muscle starts (sometimes referred to as the origin) and finishes (the insertion) increases and the muscle lengthens. This change in muscle length influences the ability of the muscle to exert forces and contract with velocity.

This change appears to be because of the number of cross-bridges available for attachment between the actin and myosin filaments in the muscle. When the muscle is at its shortest, many cross-bridges seek the same attachment sites as the actin filament is pulled far across the myosin filament in the sarcomere. Indeed, the cross-bridges may interfere with each other, reducing the tension created in the muscle and therefore the force output generated. Conversely, when the muscle is stretched, the distance between the attachment sites for the myosin heads is maximized, meaning that few cross-bridge attachments are achieved because the sites are too far apart. This also means that the sarcomere has little ability to develop force through high muscular tension.[3]

But as figure 5.15 shows, at optimum sarcomere length, many opportunities are available for cross-bridge attachment and, hence, optimal muscular tension and force-producing capabilities. This phenomenon applies to whole muscles and muscle systems as well as within single and isolated muscle fibres.[5]

In the earlier example of the biceps curl, pronating the wrist altered the relative lengths of the biceps brachii and brachioradialis muscles, changing the most efficient means for the neuromuscular system to perform the work during the biceps curl. Hence, joint positioning influences muscular recruitment patterns.

Muscular recruitment can also be influenced by the resistance that the muscular force is required to overcome. The force–velocity (F–V) curve of single-muscle-fibre contraction is best described as a hyperbolic curve (figure 5.15), the curvature of which depends on the tension in the muscle and the resistive load applied.

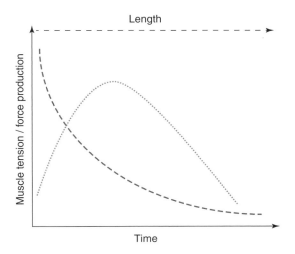

**Figure 5.15** Length–tension and force–velocity relationships in muscle fibre contraction.

This single-fibre relationship between velocity of contraction and external force-producing capabilities is mimicked, if not mirrored, in total-body movements. Although not all muscles have the same makeup of fibre types (Type IIx can produce more force with greater contractile velocity than Type I) and the range of muscles involved will all be at different lengths, the curvilinear relationship can still be described by the same-shaped curve.

This point is important for two reasons. First, exerting large forces in very fast movements is impossible. Therefore, if the first phase of a sequential movement is too rapid and insufficient forces are produced, the force deficit cannot be made up in subsequent phases of the movement. This consideration is important in throwing or lifting movements, such as when large forces are generated in the initial phases of the movement and transferred into higher velocity phases at subsequent stages of the action. For example, during the clean, in the first pull phase, high forces are developed through relatively slow velocities compared with the rest of the action as inertia is overcome to set the bar into a position. Following the stretch-shortening actions that occur in the transition phase, high forces and high velocities are achieved in the second pull phase. This exercise and relative bar velocities at each stage of the lift are detailed in chapter 10.

The second reason it is important to understand this concept is that the equation that determines the gradient of the hyperbolic curve is reasonably fixed in human motion. Therefore, to increase the athlete's ability to generate velocity at a given resistance in the middle range of the curve, he or she first needs to increase the ability to generate maximal forces. Doing so raises all ranges of the F–V power curve, meaning that the athlete is able to harness an increased range of power-producing capabilities, but the overall gradient of the curve does not change. The interpretation of this into accessible strength progressions is also presented in chapter 10.

The examples of the muscle length–tension and velocity relationships are all taken from studies of the fibres of single muscles. In a sporting context, the human body is an intact multijoint and multimuscle system. Even so, similar principles apply, and skilled movement patterns are the result of placing the joints in the optimum positions to enable peak muscle tension (or the required percentages thereof). Therefore, the corresponding muscle output forces (i.e., expressed strength) and limb contractile velocity are a function of the interaction of numerous sarcomere lengths and the mechanical attributes of the bone lever system.[5]

# Human Lever System

Levers often are referred to as machines that operate according to the principles of torques. People use them in daily life to make everyday tasks easier, either by enabling the overcoming of a resistance that is greater than the force directly applied (for example, in lifting an object with a crowbar) or increasing the speed and range of motion through which an object can be moved (for example, hitting a tennis ball with a racket or a baseball with a bat; figure 5.16).

The human body contains a complicated arrangement of levers that work together to optimize the mechanical advantage to the body during skilled movement. Mechanical advantage can be thought of as the measure of force or velocity multiplication that results from using a lever system (or machine) to do

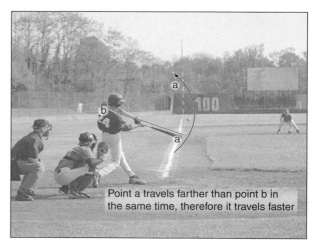

Point a travels farther than point b in the same time, therefore it travels faster

**Figure 5.16** Speed-multiplying levers in striking a baseball.

the work. It is a measure of increasing work done against the energy cost (or indeed system capabilities) for performing that work.[7]

Muscles produce pulling forces to the rigid lever skeletal system. Torques are rotational, or twisting, forces that occur as an object is rotated about an axis or pivot. Torques (or moments) are proportional to the distance between the pivot multiplied by the force applied at the end of the lever (moment equals force times distance). In the human body, the bones can be considered the rigid lever arms of the lever system. Different bones have different lengths and different leverage potentials, although because the relative positioning of bones to each other will change during a movement, the relative lengths and lever arms may also change. Joints are the pivots, muscles produce the force that moves the lever arms and resistive loads are determined by the work required to be done. This work can be ground reaction force, an external weight, gravity or a collision with an opponent, and it must include the system mass (e.g., the weight of the body or body segment that is being moved) as well as any external load or resistive force.

A change in length of the force arm alters the magnitude of force required to overcome a resistance. Although this point may seem logical when discussing a crowbar (for example), it initially takes some thought when applied to human movement. Because the length of a bone doesn't change, why isn't the moment always the same throughout a movement? This problem can be explained by relating back to the example of the biceps curl. (Note that this movement is not often used in functional sport training, but it is highly useful in explaining physio-mechanical concepts.) As with most major limb movements, this action is an example of a third-class lever (table 5.4).

In the biceps curl, as the dumbbell is lifted, the length of the moment arm (the distance between the pivot and the insertion of the biceps brachii tendon to the ulna) changes. During the lift, the muscular force (torque) that is required to lift the weight changes, and the external work that is performed changes. The conclusion is that a relationship exists between the angle of a joint and the torque that the muscles can produce (figure 5.17). When teaching techniques, coaches should emphasize joint positions that optimize not only the force–velocity potential of the muscle fibres but also the ability to produce muscular torques in the lever systems.

Because the muscles are required to produce relatively large forces to gain the speed

**Table 5.4** Lever Systems in the Human Body

| Classification | Definition | Benefits | Example |
|---|---|---|---|
| First-class lever | Pivot is between the required muscular force and the resistive load (as in a see-saw). | Can act as a lever, providing both mechanical advantage and speed advantage depending on the position of the fulcrum. | Extension of the elbow with the wrist pronated. |
| Second-class lever | Muscle force and resistive force are on the same side of the fulcrum, and the resistive mass is between the resistive force and the pivot (as in a wheelbarrow). | Acts at a mechanical advantage in terms of force. It magnifies the effect of a small force, and less effort is required to move a large force. | Plantarflexion of the ankle. |
| Third-class lever | Muscle force and resistive force are on the same side of the fulcrum, and the resistive force is between the resistive mass and the pivot (as in a pair of tweezers). | Acts at a force disadvantage and a speed advantage. It enables speed and range of motion at the expense of force. | Flexion of the elbow. |

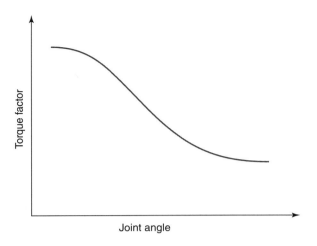

**Figure 5.17**    The relationship between joint angle and torque production.

advantage offered by the lever, actions involving these lever systems have been demonstrated to be associated with higher instances of injury to athletes. Understanding lever systems also helps in making informed decisions about exercise selections and the potential implications for performance enhancement. To illustrate the concept, consider a comparison between the good morning and the stiff-legged (or Romanian) deadlift, both of which are commonly prescribed exercises for strengthening the hamstrings, particularly in terms of generating eccentric strength.

As figure 5.18 illustrates, the movement of the trunk in these exercises is similar, and, without the load being present, the demands placed on the hamstrings to resist trunk flexion and cause trunk extension would be similar. Indeed, without considering the external load, the moment arm of muscular force would involve a third-class lever system in both movements. The resistance moment arm, however, causes the exercises to be significantly different.

Placing the load on the shoulders in the good morning movement significantly increases the resistance lever arm. This aspect has two potentially negative effects on the athlete. First, in a lever system that is at a force disadvantage, the hamstring muscle must work harder to achieve the trunk extension as the load is raised. In this instance, with a large resistance arm and small muscle force arm, the body is at an extremely disadvantaged position mechanically. Although this point may be considered an advantage in terms of training, coaches need to recognize that the exercise may rapidly overload the hamstrings and cause the athlete to use other muscles in the lumbar spine (for example, the erector spinae, which are assistors in this trunk extension movement) as prime movers. This itself is an injury risk.

Of greater potential concern, however, are the shear stresses that the lumbar vertebrae

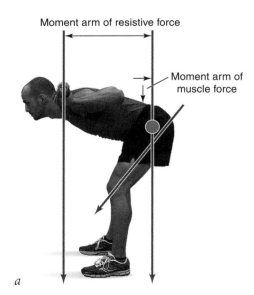

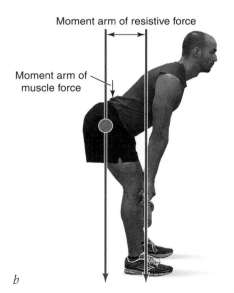

**Figure 5.18**    The moment arm of resistive force in the *(a)* good morning and *(b)* stiff-legged (or Romanian) deadlift movements.

are subject to in a movement such as this that has such a big (long) resistance movement area. Thus the stiff-legged deadlift, with a much smaller resistance moment arm, is a much safer and arguably more effective exercise for developing force-generation potential in the hamstrings. Another consideration for choosing between the two exercises is a more practical one. If the athlete fails the lift and cannot return the load to a standing position during the stiff-legged deadlift, the athlete can simply drop the bar. Conversely, during a good morning, the bar cannot be easily dumped unless it is rolled over the neck.

## Posture and Centre of Pressure

A concept that hasn't been discussed yet but that is central to the concept of athletic movement is how forces, especially impact or ground reaction forces, are distributed. This idea relates to the concept of pressure, which can be calculated as the magnitude of a force divided by the area over which the force is distributed.[8] When coaching movement, however, the amount of pressure is often not of as much interest as the area through which the force is concentrated. This area is known as the centre of pressure. This coaching concept is important, because where the athlete exerts or experiences pressure can determine the resultant movement pattern. The centre of pressure is often an important coaching cue that can be used to determine whether an athlete is performing a movement correctly.

One application of this force distribution (remembering that force is a vector quality) is seen in directional change. This idea is illustrated in figure 5.19, in which the athlete is performing an angled backpedal. As will be illustrated in the coaching progressions in chapter 8, this skill is particularly useful for athletes who need to look forwards while tracking backwards and to the side. The skill involves learning to push off from different parts of the feet to produce a resultant movement pattern.

As the athlete moves at a 45-degree angle backwards, the feet, hips and upper body should stay facing forward (square). This

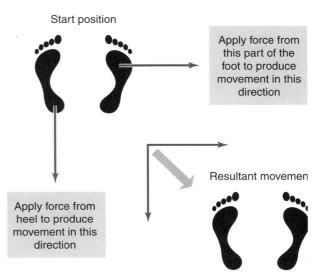

**Figure 5.19** Pressure through different parts of the foot to produce an angled backpedal.

orientation permits the athlete to respond to any necessary stimuli and change direction by pushing off from the relevant parts of the foot. If the hips point in any direction other than forward, the athlete will not be able to respond rapidly to any required directional changes, which opens up the opportunities for an opponent to pass the athlete on the inside (the side that the body has turned away from).

The concept of centre of pressure and adjusting the posture to control (or adapt) it is important in a range of locomotive skills, such as running, jumping and many direction change skills such as cutting actions. This point can be simply illustrated by the following practical task.

Have the athlete stand with his or her toes on a line. Instruct the athlete first to jump by 'forcefully pushing the feet into the floor so that you end up on your toes' (be specific in this coaching cue; figure 5.20). The resulting centre of pressure through the feet will result in a force vector that sends the athlete upwards and slightly forwards (i.e., he or she will land from the jump in front of the line). After the athlete resets on the line, instruct him or her to jump by 'extending your hips forcefully so that you end up on your toes before leaving the ground' (figure 5.21). The resulting force vector is upwards and slightly backwards, so that the athlete lands slightly behind the line.

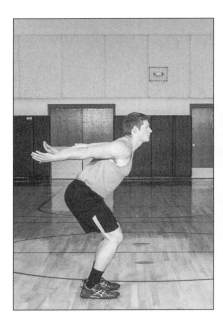
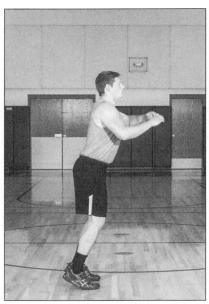
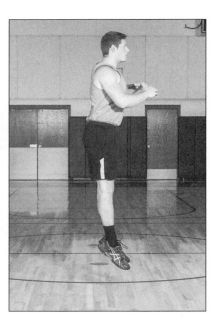

**Figure 5.20**   Centre of pressure in influencing movement through a vertical jump: 'Forcefully push your feet into the floor so that you end up on your toes.'

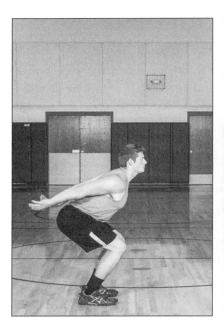
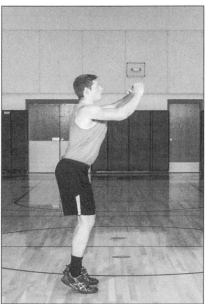
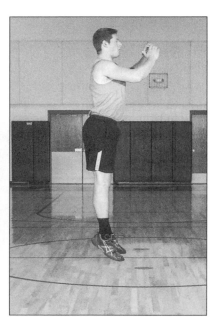

**Figure 5.21**   Centre of pressure in influencing movement through a vertical jump: 'Extend your hips forcefully so that you end up on your toes before leaving the floor.'

Landing from a vertical jump is another example of the importance of centre of pressure. Application of this forms the basis for most coaching of athletes who are moving towards multiple jump progressions. The aim in teaching this skill is to have the weight evenly distributed through the middle of the foot (figure 5.22), which optimizes load distribution and puts the legs in a position to use the stretch reflex to produce powerful reflex jumping actions (chapter 9).

The analysis of an athlete's running stride is known as gait analysis. Coaches typically are interested in how an athlete runs (for

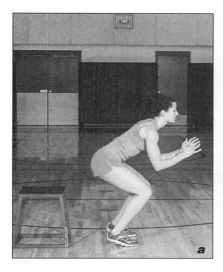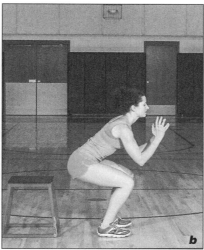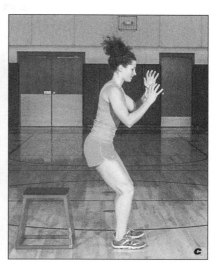

**Figure 5.22** Pressure distribution in a two-footed landing: *(a)* weight distributed too far forwards; *(b)* weight distributed evenly through the midfoot; *(c)* weight distributed too far towards the heels.

example, with a heel–toe action or a midfoot strike pattern) and how the running pattern changes with the relative intensity or speed of the action. Physiotherapists are similarly interested in analysing the centre of pressure when someone walks or runs. The deviations of the centre of pressure towards either the middle of the foot (known as overpronation, when the foot rolls too far internally as the athlete transfers weight through the foot) or the outside of the foot (known as eversion) can influence the joint and muscle actions farther up the kinetic chain. In the long term, these deviations can cause conditions such as plantar fasciitis (a painful inflammation of the fascia along the side of the foot) or other chronic conditions within the knee, hip or back.

## Summary

Skilled movement performance in sport depends on a number of factors coming together in a given time. Dynamic postural control is a central feature of skilled movement. Skilful movement requires control of actions in a number of planes because functional activities or practical movements in sport never occur in one plane. An athlete who is moving forwards (in the sagittal plane) is also controlling rotations and forces that act on the body in the frontal and transverse planes. All total-body movement is a combination of many movements, and the posture (how an athlete gets into a certain position) is critical to achieving the required blend of mobility (the range of movement required) and stability (within the given range of movement) to execute the skill.

The aim of the athlete development professional is to develop movement competence in a range of contexts, either within a sport or across a number of sports. For example, in a team sport such as soccer, most of the actions and manoeuvres in performance situations are executed with submaximal force and velocity but high accuracy and purposefulness. The most successful actions in games are seen when the outcome of an action is unique and the accuracy, speed and use of force are at a maximum.

In general, the total force experienced by an athlete in action is a sum of several forces produced by internal (muscular force) and external (reaction force, impact force, air resistance and so on) forces. The force generated is the result of the successive use of body segments from initiation of movement through the action phase. As figure 5.23 shows, the forces from each joint action are summated as muscle force is transferred from the large- to small-muscle groups through the action phase of a skill.

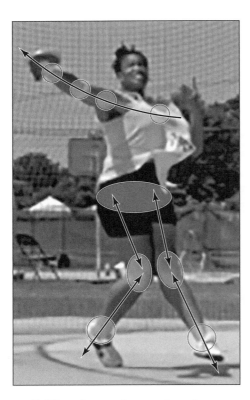

**Figure 5.23** Ground reaction forces travel through the posture in sequence.

The discus thrower initiates movement with the large muscles in the hips and legs. Ground reaction force is transferred up the body from the ground through the ankles, knees and hips in sequence. Forces generated through ground reaction at the centre of the body travel from the hips through to the spine and along the arms to the implement (discus). Forces are generated from large muscles and then transferred in coordinated sequence to smaller muscles.

For these forces to be applied at the correct time and in the desired direction, the sequence and timing of this force transfer has to be optimal and must rely on a stable base of support from which summated forces can be generated. The summation occurs through the skilled timing of sequential joint involvement in the movement execution. For example, in the well-timed shot put release, the hips begin to accelerate just as the leg drive ceases acceleration, the shoulder action commences as the hips begin to decelerate and so forth.

But skilled execution, even in a high-force event such as the shot put, is not solely about force production; it also is about movement velocity. In the human body, the velocity for the distal body parts (foot, hand, head) is produced through the human lever system of the joints. The linear velocity of the distal body part depends on the length and angular velocity of the respective lever (lower leg, thigh and so on). The relative angular velocities for each body part are produced through the respective muscle group (knee extensors, dorsiflexors and so on), and the joint must be in the correct position to have the moment arm of muscular force in the optimum position. As with force, there is then a successive generation of each link of speed from the centre of the body to the extremities through the postural or kinetic chain. All participating muscle groups begin contractions from maximum length (regardless of whether the required action is eccentric or concentric in nature) to optimize the stretch-shortening potential of the muscle.[9]

So in any movement skill, several lever systems in the body contribute to the final force application and therefore the resulting movement speed. The athlete must develop a consistency of pattern and movement that enables performance outcomes that are the result of complex multimuscle, multijoint movements. The muscles must co-act with each other to produce a stable structure that enables multiplanar forces to be produced through efficient movement patterns. As figure 5.24 illustrates, however, emphasizing performance outcomes rather than reinforcing movement techniques may result in the athlete having a perceived movement competence that achieves performance gains in the short term but limits performance and increases the potential for injury if that movement or postural patterning becomes ingrained.

The next chapter further explores the importance of posture by introducing the concept of postural analysis and corrective exercises that may aid the athlete in achieving mechanically correct postures when performing movement skills.

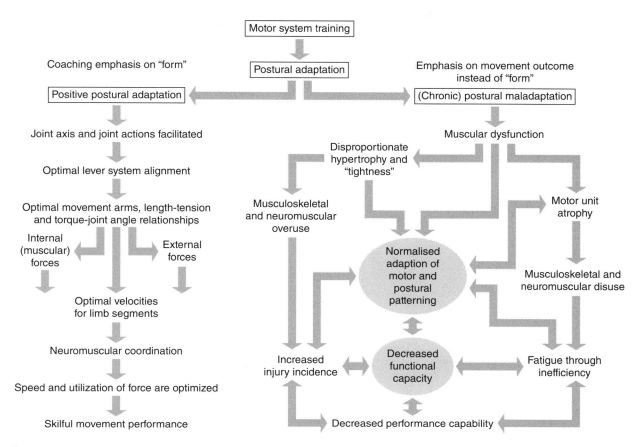

**Figure 5.24**   Importance of positive postural adaptation to efficient movement skill development.

# CHAPTER 6

# Evaluating Posture

Previous discussions highlighted that a central tenant for enhancing an athlete's movement efficiency is the ability to produce and control forces through the maintenance of effective posture. As discussed in chapter 5, imbalances and asymmetries in the athlete's body, whether between the front (anterior chain) and back (posterior chain) or between the left and right sides of the body, lead to movement inefficiencies, which in turn limit the movement options available to the athlete to solve problems presented by his or her sport. Credible evidence also demonstrates a strong correlation between poor posture and subsequent injury in contact sports.[1] Therefore, practitioners need to assess an athlete's postural limitations so that they can understand the athlete's potential limitations and, more important, create strategies for intervention to correct the deficiencies identified. This chapter describes the basic principles and some strategies used to assess and quantify the postural control of an athlete.

In the coaching process, observational analysis is the core skill in problem identification. The practitioner needs to quantify the problem (i.e., obtain some data) and record or understand the athlete's ability (or inability) to execute a task. Such data shouldn't merely quantify the athlete's training state; the records should be structured to inform and guide prescription to the athlete's best advantage. This method enables the evaluation of the effectiveness of the designed intervention after the requisite time has passed, when the athlete can be reassessed to determine the rate of improvement. The basis for intervention is to improve body mechanics and thus improve performance and reduce injury risk. Therefore, an important goal is to determine the success level of the programme.

Quantification doesn't always mean that an objective number has to be attached to the test. Experience has shown that this is especially important in analysing posture, in which notes and observations are arguably as important as any scoring system. Indeed, a number of postural screening tools enable the practitioner to apply a numerical score to the postural assessment, but the basis of many aspects of these tests is a subjective one; that is, the practitioner decides whether the athlete has achieved the objective criteria for scoring a 1 or a 2 on a particular test. Some tests allow objective monitoring of aspects of movement control (for example, goniometry measures range of movement around a joint), but the importance of observation in monitoring postural control cannot be underestimated or underplayed. Experienced practitioners often do not require assessment protocols to analyse an athlete's postural control. They are able to identify an athlete's postural limitations by watching the athlete perform everyday movement tasks.

In scoring or monitoring systems for posture, or even for specific joint movements, a useful approach is to refer to the concept of what is optimal for the athlete rather than what is normal for a population. Many researchers have published norms for the range of movement of a joint, but these data often are produced in a manner that is not representative of a specific population. For example, if you consider the ranges of movement required in a joint or series of joints such as the spine (figure 6.1) in the high jump (figure 6.2) and compare these to what is deemed a normal range of movement for the spine, then the concept of normality is really challenged. The questions the practitioner should ask are, 'What are optimal for this athlete and the demands that he or she is subject to within his or her sport?' and 'Does the athlete have adequate motor control (muscle activation sequences, force production) through the full movement range?' These questions are important to consider in screening an athlete, because moving through a full range without the necessary strength to facilitate control is a recognized precursor to injury.

Throughout this text, discussions about posture have revealed the importance of the interrelationship between the body segments and the neuromuscular structures that facilitate their movement throughout the kinetic chain. Identifying areas of inefficiency in the athlete's kinetic chain allows correction in areas of weakness, which in turn leads to the reduction of other compensations throughout the kinetic chain.

This idea can be exemplified through reference to injury predispositions in the leg that may occur because of dynamic postural control deficiencies. Hamstring tightness and weakness are particular concerns to athletes across a range of sports, especially those based on single or repeated maximal sprints. The biomechanics of hamstring strains typically result from generation of a large knee extensor moment at the terminal swing phase in sprinting (see chapter 8), which causes a large eccentric load on the hamstrings.[2] If the extensor moment created by the quadriceps exceeds the eccentric capability of the hamstring, failure will occur.

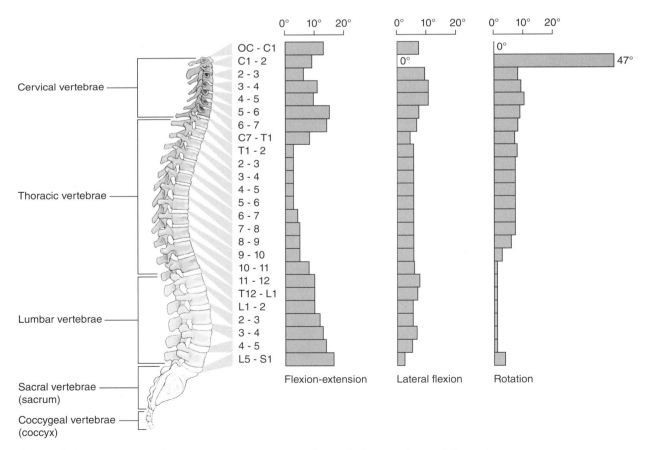

**Figure 6.1** Normal triplanar movement ranges through the sections of the spine.

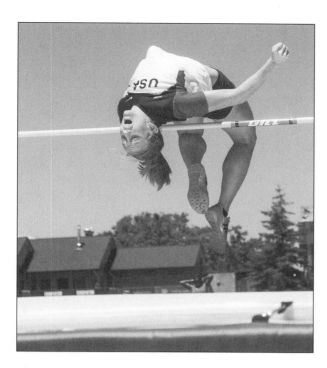

**Figure 6.2** The required ranges of spinal movement for certain techniques in sport (for example, the flop technique in high jump) far exceed what might be considered normal.

# Role of Postural Assessment

Recently, a plethora of methods have been proposed for assessing the functional movement of athletes. Each of these models proposes a number of tests designed to assess various aspects of joint movement and postural control, potentially to enable those working with athletes to derive information about the athlete's movement abilities. But the published literature offers little consensus about whether such testing batteries or screens achieve their stated aims, especially when they are undertaken in isolation of other programme considerations such as the physical demands of the sport or the athlete's injury history, training age or background. Being data rich but analysis poor is not a sound basis for the development of a successful programme in any context.

A practitioner who integrates a testing battery into the programme must have a fundamental objective for that battery, regardless of what aspect of fitness, psychology or lifestyle is being assessed. That objective must be to gather data that is valid, reliable and interpretable and, most important, forms a basis for a monitored intervention. Many coaches and sport scientists are highly capable of gathering large amounts of data about the athletes they work with, but often the data do not translate into an action plan.

All successful athlete development programmes are based on informed decisions, that is, decisions with a sound evidential basis. Although it may sound simplistic, test or observational data need to form the baseline measurement against which an intervention programme is designed. Ongoing monitoring and ultimately a timely retest determine the success of the intervention. Common sense dictates that if analytical data are to be collected, they should have a meaningful purpose in influencing programme development. Unfortunately, common practice is to incorporate testing (including movement screens) without using the data for meaningful purpose. This practice is a waste of the athlete's time and the programme resources. Most athletes, at all levels, willingly participate in testing batteries, providing it is clear how, when and why the gathered data will be used.

For a test to be valid, it must measure what it purports to measure. For example, the in-line lunge has potential to reveal asymmetry between the left and right sides of the body in a fundamental movement pattern. The in-line component of the movement (figure 6.3) establishes a narrow base of support, challenging balance through a full (maybe even extreme) movement range that requires mobility. With contralateral hips in extension and flexion, the action also requires the athlete to maintain pelvic stability and therefore trunk alignment.

The athlete holds a broomstick or dowel rod across the back of the shoulders on the shelf made by retracting the shoulder blades (figure 6.3a). The hands hold the stick in an overhand grip slightly wider than shoulder-width. A line of tape is placed on the floor between the athlete's legs. The athlete's feet are spaced so that the heel of the front leg remains flat on the floor and the knee of the rear leg touches the heel of the front foot (figure 6.3b). The toes of the back leg remain on the tape. The athlete should be able to extend and flex the hips and knees repeatedly without moving the feet and while maintaining balance (i.e., the shoulders remain level) and holding the trunk upright.

The first role of an athletic development practitioner is to be a movement coach. Therefore, an athlete's quality of movement should be assessed. But if an athlete performs an in-line lunge sequence in training with the dowel placed in a different position[3] (for example, held so that it runs vertically along the spine; figure 6.4), the outcome of the movement, and therefore the potential observations and interpretations, may be different. In this context, movement may be limited by shoulder or thoracic spine mobility rather than hip and lower-limb mobility or control. The point of this illustration is to show that for a test or observation to be valid, it must test what it is designed to get rather than be limited by a conflicting or mitigating factor.

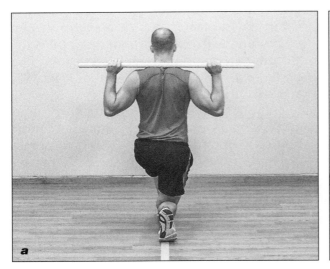
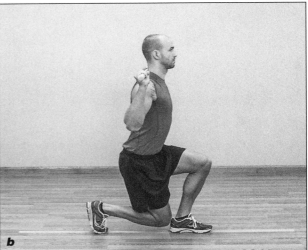

**Figure 6.3**   In-line lunge with stick across back of shoulders: *(a)* starting position, back view; *(b)* lunge position, side view.

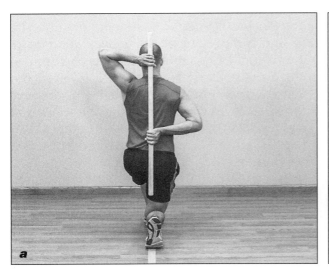
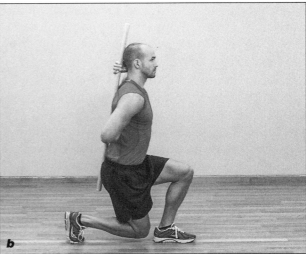

**Figure 6.4**   In-line lunge with a potentially conflicting protocol: *(a)* starting position, back view; *(b)* lunge position, side view.

Similarly, the observation should be valid for the population that the practitioner is working with. Although it can be argued that exercises within a battery designed to assess functional movement should be generic (i.e., nonspecific for all sports), certain athletic populations will not be able to perform some commonly proposed tests. For example, a commonly used test of static shoulder flexibility requires an athlete to hold a dowel behind the back with an overhand grip with one hand high and one hand low (figure 6.5); the distance between the hands represents the range of mobility (the smaller the distance, the greater the shoulder mobility).

Such a test assesses the athlete's shoulder mobility, but the validity of such a test without assessing stability at the same time is questionable in terms of functionality. A joint that has mobility without stability is prone to injury, especially when forces are high, such as in catching, throwing or pulling movements. Conversely, when an athlete has stability without mobility, movement restrictions in some planes can occur. How important is this to all athletic populations? Interestingly, once the test is conducted without the dowel, then it can be argued that motor control is being assessed, which may present a slightly different assessment of the available shoulder range of movement.

For example, in contact sports such as rugby and football, athletes have tremendous stability (strength and control) as well as muscular bulk around the shoulder joints as a protective mechanism against impact forces (in excess of 15 times body weight) that go through the joints. Ranges of movement beyond 50 degrees for internal rotation and 90 to 100 degrees for internal rotation are not required for these athletes, although movement restrictions within these ranges have been shown to increase the chances that the athletes will sustain shoulder injuries.[3] Such ranges of movement can be assessed by accepted mobility and stability tests if they are a specific consideration for the athlete in question. The counterargument is that any athlete must have the appropriate balance of stability (strength and control) and mobility (range of movement) and that that this consideration isn't necessarily sport specific.

# Key Principles of Assessing Posture

When considering the tests available, the practitioner needs to be able to determine the principles that underpin the developed test battery. A practitioner who understands the *what* and the *why* of the assessment methodology will be able to incorporate or adapt it to the requirements of the respective programme.

Leading sport physiotherapist Andrew McDonough[4] consistently advocates the importance of analysing gross static posture as the basis for any decision-making process. Using the reference markers for sound posture as described in chapter 5, the practitioner can record his or her observations about the athlete's standing posture (figure 6.6).[5] The implications of conditions such as kyphosis or lordosis for effective movement mechanics have been clearly identified and the implications described.

The practitioner should be looking for symmetry between the left and right sides of the body. To identify symmetry, he or she should look at the key anatomical markers of the shoulder, hip and knee, which should be level in standing. Some aspects of balance are

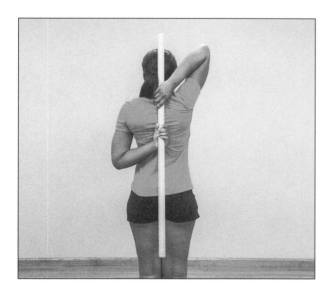

**Figure 6.5** Static shoulder flexibility test.

**Posture**

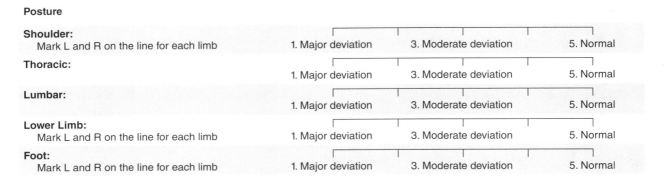

| | | | |
|---|---|---|---|
| **Shoulder:** Mark L and R on the line for each limb | 1. Major deviation | 3. Moderate deviation | 5. Normal |
| **Thoracic:** | 1. Major deviation | 3. Moderate deviation | 5. Normal |
| **Lumbar:** | 1. Major deviation | 3. Moderate deviation | 5. Normal |
| **Lower Limb:** Mark L and R on the line for each limb | 1. Major deviation | 3. Moderate deviation | 5. Normal |
| **Foot:** Mark L and R on the line for each limb | 1. Major deviation | 3. Moderate deviation | 5. Normal |

**Figure 6.6** Checklist for standing posture.

more subtle. For example, although observing someone leaning weight on to one leg may be easy, the distribution of weight between both feet (or indeed through the whole foot) may not be so easy to observe.

Using the reference markers for sound posture described in chapter 5, the practitioner can record observations about the athlete's standing posture. This simple process is based on the known relationship between increased lumbar lordosis and lower-limb injury in dynamic movements.[1]

Postural assessment photos (figure 6.7) are a common tool for evaluating and recording an athlete's standing posture. Taken from the front, rear and both sides, the change in an athlete's physique and standing posture can be easily assessed using pictures that form a permanent record of the athlete's progress or regression.

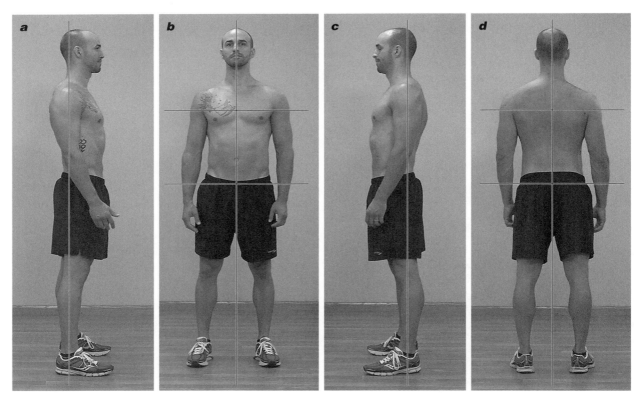

**Figure 6.7** Postural assessment photos provide a means of recording an athlete's standing posture: *(a)* right side; *(b)* front; *(c)* left side; *(d)* back.

The athlete should ideally be barefoot for this assessment so that the practitioner can gain a better understanding of whether the athlete is comfortable balancing on the foot and distributing weight evenly or whether the athlete needs to use strategies (probably subconsciously) such as redistributing the weight through the foot or clawing the big toe to maintain an upright position. Such compensation strategies will cause the medial arch of the foot to collapse as the foot rolls inwards and is indicative of poor proprioception or motor control.

One easy trick indicative of the weight distribution in standing is the ability of the athlete to have a big toe lifted by a practitioner. The toe should come off the floor easily when lifted and moved through range in standing without undue resistance. A stiff big toe is associated with a range of lower limb pathologies relating to the Achilles tendon, tibialis posterior tendinopathy and shin splints, because of its influence on running and walking mechanics.

Because the knee has only a small range of rotation (approximately 15 degrees), any inward (valgus) or outward (varus) movement of the knee in a single leg is an indicator of potential control problems at either end of the lower limb. Excessive lateral knee movement may be associated with poor gluteal strength, especially if the hips can be seen to tip away from the standing leg, or poor ankle proprioceptive control if the athlete performs a lot of adjustment movement at the ankle in attempting to maintain the static position.

# Dynamic Posture Assessment

Although static postural assessment is useful, dynamic (moving) postural assessments are generally considered more reliable, especially in terms of predicting injury, than static postural assessment because dynamic assessments incorporate multiple variables such as strength and proprioception within movement contexts. These qualities underpin all movement skills, and deficiencies in these qualities are associated with movement inefficiencies, dysfunctions and most common injury pathologies.

The first thing to observe is the athlete's walking stride. Podiatrists with specialist equipment can assess specific aspects of foot mechanics throughout the walking gait to see whether the athlete overpronates (excessively rolls the foot outwards) or supinates (excessively rolls the foot inwards) during the normal walking stride.

One aspect of movement that doesn't require any specialist diagnostic tools is hip positioning throughout the stride; simple observation is sufficient. The hips should remain level as the athlete transfers weight from one foot to the other. A Trendelenburg gait (figure 6.8a) occurs when, in the stance phase of walking, weak abductor muscles (gluteus medius, gluteus minimus) allow the pelvis to tilt down on the opposite side. To balance this tilt, the trunk lurches to the weakened side in an attempt to maintain a level pelvis throughout the gait cycle. A similar compensatory motion can be seen within a coxalgic gait (figure 6.8b), in which the athlete shifts the trunk excessively towards the standing leg without the associated contralateral hip drop.

A simple body-weight squat (figure 6.9) can tell a practitioner a lot about the athlete's dynamic posture control through a full movement range. The coaching progressions towards this important strength exercise are discussed in chapter 10, but in terms of assessing postural control, much can be learned from analysing this fundamental movement.

Throughout the movement, the athlete should maintain the natural lumbar curve. The correct curve should be evident at the bottom position; the chest is pointing upwards, and no hinging should occur at the lumbosacral or lumbothoracic junctions (figure 6.9a). Essentially, the pelvis controls the amount of curve in the lumbar spine (lower back). When the pelvis tips too far in an anterior direction, the arch in the lower back increases significantly (figure 6.9b). More common is a posterior pelvic tilt (often observed as a tucking under in the squat), in which the lumbar curve disappears (figure 6.9c).

In training, the depth of the squat is important. At some point after the hip drops below the level of the knee (the rationale for this depth of movement as a marker is presented

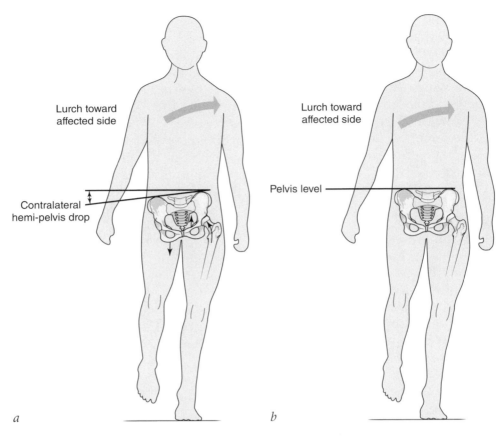

Figure 6.8 Gait assessment: *(a)* Trendelenburg and *(b)* coxalgic gait patterns are the result of weakness in the hip abductors.

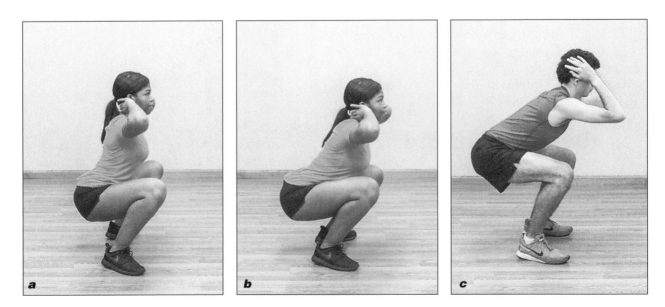

Figure 6.9 Bodyweight squat: *(a)* natural lumbar curve; *(b)* anterior pelvic tilt; *(c)* posterior pelvic tilt.

in chapter 10), maintaining the desired lumbar curve throughout the descent becomes exponentially more difficult. Therefore, the typically described butt-to-floor movement often prescribed for a squat may not be realistic for any but the most flexible athletes. Consequently, movement range is determined by the athlete's ability to maintain normal lumbar lordosis through the squat. The desired or acceptable minimum range is determined by the line of the femur (demarked by the centre of the hip and knee joints) breaking parallel.

Progressive and repetitive anterior or posterior pelvic tilt as the athlete ascends and descends during the movement may cause compressive actions on the intervertebral discs. The resultant compressive and shear forces increase the risks of a herniation in the disc.

In an athlete with no associated pathology for lumbar dysfunction, the athlete may tuck under for four reasons (a posterior pelvic tilt at the base of the squat is more common):

1. The hamstrings may be shortened or tight. As the athlete nears the bottom of the squat, the hamstrings stretch. If hamstring mobility is limited, the insertions of the hamstrings on the tuberosity of the ischium (pelvic bone) will cause the pelvis to tilt posteriorly.

2. If the athlete is unable to initiate the movement with a coordinated and simultaneous flexion of the hips and knees, the pelvis often anteriorly rotates, elongating the hamstrings at the start of the movement. Often this is mistakenly taught as a deliberate action. The result is that the hamstrings become more stretched through the descent and therefore have no elastic capacity as the hips near the bottom position, resulting in a posterior pelvic tilt.

3. The athlete may not be activating the gluteal muscles or maintaining the braced activation of the trunk muscles through the exercise. Coaching to maintain the activation in the back muscles and the abdominal brace will aid this, as will pushing outwards through the heels.

4. Sometimes, especially in novice athletes, the kinaesthetic mechanisms within the muscles are not sufficiently trained to the correct motor patterning of the movement, and the athlete is not aware that he or she is adopting a maladaptive position. Simply increasing the athlete's awareness prevents the athlete from learning a compromised movement pattern. The coach should ensure that the athlete can tilt the pelvis and distinguish between hip and lumbar spine actions in an unloaded situation before correcting this during the squat.

The athlete's knees should track along the line of the second toe. A common fault seen during the descent phase of the movement is that the athlete brings the knees inwards into a valgus position, which significantly increases the risk of collapsing inwards and injuring the knee ligaments. This inwards movement of the knees may indicate a weakness in the hip abductors. Alternatively, the athlete may be exerting pressure through the inside of the foot (the instep) rather than through the entire foot. If this is a motor control issue, strategies to overcome this problem include actively encouraging the athlete to push the knees outwards during the descent and reinforcing a 'rip the heels sideways' action (increased gluteal action encourages external rotation of the hip). Specific remedial gluteal strengthening exercises are introduced later in this chapter.

At the base of the movement the weight should be distributed towards the heels so that the foot remains flat on the floor; the weight moves towards the heels from the midfoot as the athlete descends. The relationship between foot position and weight distribution is important. If the athlete's centre of mass remains directly above the midpoint of the foot (facilitated by an upright trunk position), weight distribution through the foot will be correct. But if the trunk leans forward either through excessive hip flexion or thoracic flexion during the descent or in the bottom position, the weight will be distributed towards the front of the foot. This forward lean often causes the athlete's heels to leave the floor at the base of the squat (i.e., heel raise is the symptom; trunk lean is the cause).

Understanding an athlete's anatomy is paramount in analysing squatting movement. Remember that this is exactly what movement analysis or screening is about—understanding what the athlete does in key movements and why so that corrections or reinforcements can be planned and delivered.

Although the focus of the movement analysis is on the actions of the hip, knee and ankle in the sagittal plane, the hip movement in the transverse plane is also important during the squat. Using the lateral rotator muscles of the hip (piriformis, gemellus superior, obturator internus, gemellus inferior, quadratus femoris, obturator externus and the lower fibres of the gluteus maximus), the athlete can rotate the femur at the articulation with the pelvis. This rotation allows the hips to move forwards slightly, which moves the centre of mass back within the base of support, allowing the athlete to maintain a stable and balanced position. This action can be prompted by asking the athlete to push out sideways through the heels whilst descending through the squat. This prompt is also useful in correcting an athlete who demonstrates a knee valgus (inward rotation of the femur) during movement descent.

Using a scoring system such as the one used for the squat encourages two things. First, the checklist (figure 6.10) provides the practitioner with a series of technical points to guide the observation process during the movement. A scoring system is especially important when the practitioner is developing experience in movement observation. The sliding scale also enables the practitioner to record what is wrong with the movement, providing a basis for

constructive and corrective intervention and a permanent record that, in review, will enable the recording of technical progression. The extent to which the identified movement may be problematic can also be determined using this method. For example, if the athlete displays a slight anterior pelvic tilt during descent, the mark on the scale may be closer to the midline than if the athlete has a pronounced anterior pelvic tilt, in which case the mark on the scale will be further to the left end of the scale.

Looking at the interaction between the technique variables as well as each point in isolation is important. For example, if the athlete is able to move the hip below parallel only with an anterior pelvic tilt or forward trunk lean, this issue should be identified by cross-reference to the information recorded on the scales. The practitioner would observe the athlete move until, for example, the athlete could not maintain a neutral pelvic position (normal lumbar curvature), and then record the depth at which this occurs.

Some criticize such sliding scales as being subjective rather than quantitative. But even movement screening tests that record numbers often rely on the practitioner's ability to make qualitative assessments of the movement and then attribute numbers to the observation. This practice is arguably no less subjective and provides little in the way of a permanent record of exactly what the observations were.

Some movement assessment screens use a sliding scale of major problem or deviation,

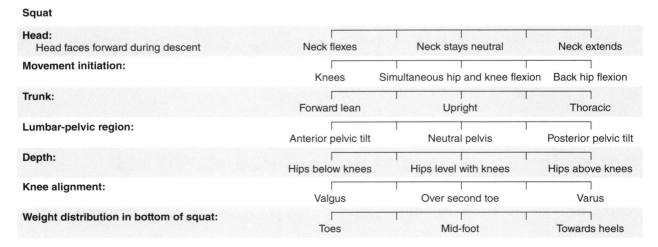

**Squat**

| | | | |
|---|---|---|---|
| **Head:** Head faces forward during descent | Neck flexes | Neck stays neutral | Neck extends |
| **Movement initiation:** | Knees | Simultaneous hip and knee flexion | Back hip flexion |
| **Trunk:** | Forward lean | Upright | Thoracic |
| **Lumbar-pelvic region:** | Anterior pelvic tilt | Neutral pelvis | Posterior pelvic tilt |
| **Depth:** | Hips below knees | Hips level with knees | Hips above knees |
| **Knee alignment:** | Valgus | Over second toe | Varus |
| **Weight distribution in bottom of squat:** | Toes | Mid-foot | Towards heels |

**Figure 6.10** Checklist for squat.

minor problem or deviation and normal or no problem. This scale enables the practitioner to record observations in relation to his or her perception of how problematic an observed movement dysfunction appears to be. For example, studies have found that tennis players had on average 43.8 degrees of internal rotation and 89.1 degrees of external rotation on the racket arm compared with 60.8 degrees of internal rotation and 81.2 degrees of external rotation on the nondominant hand as a function of their play and practices.[6] Unsurprisingly, similar asymmetrical patterns have been found in other activities such as baseball pitching.[7] In elite rugby players, limited internal ranges of movement (less than 60 degrees) have been linked to increased risk of shoulder injuries, as has reduced eccentric strength in internal rotation activities.[4]

Scoring systems based on deterministic analyses of each symptom of a movement dysfunction (such as the one used for the squat) are highly preferable to systems that allocate a single numerical score to an exercise within a screening battery. For example, Cook[3] suggests five conditions for the in-line lunge movement that must be met if the exercise is to score 5/5:

- The feet must remain in contact with the taped line on the floor.
- The heel of the front foot must remain in contact with the floor.
- The back knee touches the floor immediately behind the front knee.
- The trunk does not flex forward at the hip or thoracic spine.
- Balance is maintained (the dowel does not dip).

One point is lost for every one of the conditions that is not met. Note, however, that for this scoring to be informative to programme development, it has to be accompanied by an observational record noting what caused the score. For example, let's imagine that the athlete's feet move off the tape as he or she loses balance when the heels come off the floor, which in all probability will also cause the dowel to tip (so the score is 2). If only the numbers are recorded without any observational notes, the score may prompt an intervention of balance training and lower-limb mobility work. Subsequent retesting may score a 3 if the athlete's heels come off the floor as the trunk flexes forward and the centre of mass moves forward. The score looks to have improved slightly over time and the symptoms of movement dysfunction are similar, yet the causes in each instant are considerably different. A change in score can indicate progress in overall athletic development, but it doesn't necessarily identify a change in the athlete's mechanical control.

Although less common than practitioners realize, another reason for the athlete's heels coming off the floor in this position is poor ankle mobility, which would be highlighted by a targeted follow-up test. This circumstance is another reason to use generic screening tools, because they often highlight areas of postural deficiency that require further investigation through more specific tests that may either quantify or rule in or out the need for specific interventions. For example, a simple follow-up test can identify whether reduced ankle mobility is what causes the athlete to lose position in the lunge. As figure 6.11 shows, if the athlete puts a foot onto a raised step (20

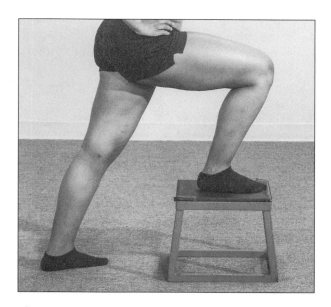

**Figure 6.11** Ankle mobility test. The athlete places a foot on a raised step and pushes the knee forward over the toe. If the knee can move in front of the toes while the weight remains through the athlete's heel, the athlete's ankle mobility typically will not limit squatting actions.

to 40 centimetres), keeps the foot flat and can push the knee forward of the toes whilst maintaining heel contact with the flat surface, ankle mobility isn't a primary focus for intervention.

But if the athlete cannot do this without the heel coming off the step, ankle mobility cannot be ruled out as a specific consideration. A further follow-up test typically is required. A common means of measuring ankle joint complex flexibility is the knee-to-wall distance test.

The knee-to-wall distance test is quick and easy to set up and use as a regular monitoring tool for athletes. Place a ruler or measuring stick on the floor, with 0 centimetres at the wall. With shoes off, the athlete stands with the foot flat against the floor and the heel touching the ground. The knee stays in contact with the wall, hip–knee alignment is maintained, and the knee tracks over the second toe. The athlete gradually slides the foot backwards until the heel can no longer maintain contact with the floor whilst maintaining knee contact with the wall (figure 6.12). At this point, the distance of the big toe from the wall is recorded. Published ranges suggest that 6 to 10 centimetres is normal, but there is little to support this as a functional requirement. What is probably more important than distance is symmetry between the left and right legs.

The single-leg squat (figure 6.13) is a useful follow-up exercise to the body-weight squat,

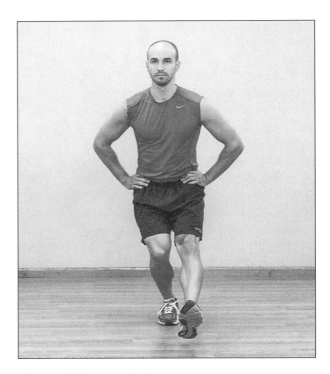

**Figure 6.13**    Single-leg squat.

because it illustrates single-limb strength in the squatting movement. The observation points remain similar to those for the normal squat. The narrowed base of support, which is offset from the athlete's centre of mass, increases the emphasis on maintaining a level hip position as the athlete descends.

During the downwards movements, the athlete should maintain the hip, knee and second-toe alignment and spinal alignment and not drop into anterior pelvic tilt or lumbar spine extension. The standing foot should be balanced, and no overpronation or excessive eversion should occur throughout the movement.

The movement should be fluid; the athlete must maintain good control throughout. As identified in chapter 4, off-centred forces cause rotations throughout a system mass. These forces need to be countered by the actions of the gluteus medius and minimus at the hip and the external obliques in the trunk to maintain a level pelvis and hip, and alignment of the knee and second toe. Similarly, the shoulders need to remain level. Rotations in the transverse plane at the shoulder (figure 6.14*a*) are symptomatic of rotations in the trunk, which

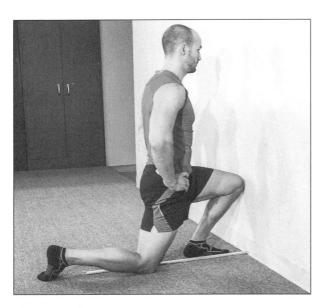

**Figure 6.12**    Knee-to-wall distance test.

the athlete may employ to counter rotations in the hip or lower limb and simultaneously maintain a balanced position. Valgus movements at the knee may also be seen if the athlete attempts to counter rotations through lower-limb rotations.

The practitioner should look at hip–knee alignment; hips and shoulders should be level and not rotated through the transverse plane. When the athlete can no longer maintain the correct alignment or movement control, the practitioner should record the depth of the movement and note observations of compensations. The line of the femur provides a good marker for recording this depth. If it is at 0 degrees in standing, then ranges of 60, 90, 120 or more degrees provide sound markers for evaluation of depth.

Also of interest is the movement strategy that the athlete adopts to maintain balance in this athletic skill. With a single (and narrow) contact point with the floor, the base of support is small and slightly off-centred. To maintain balance, the athlete must move so that the centre of mass remains above the base of support. Performing this action with a knee-first movement will cause the ankle to dorsiflex excessively and the knee to come in front of the toes (figure 6.14b). Ultimately, ankle flexibility

will limit the movement, not because the ankle is inflexible (as described previously) but because of the movement strategy adopted by the athlete. Similarly, an athlete who tries this 'knee dip' exercise by leading the movement with a rearward movement of the hips will quickly move the centre of mass posteriorly to the base of support. The trunk will then have to lean forward to redress the balance, either through greater flexion of the hip or by rounding the shoulders and flexing the thoracic spine. These compensations also may be evident in the normal squatting movement as a strategy to maintain balance.

One of the key functions of recording such movement compensations in an athlete is to inform the coaching strategy. Often, the anatomical limitations within the kinesiological chain do not limit actions; instead, the athlete does not understand how these actions should be performed. In my last professional rugby league club, in a screening process for more than 35 professional players at first-grade level, only 2 had genuine anatomical restrictions to flexion at the hip and only 1 had an anatomical restriction at the shoulder. Excellent coaches understand this indicator and adopt their movement development strategies to guide the athlete into ever more appropriate movement

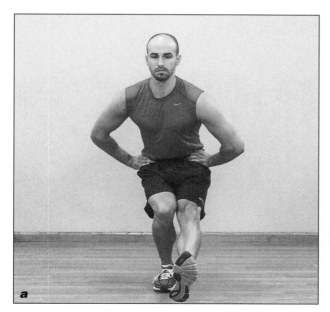 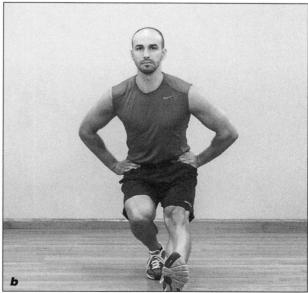

**Figure 6.14**    Common movement errors in the single-leg squat: *(a)* rotation of the shoulders in the transverse plane; *(b)* poor midsection control and associated lower-limb malalignment.

sequences. Such observation notes form the basis not just for identifying movement limitations or compensations but also for guiding the teaching strategy. This approach is not possible if the screening tool only identifies scores such as depth of movement.

As will be emphasized in chapter 9, the ability to maintain hip, knee and foot alignment (with the knee tracking along the line of the second toe) in landing actions is crucial in an athlete, especially when braking actions or multidirectional movements are central components of sport performance. For this reason, observing double- and single-leg landing movements from simple positions such as stepping off a box provides the practitioner important information about the athlete's potential robustness (i.e., injury avoidance) in these movement contexts.

Drop jump, or step down, landings can be observed from boxes that are 20 to 40 centimetres high. The athlete should be encouraged to step off a stable box or platform (figure 6.15a); actively jumping increases the vertical displacement of the centre of mass and therefore the ground reaction force on landing. The athlete should attempt a flat-foot landing that is stable

and quiet (figure 6.15b). The practitioner looks for the trunk to remain upright and stable on landing, and the hips to be square and level (i.e., one side shouldn't dip). Alignment of the hip, knee and ankle is crucial, and the knee and hip should not sink or absorb force. The athlete should be coached to stick the landing in a solid and stable position that does not change after ground contact.

As a teaching point, to facilitate a flat-footed landing, the athlete should be encouraged to pull the toes of the leading leg up towards the knee so that there is plantargrade dorsiflexion at the ankle (i.e., the flat foot is parallel to the floor) as the athlete steps forward.

After the athlete can consistently control his or her posture in a two-footed landing, the movement can be progressed to a single-foot landing (figure 6.16). Reducing the base of support makes this task much more difficult than the double-foot landing. Careful consideration should be given to the height from which the athlete steps. Depending on the competency of the athlete, reductions of 50 per cent in drop height, or a drop height of 10 to 20 centimetres in the first instance, might be considered for this action. The narrowed base of support also

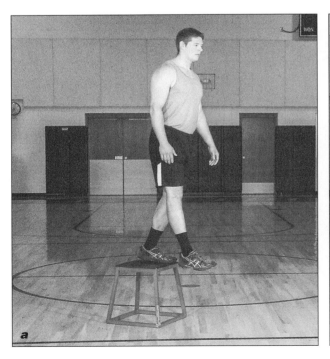
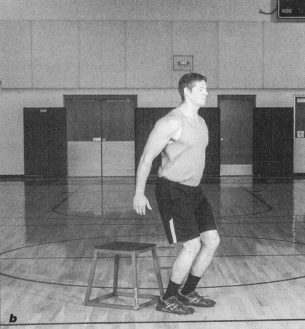

**Figure 6.15** Drop jump with a double-foot landing: *(a)* starting position; *(b)* stable flat-foot landing.

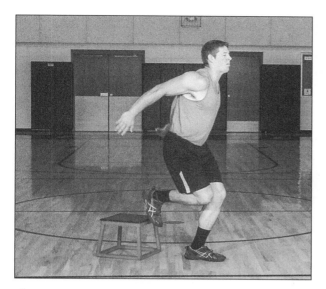

**Figure 6.16**  Drop jump with a single-foot landing.

makes it exponentially more difficult to control the hip alignment in the transverse plane (i.e., to keep the hips level), so this activity typically highlights a weakness in the gluteus medius or minimus muscles. Medial or valgus movements of the knee are a particularly strong indicator of this weakness.

This screening activity might be especially important in female athletes during or immediately after peak height velocity, because the typically increased Q-angle leads to potential for increased medial forces at the knee on landing. This alteration in the body's anatomical structure also predisposes the female athlete to the potential for asynchronous firing of the hamstrings and quadriceps muscles, a predisposition to knee instability in high-speed or high-force actions.

To gain a more complete analysis of a player's movement capabilities, screening movements should incorporate highly dynamic activities that replicate an increased physio-mechanical demand beyond what can be induced by ground-based exercises (i.e., a foot is in contact with the floor at all times). Dynamic screens test a range of athletic qualities that influence strength, skill execution and the predisposition or vulnerability to injury. This single factor significantly increases the validity of this type of screening over slower or static screening methods.

As an exercise in lower-body muscular power, the repeated tuck jump has been proposed as a qualitative test that can be used to assess the neuromuscular techniques of athletes in jumping and landing techniques.[8] The athlete starts in a standing position with the feet hip-width apart to enable optimal vertical force generation. The jumping movement is initiated with a rapid countermovement action (flexion of the hips, knees and ankles, and arms extended behind the athlete; figure 6.17a) that precedes a maximal vertical jump. As the athlete jumps, he or she reaches the arms as high (forward) as possible and brings the knees as high as possible after the feet leave the floor (figure 6.17b). The intention of the jump is for the thighs to be parallel to the ground as the centre of mass reaches its highest vertical point. Figure 6.18 is a checklist for evaluating the repeated tuck jump.

The athlete lands with an active flat foot and the knees tracking along the line of the second toe. Weight is distributed through the midfoot on landing. As soon as the athlete lands, he or she begins the next tuck jump, up to a maximum of 10 in sequence. The jumps should be vertical, with no (or minimal) horizontal trajectory. If at any point the athlete cannot control the landing posture, the practitioner should stop the athlete from repeating the movement.

The introduction of an external obstacle, such as a hurdle for the athlete to jump forward or laterally over, may provide an additional movement challenge to the athlete in terms of take-off, flight trajectory and therefore control of the subsequent landing. A small hurdle, up to 40 centimetres high, can be used. The hurdle requires the athlete to control the landing after a jump that has both horizontal and vertical quantities of force. The athlete must jump (using a double-footed take-off; figure 6.19) or hop (using a single-leg take-off; figure 6.20) over the hurdle from a set distance away and stick the landing in a balanced and controlled manner.

The distance of take-off needs to be proportional to the hurdle height and the athlete's capacities. The key observations are not necessarily about the height jumped or distance

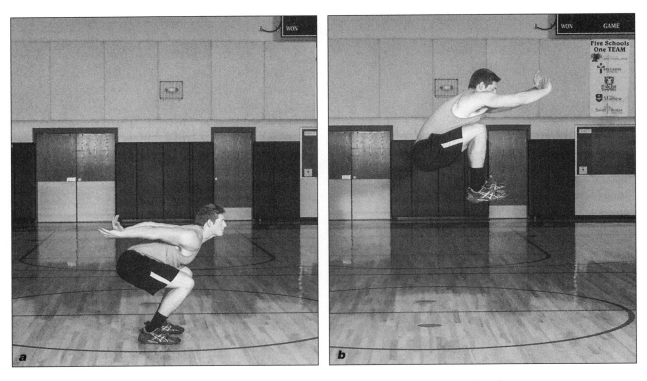

**Figure 6.17** Repeated tuck jump: *(a)* countermovement action; *(b)* jump and tuck.

**Repeated tuck jump**

| | | | |
|---|---|---|---|
| **Knee position at landing:** | Valgus | In line | Varus |
| **Timing of foot contact:** | Left foot first | Simultaneous landing | Right foot first |
| **Quality of foot contact:** | Too quick | Optimal | Slow and heavy |
| **Foot contact:** | Forefoot landing | Active flat foot | Heel contact |
| **Stance at landing:** | Narrow | Hip-width | Wide |
| **Level of feet at landing:** | Left foot forward | Level | Right foot forward |
| **Level of thighs in flight:** | Left leg higher | Level | Right leg higher |
| **Thighs at apex:** | Don't make parallel | Parallel | Break parallel |
| **Arm action:** | Left arm rises first or higher | Level | Right arm rises first or higher |
| **Arm trajectory:** | Range inadequate | Range maximal height at apex of jump | Range excessive |
| **Movement endurance:** 10 jumps | Quality deteriorates | Quality maintained | Quality improves |

**Figure 6.18** Checklist for repeated tuck jump.

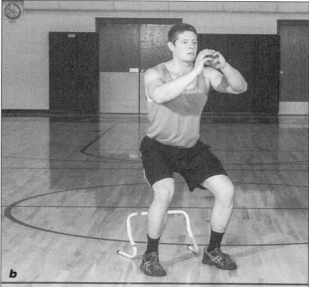
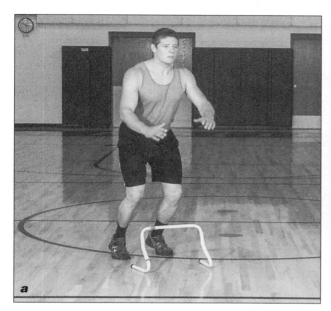

**Figure 6.19**    Hurdle jump (double-leg): *(a)* take-off; *(b)* landing.

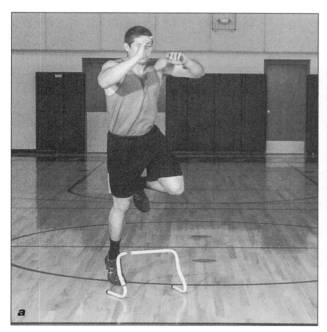
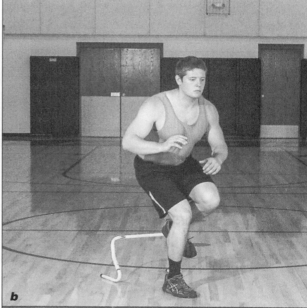

**Figure 6.20**    Hurdle hop and hold (single-leg): *(a)* take-off; *(b)* landing.

travelled, but rather how the athlete executed the jump, especially the landing. The use of a hurdle helps ensure consistency in the required jump height between observations. The observer can then draw conclusions based on like-for-like repetitions with similar take-off, flight and landing demands. The progressions for such jumping tasks are presented in chapter 9.

The transition from landing on two feet to landing on one foot will show any control issues the athlete has more than changing the number of feet used in the take-off.

To ensure that sufficient force is exerted during the single-leg take-off, the athlete should drive the take-off leg into the ground to produce enough power for the thigh (femur) to come to parallel with the floor as it clears the hurdle. An alternative strategy is to adjust the height of the hurdle to ensure that this action happens.

Most sporting actions (certainly those that require the athlete to move the feet) require a range of movements in both the sagittal and transverse planes. Because of the issues identified with postural alignment in, for example, landing and cutting actions, any analysis focused on enhancing the athlete's mechanical control should test take-off and landing from jumps with different emphasis on the ability to control vertical, anteroposterior and mediolateral forces. A simple modification of the hurdle jump or hurdle hop, changing the direction of flight from vertical and forward to vertical and lateral, permits this; movement is lateral rather than in the sagittal (i.e., forward and backward) plane. The same progressive challenges are given to the athlete; he or she is required to jump over the hurdle and stick the landing, but this time the jump is lateral (figures 6.21 and 6.22).

The coach should look for correct hip, knee and ankle alignment throughout take-off and landing. The athlete should have good control of the movement and should not need to overuse the arms or trunk to control rotations and aid the landing. The progressive approach

to analysing competency in controlling lateral landings is also recommended; a double-foot take-off progresses to a single-foot take-off with a double-foot landing. After the athlete demonstrates competence with the single-foot take-off, double-foot landing (figure 6.22b), the progression is to a single-foot take-off, single-foot landing (figure 6.22c).

As a progressive analysis tool that links sequences of maximal hops rather than isolates them as single actions, the triple-hop distance (THD) test (figure 6.23) has been found to be a reliable and valid predictor of lower-limb muscle strength, power and balance,[9] especially if it is modified so that the athlete is asked to maintain landed balance at the end of the THD and timed for stabilization (in seconds). This modification arguably enables the test to be more reliable in predicting balance deficits than static tests. Therefore, the THD should be more useful in predicting postural control and balance deficits.

The test is simple and easy to administer. From a single-leg stance on the starting line, the athlete performs three maximal hops (taking off and landing on the same foot) with the aim of travelling as far as possible. The distance hopped is recorded in metres and the time, in seconds, is taken to reach a stabilized and balanced position on landing after the third

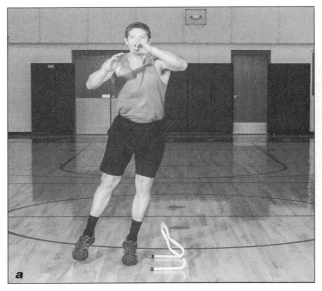
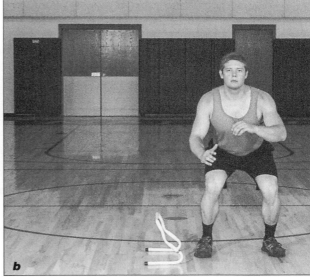

**Figure 6.21** Lateral hurdle jump (double-foot): *(a)* take-off; *(b)* landing.

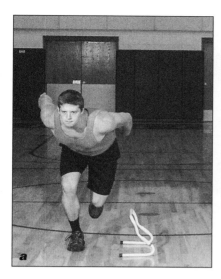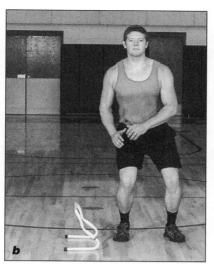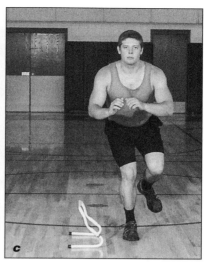

**Figure 6.22**    Lateral hurdle hop (single-foot): *(a)* take-off; *(b)* double-foot landing; *(c)* single-foot landing.

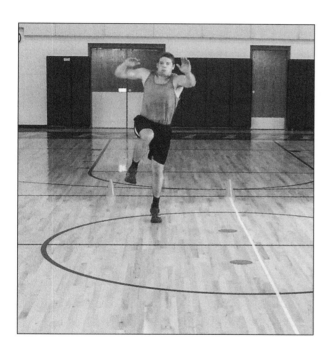

**Figure 6.23**    Triple-hop distance test.

hop (i.e., achieving stability after 1 second is better than needing 3 seconds to achieve a balanced and stable position). The practitioner can use a form such as table 6.1 to record results and comments.

Besides doing the quantitative assessment in terms of distance, the practitioner must also observe the quality of the athlete's movement in this test. For example, a tendency to land with less knee flexion and greater valgus movement at the knee will increase load on the ACL and potentially lead to failure of this structure. If possible, these movements should be recorded and evaluated using video analysis; medial deviation of the landing knee should be scored as normal, mild, moderate or severe abnormality. If kinematic analysis is available, the angle, distance or deviation can be measured quantitatively for more detailed analysis over time to measure improvement following intervention.

**Table 6.1**    Evaluation of the Triple-Hop Distance Test

|  | Distance (cm) | Time to stabilization (seconds) | Observed knee valgus (normal, mild, moderate, severe) | Observed knee flexion (normal, mild, moderate, severe) |
|---|---|---|---|---|
| Triple-hop distance left |  |  |  |  |
| Triple-hop distance right |  |  |  |  |

From C. Brewer, 2017, *Athletic movement skills* (Champaign, IL: Human Kinetics).

Most of the movement observational analysis tasks described in this chapter are based on analysis of the entire kinetic chain and consider multiple joints because most movement skills are ground based and rely on the athlete's ability to control posture. But one specific joint complex worth detailed investigation on its own is the shoulder. The shoulder complex is made up of four joint structures: sternoclavicular, acromioclavicular, glenohumeral and a false joint of scapula–thoracic. The shoulder is pivotal in upper-body sporting movements. Indeed, many actions that involve the shoulder, such as collisions in contact sports, throwing actions and hitting actions, tend to be repetitive, high velocity and high force. Practitioners who work in sports that involve such movements should consider undertaking functional assessment of this complicated structure as part of their athlete needs analysis.

The tests in this chapter offer some easy, quick and relevant opportunities for screening athletes for potential postural and movement dysfunctions that may limit their potential, but these tests are by no means the only ones. For example, there is pervasive argument that screening protocols should include tests that look at the shoulder complex, trunk strength and trunk strength endurance.[10] More important, screening provides recorded notes that can be used to structure training interventions that target areas of necessary improvement.

# Address Areas of Identified Need in an Athlete

Many areas of improvement may be addressed using the movement and strength development progressions discussed in the following chapters. Progressive training that enhances performance is fundamentally similar to training that corrects problems. The difference is one of progression based on where the athlete lies on a continuum between basic and advanced stages.

This chapter identified two areas for remedial work commonly associated with movement skill execution in athletes across a range of sport. These areas are associated with the hip (for example, underactive gluteal recruitment) and the foot and ankle. Corrective exercises can be identified to address dysfunction in these areas, exercises that are simple to add to any programme or perform in any exercise setting.

In exploring these exercises, practitioners will learn concepts of prescription and exercise supervision to enhance their understanding of exercise objectives, including when to use such exercises and why they might be beneficial. One clear principle must be adhered to throughout these exercises: Because athletes can develop movement compensations if form is not corrected, the person supervising the athlete must not tolerate nonoptimal postures or movement sequences during execution of corrective exercises.

Joint positioning determines function. Movements done correctly develop the neuromuscular system. The athlete needs to feel the movement and use sensory and motor nerves to establish so-called muscle memory of how a movement should be executed. Doing the exercises is easy; feeling the movement is conceptually different even though it may look the same! Quality movement is required at all times, a concept that requires commitment from both the athlete and the practitioner. Examples to reinforce this concept are found throughout this book in a variety of concepts or settings.

# Gluteal Activation

In most sporting movements, power is generated through the forceful extension of the hip joint with the pelvis in a neutral position and the lumbar spine maintaining its normal curvature. This action requires activation of the gluteus maximus and synergistic coactions in the gluteus medius and minimus. Often forgotten is that many sporting actions, and therefore training movements, occur in the sagittal plane. Although many total-body movements also occur in the transverse plane, this frequency of action is often not transferred into a training context. Often, this approach leads to inadequate recruitment of the gluteus muscle complex in training actions, leading to underpowered actions and overuse of other muscle groups, such as the quadriceps, hip flexors, quadratus lumborum and tensor fasciae latae in movement compensation.

## Clam

Some practitioners attempt to correct this muscle recruitment problem as a way to correct the observed movement pattern. Clam exercises are often prescribed. For the clam, the athlete lies on his or her side with the knees bent to approximately 90 degrees and the hips at approximately 135 degrees (figure 6.24a). The ankles, knees and hips are together. From this position, the athlete slowly raises and lowers the top knee (figure 6.24b) under direct control of the external rotators in the buttocks (gluteus medius). Athletes should be coached to feel this muscle working.

This basic exercise can be progressed either by adding an external resistance such as a resistance band to the abduction movement in the hip or by increasing the lever arm of the leg being raised by straightening the leg. This progression changes the activity into a lying hip abduction (figure 6.25). In this exercise, the athlete starts on his or her side with the knees fully extended and ankles dorsiflexed (toes pulled up towards the knees). The athlete raises the straight top leg to the end of his or her range.

A sound coaching point to encourage the correct movement is to coach that the 'Heel bone should lead the movement,' or 'Imagine you are trying to pour water out of your toes as your foot gets higher.' This movement ensures that the femur isn't externally rotated as the leg lifts to increase the range of movement possible around the hip. This simple compensation changes the movement from one of hip abduction to one of hip rotation. Because the foot isn't fixed (i.e., in contact with the floor) or resisted, the recruitment pattern changes from being led by the gluteus medius and minimus

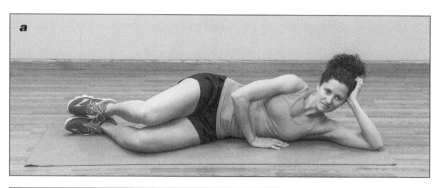

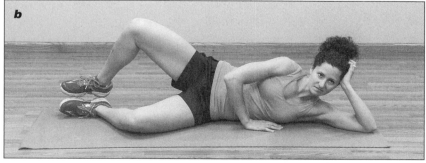

**Figure 6.24**   Clam: *(a)* starting position; *(b)* raise knee.

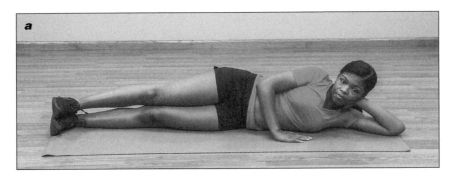

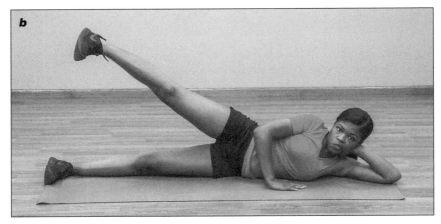

**Figure 6.25**    Lying hip abduction: *(a)* starting position; *(b)* raise leg.

to being dominated by the piriformis, quadratus femoris, internal and external obturators, and superior and inferior gemellus.

## Crab Walk

The clam and lying hip abduction are commonly prescribed remedial exercises, but many practitioners question the rationale of using a lying exercise to recruit muscles instead of training a movement that can develop the same movement recruitment patterns. The question involves the functionality or transfer of training benefits between these two distinct contexts. This issue of exercise functionality is dealt with comprehensively in chapter 10.

The same principles of joint movement and positioning can be applied to a ground base exercise commonly known as the crab walk (figure 6.26). These exercises are commonly performed with a resistance band. This approach is useful, because the resistance can be easily increased (by using a higher-tension resistance band) and it is not accommodating

to the effort. As the range of movement increases, more force is required to overcome the resistance of the load. The athlete can really be tasked with feeling the movement and the action of the muscles.

Crab walks are usually performed in the transverse plane; the athlete is in a two-footed stance, has the knees slightly flexed and is ready to move sideways. The resistance band is looped around the athlete's ankles. A common coaching point is to 'Lead the movement with the ankle bone.' Flexing the knees and hips slightly (figure 6.26a) increases the athlete's stability and the recruitment of the gluteal muscles. From this position, the athlete abducts the lead leg, lifting it slightly and moving it sideways in the intended direction (figure 6.26b). This action requires the gluteus medius and minimus to abduct the femur and move it away from the body. The athlete then adducts the other hip to complete the step in this cyclical action.

Although the crab walk may provide the athlete with a stimulus for recruiting the

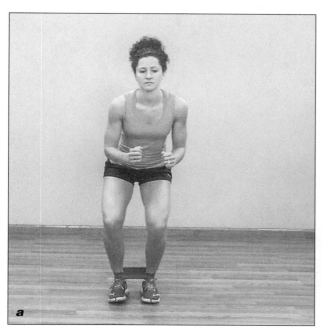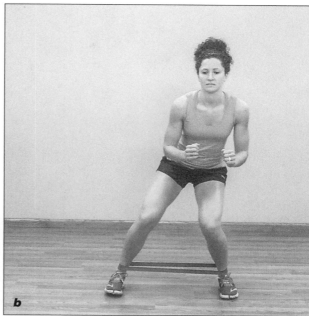

**Figure 6.26**    Crab walk: *(a)* starting position; *(b)* step to the side.

muscles to action, debate continues about whether this exercise is representative of desired sporting movement patterns. Movement direction and efficiency is subject to the laws of Newtonian physics. During a sporting performance, a side step to the left isn't led by the left foot moving sideways; if it were, deceleration would occur. First, there is no lateral push to move the centre of gravity in the desired direction of movement. Second, by leading with the left, the athlete effectively widens the base of support, which increases stability inversely proportional to the movement capacity of the athlete's system.

Therefore, to move to the left (and incorporating Newton's second law of motion), the athlete pushes into the floor with the right foot so that the force vector into the ground moves the centre of mass to the left. The athlete pushes with the inside of the foot as it maintains contact with the floor. As the system begins to move laterally, the athlete pushes outwards with the left leg, leading the movement with the ankle bone so that the left femur adducts at the hip. Because the powerful lateral movement of the right foot overcomes inertia, momentum is transferred to the left leg. Performing the crab walk in this manner is more

dynamic, but to achieve the learning benefit in terms of gluteal recruitment, the elastic resistance around the leg needs to be increased. A practical and constructive teaching progression for an athlete who needs remedial education in the recruitment of the gluteal muscles may be to begin this process with the former version of the exercise (leading with the left to step left). As neuromuscular recruitment becomes more efficient and the athlete learns to recruit the muscles more effectively, the movement can progress to become more forceful and indeed functional (moving to the left by pushing with the right foot).

The crab walk can also be developed to incorporate a sagittal plane movement component (figure 6.27). The athlete moves the leg forwards and sideways as he or she moves forward. The toes point forwards or are turned slightly inwards to maintain the hip abduction focus of the exercise. Otherwise, the moment becomes resisted hip flexion, possibly with accompanying external rotation. Indeed, in sprinting motions, maintaining the hip position is a key function of the gluteus medius and minimus, because they control pelvic rotations on the (unsupported) swing (as explained in chapter 8).

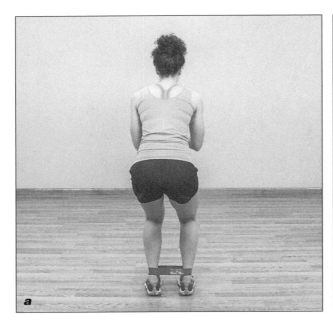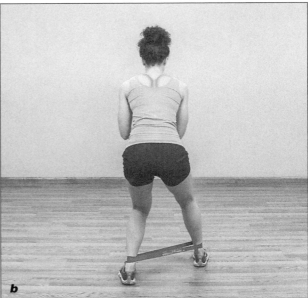

**Figure 6.27**    Crab walk with sagittal plane movement: *(a)* starting position; *(b)* step forwards and sideways.

## Glute Bridge

A number of exercise progressions can be used to develop the hip extensor function of the gluteus maximus. The simplest is the floor-based glute bridge.

The athlete lies on his or her back, with feet hip-width apart and knees bent to 90 degrees (figure 6.28*a*). The easiest form of the exercise begins with the athlete's arms on the floor to improve stability by increasing the surface area in contact with the floor. Exercise difficulty can be increased by raising the arms off the floor. The athlete braces the trunk muscles, squeezes the gluteal muscles together to lift the pelvis from the floor and pushes sideways (laterally) through the heels. With the feet fixed, this sideways push will activate the gluteus medius as a synergist to maintaining the lateral stabilization of the pelvis. The lifting action ceases when the shoulders, hips and knees form a straight line. The athlete maintains the stable top position (figure 6.28*b*) for 10 to 15 seconds, releases the position and repeats.

Athletes who feel pain or acute discomfort in their hamstrings or lower back during this movement typically are not using the gluteal muscles to facilitate hip extension. The movement and verbal cues for the initiation of this action are important. If the athlete focuses on the outcome, that is, the raising of the pelvis, the resultant action is often one of lumbar

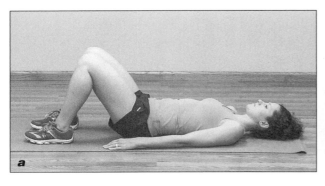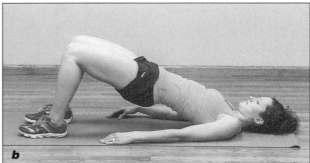

**Figure 6.28**    Glute bridge: *(a)* starting position; *(b)* hip lift.

spine hyperextension, a completely different movement outcome. The athlete needs to be coached to initiate the action from the buttocks.

Many seek to progress this exercise by adding an external resistance such as a barbell or weight disc laid across the hips. The added weight might increase the force requirement from the hip extensors, but that would be the only additional quality provided. A more appropriate progression is towards a single-leg glute bridge (figure 6.29). The movement is similar to the double-leg movement, and the athlete can perform it with the arms on the floor or in the air, depending on competency. This progression is real in terms of motor control. First, the load is effectively doubled because the same body mass now must be lifted by one leg only. More appropriately, because the base of support is reduced and is effectively off centre to the centre of mass, the athlete has to recruit the gluteus medius and minimus as well as the bracing muscles in the trunk to keep the pelvis level as the hips extend. Failure to do so will result in the unsupported hip dropping as extension occurs.

Practitioners can make the single-leg glute bridge easier or harder by altering the amount of hip and knee flexion in the unsupported leg. A shorter lever arm relative to the fulcrum or pivot (a bent unsupported leg) requires less force to move than a longer lever (an extended unsupported leg).

## High-Box Step-Up

Following the principle of transference of exercise benefits to training, the benefits of the glute bridge can be transferred to a standing action through single-leg actions such as a high-box step-up and single-leg squat.

The key to executing a high-box step-up is choosing the correct box height. To ensure that the gluteus maximus is the prime mover, the hip must be well below the knee in the starting position (figure 6.30a). If the box is too low, the athlete will execute the step-up through a quadriceps-dominated movement pattern in which hamstring activation also plays a large part in extending the hip. A very high box will position the joints so that knee flexion cannot lead the movement.

The athlete places the support leg on the box so that the whole foot is flat on the surface and the heel is in contact. The athlete's trailing leg must not initiate the movement. In such a mechanically disadvantaged position, the tendency is for the athlete to perform the step-up with an explosive contraction of the calf muscles in the trailing leg, which would plantarflex the ankle and drive the athlete upwards. By starting with the ankle of the trail leg already plantarflexed (i.e., starting on the toes of the trailing leg), the athlete cannot use this action.

The athlete initiates upward movement by forcefully pushing down through the heel of

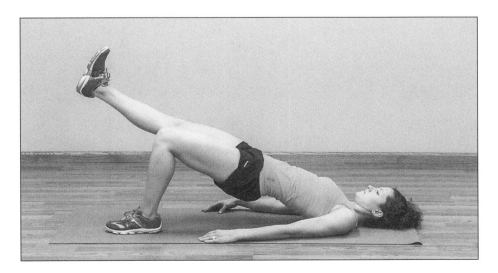

**Figure 6.29**  Single-leg glute bridge.

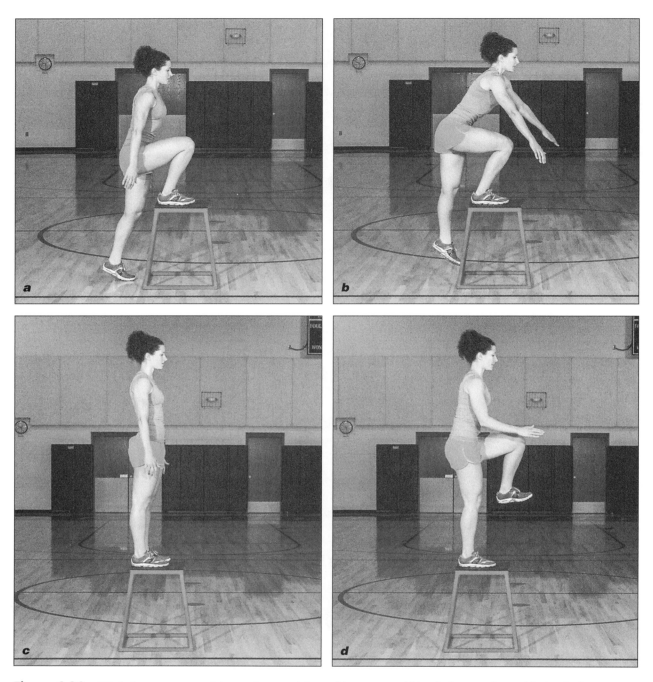

**Figure 6.30**   High-box step-up: *(a)* starting position; *(b)* step-up; *(c)* both feet on box; *(d)* single-leg stance with trailing leg in front of body.

the support leg to generate enough force to extend the hip (figure 6.30*b*). In this mechanically disadvantageous position, the athlete must create forceful contraction of the gluteal muscle complex. Watch for the athlete who is trying to bend the back knee and load it to initiate the upward drive. Stronger athletes

who do this should try starting the movement with the toes of the back foot pulled up towards the knee, which remains straight. The heel is in contact with the ground, which makes it exceptionally difficult for the athlete to load the back leg to begin the vertical movement. At all times the trunk should be kept upright.

A common compensation is for the athlete to lean forward at the trunk, causing forward movement as the centre of mass moves anterior to the base of support. Also pay attention to the lumbar spine, especially during the lowering phases. Ensure that the athlete maintains the normal curvature in the lumbar spine.

The movement continues until the athlete is fully upright, with either both feet on the box (figure 6.30c) or in a single-leg stance with the trailing leg flexed at the hip in front of the body (figure 6.30d). The single-leg stance is a more unstable position because of the reduced base of support; the gluteus medius must be active to keep the hip level. Further means of increasing the difficulty of this movement are explored later, the principles of which can be easily applied to this or any other exercise challenge. Performing two or three sets of 10 repetitions on each leg and allowing for recovery between sets on each leg should be adequate to ensure progression.

## Single-Leg Squat

The single-leg squat has a number of variations that can be used, depending on the required outcome and the athlete's movement competency.

Lateral single-leg squats (figure 6.31) target both the hip extensor function of the gluteus maximus and the key role that the gluteus medius and minimus play in athletic movements—preventing the hip from dropping in unsupported actions (i.e., when the foot is not in contact with the floor).

The athlete stands on a short box, typically 10 to 20 centimetres in height initially. One foot is flat on the box, and the other is suspended to the side (figure 6.31a). The athlete simultaneously flexes the hip and knee of the standing leg sufficiently to allow the heel of the nonstanding leg (which has toes pulled up towards the knee) to descend and touch the floor (figure 6.31b). The hips must remain level throughout the exercise. The athlete performs two or three sets of 10 repetitions on each leg. The exercise can be performed with or without a dowel to aid balance and trunk positioning or an Olympic bar, which provides additional loaded resistance. Before loading the movement, the exercise can be progressed by increasing the box height to increase the range of movement required in the depth of the squat.

Single-leg squats are ideal for strengthening the hip muscles. As with all exercise

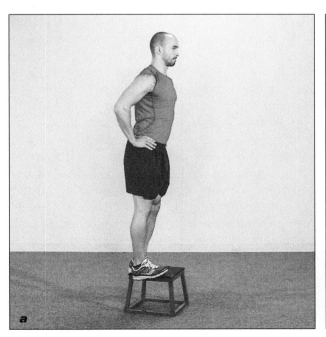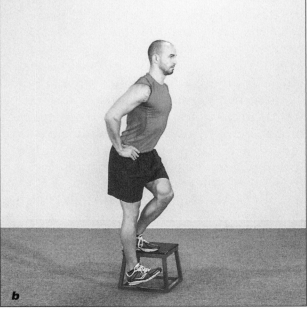

**Figure 6.31**    Lateral single-leg squat: *(a)* starting position; *(b)* squat.

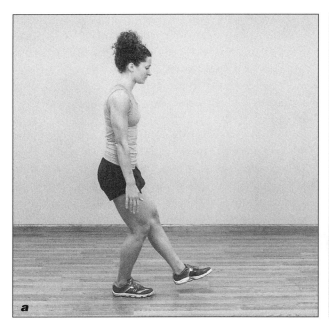 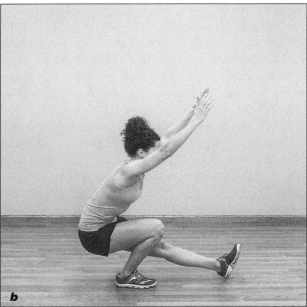

**Figure 6.32** Pistol squat: *(a)* starting position; *(b)* squat.

progressions, the exercise difficulty should be matched to the athlete's movement competency. If the exercise is too difficult and the athlete cannot execute it correctly, movement compensations will occur. Appropriate progressions for the development of a single-leg squat are presented in chapter 10.

The full single-leg squat, or pistol squat (figure 6.32), is the final level of difficulty in progression in terms of a remedial exercise. Later chapters show how this movement can be made more or less challenging by adding external loads in various positions. As chapter 10 describes, achieving full ranges in this exercise really tests the gluteal complex as well as much of the musculature around the hips and groin. Note that the full-depth pistol squat is nearly impossible to achieve without tucking under the pelvis at the bottom of the movement. This concern isn't necessarily significant for the athlete, because there will be no axial load to promote compromising shear forces to the intervertebral discs in the lumbar spine. If loading is used as a specific strengthening movement, the recommended approach is to compromise the range of motion to ensure the integrity of the normal lumbar curve.

# Ankle Joint Stability

At the other end of the lower limb is the ankle, which might be associated with poor movement control. The first thing the athlete should practice is setting the foot: standing and holding the position, first bilaterally and then on one foot with a neutral medial arch. This action requires slightly gripping with the toes, but it should not be forced or exaggerated.

The cocontraction of the peroneus longus and tibialis posterior increases stability and control. After the athlete achieves a stable, balanced position, distractions are added—simple challenges designed to move the athlete's arms or trunk and thereby displace the centre of mass. The athlete might be required to touch the end of a dowel that is moved around him or her or catch balls of various weights, thrown at different heights or at different speeds. Removing the athlete's vision also significantly increases the emphasis that the proprioceptive and neuromuscular systems have in maintaining the balanced position.

Another way to increase the level of difficulty is to introduce a moderately unstable or uneven surface, such as a cushion or pillow. Although strength cannot be significantly improved by working on unstable surfaces (as explained in chapter 10), this type of work enhances the proprioceptive capabilities in the ankle. Adding increasingly complex movements such as a knee dip also can be used to enhance this exercise.

# Summary

Quality athletic development programmes are based on the athlete's objectives. Many of these objectives should be based on needs identified through screening. Although many wide-ranging screening processes are available, this chapter has identified a series of practical and easily implemented protocols that will show how the athlete is able to control posture in both static and movement situations. Qualifiable observations of these tests can guide programme development.

Most postural control dysfunctions are related to movement compensations, and they affect more than one area of the posture. For example, tight hamstrings and tight hip flexors are associated with quadriceps-dominated running actions, which in turn are linked with underutilization of the gluteal muscles. Basic remedial exercises can be progressively introduced to an athlete's programme to address these issues. The next chapter looks at principles that the coach can apply to develop and progress programmes effectively from sound foundations.

# CHAPTER 7

# Designing a Progressive Curriculum: Considerations for Movement Skill Learning and Physio-Mechanical Training

A motor skill development programme should be based on an inclusive process that encourages athletes, especially children, to become competent in the foundational skills that underpin both sport and lifelong physical activity. Systematically, the process should connect and integrate movement education programmes with sport-specific programmes so that the athlete is doing the right things at the right time for long-term development, rather than for immediate success or gains. The focus should be on what the athlete can do rather than what he or she can't or shouldn't do!

The precise nature of skilled performance varies from sport to sport and ultimately involves the performer making the best decisions based on the information available at the time.[1] The athletic development programme promotes dynamic physical qualities that enable the athlete to execute the appropriate solutions to problems presented in the sporting context.

In this respect, training or practice should always be equated to learning because the programme instils a more or less permanent change in the athlete's motor patterns. Skill acquisition is the process of acquiring new skills through practice; skill retention is the developed ability of the performer to retain the learned skill over time. Motor skill retention requires progressive overload of the athlete's motor system (as explained in chapters 1 and 2), consideration of the athlete's needs (chapter 3), the use of core movement skills (chapters 8 through 10) and, with increasing levels of specialization, specific knowledge relating to the demands of the sport itself (see chapter 11 for examples).

A practitioner planning an athletic development programme needs to know how to deliver a planned curriculum that progresses core skills towards meeting the demands of specific sports. To deliver developmentally appropriate practices for athletes, the practitioner must understand three key areas of need:

1. Task: understand the movement requirements of a sport or a range of sports and

be able to relate these to developmentally appropriate technical and tactical principles

2. Individual: understand how athletes learn and how they develop biologically, psychologically and socially

3. Environment: establish the learning climate through coaching practices, programme structures and participant and possibly parental support

Combining these keys with the technical information about specific movement and postural-strengthening skills in the following chapters enables a practitioner to develop a progressive movement programme that will enhance movement skills, regardless of the athlete's level of sporting performance. This chapter introduces practical examples of progressing skills and some fundamental concepts of how to coach, many of them grounded in the best practice from physical education.

A movement skill can be considered a series of related movements integrated into an observable performance executed with accuracy, precision and intent. This movement skill may be generic, such as running or jumping, or highly specialized, such as an outside foot cut. The skilled practitioner can identify when an athlete is ready to progress from fundamental movements into more advanced ones and knows how to introduce specialized skills to give the athlete the best chance of learning and applying them in a sporting context. This progression explains the references in earlier chapters to the concept of physical literacy. The programme, or curriculum, is like the building blocks of words that can form sentences, paragraphs and stories so that information can be processed or transferred into any required communication (or sporting) context successfully.

## Building a Holistic Curriculum

Many practitioners start movement education programmes from a specific sport perspective by identifying the demands of the sport that the athlete currently plays. This approach often undermines the progressive development of the person and leads to bias in training. Indeed, a major limitation of this specialization approach is that practitioners often underestimate the generic physical competences that underpin sport-specific movements. They also often overestimate the generic movement experiences that an athlete may have experienced in other sporting or educational environments, such as physical education classes in school. Many Western societies have moved away from well-implemented and specialized physical education classes that emphasize fundamental skills and postural control to programmes that are more sport specific. The learning experiences for athletic ABCs (agility, balance, coordination and speed), the basics of athleticism (running, jumping and throwing) and the basics of sporting skill (body awareness, gliding, catching and striking) are not taught to many children in a structured or systematic manner. Often, a skills gap needs to be identified and bridged by an athletic development programme that is external to the school environment, especially when sport-specific coaching tends to focus on the skills required for a particular sport rather than the development of physical literacy and fundamental skills.

The other consideration for the early over-specialization of sport-specific movements is that the athlete is subjected to repetitive movement patterns and muscular actions that often lead to overdevelopment or excessive fatigue in certain neuromuscular groups and underdevelopment (lack of recruitment, force-producing or endurance capability) in other muscles. Ultimately, this shortcoming may limit the athlete's performance capacities. Muscle recruitment imbalances between synergistic muscle groups can lead to tightness in the muscles and maladaptive patterns of muscle recruitment. The result may be the large number of injuries associated with repetitive high-force or high-velocity action in adolescents within certain sporting populations. Such conditions include Sever's disease in the ankle, in which repetitive loading of the heel or excessive traction forces through the tendon cause inflammation in the calcaneus (heel bone). Similarly, in adolescents, repeated stress from contraction of the quadriceps is transmitted through the patellar tendon to the immature tibial tuberosity, which can cause multiple subacute avulsion fractures along with inflammation of the tendon, leading to excess bone growth in the tuberosity and producing a visible lump that can be quite painful.[2] This condition, known as Osgood-Schlatter syndrome, has been reported in 21 per cent of young people participating in sport (compared with only 4.5 per cent of nonathletic young people).[3]

Skilled performance can be regarded as the forceful application of technique under pressure. Ultimately, high-level sport participation requires the complete and coordinated development of the neuromuscular and musculoskeletal systems so the large forces needed for acceleration and deceleration in running, jumping, throwing, kicking and twisting can be achieved. Similarly, the efficient mechanical actions (techniques) of these particular movement and sport-specific skills need to be ingrained so that the athlete can successfully replicate them in performance. An athletic movement curriculum must provide a balanced approach to developing the necessary movement skills that enable an athlete to execute sport-specific skills and the required physical qualities (strength, speed, endurance and so on) to make this skilled execution effective. Too often, the focus is on the physical qualities of performance, not the movement competencies that underpin these qualities.

To put this concept into context, consider that an adolescent soccer player must produce a number of running, jumping, throwing and kicking actions in a game. Each action requires the player to possess both technical and physio-mechanical qualities to execute the technique and adapt it appropriately to the environmental demands of the specific game situation. For a specific example, to jump and head the ball, a player may be required to jump from one or both feet, may be required to transition from moving forwards or backwards and may be required to compete for the ball in the air under time and space pressures

from other players. The range and nature of the heading skills that a player may be required to exhibit during a game also require differential physical qualities. For example, a defensive clearing header requires distance (increased force from the trunk and neck), a directional attacking header requires lateral power production through the neck and a passing header (for example, heading a ball back to the goalkeeper's arms in a defensive situation) requires absorption of force from the ball through the kinetic chain.

In invasion games such as soccer, most skills are executed chaotically, determined by responses to the movement of the ball or other object and the opposition. The nature of movement is chaotic, and movement skills are often linked (for example, running and jumping, landing and accelerating, decelerating and accelerating). Chaotic movement requires a range of considerations (as illustrated in figure 7.1) to be built into the physical curriculum so that the athlete can learn these skills and effectively apply them to the dynamic movement context or particular sporting challenge.

Training methodologies can be implemented that address each of the areas identified in figure 7.1. For example, linear acceleration drills develop linear acceleration mechanics (chapter 8), functional strength training develops postural strength and leg flexor and extensor strength (chapter 10), and specific plyometric technique enhances the rate of force development in triple-extensor and triple-flexor actions (chapter 9). Each method, if used in isolation, may produce short-term changes in the athlete's chaotic speed and induce specific adaptions within the human body. The use of such methods, however, induces both short-term and residual fatigue that limits the athlete's motor capacity at any given time. This fatigue can interfere with specific adaptions from subsequent training sessions and may limit the potential for training methods to be performed safely in the first place.

The focus of effective programming should not simply be about understanding and presenting training methods. Presenting a series of exercises without a specific objective does not

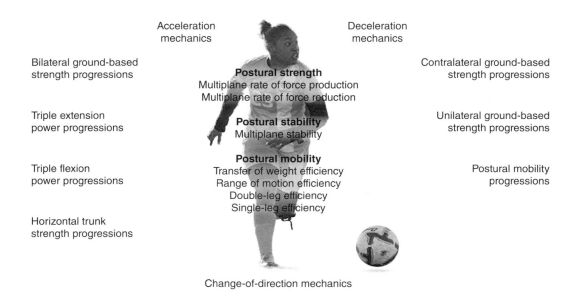

Acceleration
mechanics

Deceleration
mechanics

Bilateral ground-based
strength progressions

Contralateral ground-based
strength progressions

**Postural strength**
Multiplane rate of force production
Multiplane rate of force reduction

Triple extension
power progressions

Unilateral ground-based
strength progressions

**Postural stability**
Multiplane stability

Triple flexion
power progressions

**Postural mobility**
Transfer of weight efficiency
Range of motion efficiency
Double-leg efficiency
Single-leg efficiency

Postural mobility
progressions

Horizontal trunk
strength progressions

Change-of-direction mechanics

**Figure 7.1**    Multidirectional (chaotic) movement curriculum considerations: desired training outcomes and required training inputs.

make an effective training session; similarly, presenting a series of training sessions does not make a programme. A strategy that identifies a specific outcome and uses an appropriate and effective method to achieve this outcome is needed. But more than this, the effective programme is based on the understanding that each method has some prerequisites that need to be developed for that methodology to be effective and safe.

Returning to figure 7.1, the strategic outcome is to develop chaotic speed. The physiological qualities needed to achieve this outcome are postural strength, postural stability and postural mobility. To develop these qualities, the technical (mechanical) areas for refinement are acceleration mechanics, deceleration mechanics and directional change mechanics. The physical characteristics that can be expressed through the mechanics include eccentric and concentric force-producing capabilities throughout the postural chain, especially in the hip, knee and ankle flexors and extensors. An essential quality that underpins the ability to express rate of force development through an acquired technique is the stretch-shortening cycle, which is best developed using plyometrics.

The practitioner needs to identify how competent an athlete is to perform a particular

methodology and then develop specific sessions to target a specific outcome (e.g., acceleration mechanics) based on the athlete's needs and abilities. Similarly, the practitioner needs to develop other sessions or units of work within the same session for the other areas of need (postural strength, single-leg strength, rate of force development and so on), making the most of the method with respect to the individual athlete's needs and capacities. Then sessions need to be put together into training weeks and longer blocks of time that are integrated so that residual fatigue and training interference are minimized. Examples are in chapter 11.

Similarly, prerequisite physical and technical qualities (identified in the following chapters) need to be sequenced appropriately to ensure that training is actually beneficial in progressing the athlete towards the identified aims. Occasionally, a skill component may need to be regressed to ensure that the correct movement capabilities are challenged, apparently going backwards to move forwards.

While following this process, the practitioner must constantly refer back to the principles of biomotor ability and capacity development highlighted in chapters 1 through 3. Effective programming requires an understanding of human form and function beyond certain exercises. The practitioner must understand the biomotor systems, the way in which they develop and work, the adaptations they induce and produce, and the various physio-mechanical qualities and the way in which they adhere to principles of adaptation with their implementation.

Targeting training strategies to the athlete's developmental stage and training age and status is an important part of the programming process. The same programme cannot be applied to a child and an adult. Similarly a 25-year-old ex-college athlete transferring from one sport programme to another cannot expect to progress if he or she is trained in the same way as a 35-year-old office worker who cycles leisurely for 20 minutes three times a week.

Physical capacities can underpin sport performance only if they can be effectively transferred into the sporting context. The development of physical qualities without looking at when and how they will be integrated into development of sport-specific skills is a fundamental error. The athlete needs to be at the centre of the process. The athletic development professional makes the athlete a better performer by asking, 'What physical qualities does the athlete need to do this, and how can I best develop these qualities?'

For example, consider a good sprinter who is identified as not having an adequate power-to-body-weight capability; the athlete cannot exert sufficient force into the ground with each stride to propel his or her mass forward, typically limiting the ability to generate accelerations and maintain maximum velocity while running. A programme needs to be developed that will enable the athlete to increase his or her force-producing capabilities and then express these within his or her running technique to enhance speed. Strength training that cannot be transferred into linear sprinting may have the undesired consequence of slowing down the athlete! Table 7.1 shows how this goal might be achieved; specific movement and force development considerations are explored in later chapters.

A holistic programme also aims to develop young athletes who have the capability to develop their range of physical competencies as their sport careers progress. They will be physically competent to solve a greater range of environmental problems within the context of their performance. In short, athletes must be able to learn physically on an ongoing basis and thus become physically adaptable. Those who constantly seek the same solutions to new problems (i.e., they are physically unadaptable) will not be able to progress in their performance. This result often happens with athletes who are highly specialized in their athletic training at too early a stage in their development.

Indeed, a good amount of evidence supports that diversification of athletic experiences enhances athletic aspects of performance as well as many technical and tactical aspects. For example, perceptual elements of performance are based on the athlete's interpretation of

**Table 7.1**  Medium-Term Programme Outline for Strength and Speed Improvement in a Sprinter

|  | Block 1: Force production | Block 2: Application | Block 3: Realisation |
|---|---|---|---|
| Strength emphasis | Multijoint, multimuscle high-force actions | Strength and speed emphasis; high rate of force production; lactic power | Speed and strength emphasis; reactive strength; alactic power |
| Technical emphasis | Acceleration and maximum velocity mechanics | Acceleration to transition; build into transition to maximum velocity | Maximal speed |
| Conditioning | Incomplete recovery intervals to increase phosphate turnover |  |  |

environmental information to make performance decisions. This skill is learnable across a number of environments. For example, soccer and basketball both require spatial awareness and the ability to identify the actions of an opponent. Consider the quick transition from offence to defence in basketball that many soccer coaches wish their defensive players could adopt. Conceptual elements refer to the athlete's tactical appreciations of a context, whether this is rules or strategies to achieve success.

Simple principles of training progressions should govern integrated programme development. Before exploring this idea further, recognize that the athlete's individual needs are key in this programming, even within a group coaching environment. Programme delivery should always be athlete-centred, based on an individual and educational approach and founded on a desire to make a long-term difference to the athletes. These objectives should be reflected in the planning, delivery and evaluation of the programme.

# Competency-Based Approach to Developing Skills

Skilled performance in any context is ultimately based on a foundation of movement control or technique. This foundation takes many years to develop and will ultimately take place across a number of different environments. The process of growth and movement skill development is reasonably predictable in terms of universal principles and sequential progressions as children develop higher levels of functional competence. The key to successful coaching with both children and adults is to programme the appropriate progressions and use the appropriate methodologies to match these sequential, development progressions in a fun and imaginative way that keeps the participant interested in getting better.

Planning for long-term development involves the logical and systematic sequencing of training factors to optimize specific training outcomes at predetermined times.[4] The identification of progressive outcomes is key in this process. A fundamental part of programme development in respect of any aspect of physical conditioning is that the content or element of a programme is fundamentally determined by the objective that the practitioner seeks to achieve. The best methods can be adopted to achieve the outcome.

## Progression

Competence is a major theme in programme development because it would typically form the basis for progression between different levels of task complexity. For example, as illustrated in chapter 9, a person shouldn't undertake relatively high-intensity plyometric tasks until he or she can demonstrate competence at controlling the posture during various landing tasks and has achieved the strength required to execute the task. Movement competencies grow through experience, and because movement takes place in various sporting contexts, the athlete would need to be presented with the movement task in a number of situations to learn and demonstrate competency. The athlete would be able to interpret the required movement in the situational context and have mastery of the tools—the techniques—to take the most effective action (or movement response) in a given situation.

This concept can be illustrated through reference to a potential teaching progression for the clean weightlifting movement. Weightlifting is regarded as a closed skill, which means that the execution of the intended movement is entirely within the control of the individual and that no outside agents such as weather, opposition, a moving object or a moving target can influence the athlete. As a multijoint, multimuscle exercise that requires the development of high rates of force from a dead-stop starting position, the clean (and derivate movement components) may be regarded as a cornerstone exercise within a functional strength-training programme, as discussed in chapter 10.

Although the clean is a closed skill, the joint movement sequencing and intramuscular coordination that are required to execute the overall movement are reasonably complex. The coordination of the posture with the progression of the bar and the various movement velocities that are achieved in the bar at different stages of the lift mean that the movement typically isn't easy to master. Although there isn't one correct way to teach a technique, breaking the executive movement down into smaller movements (subroutines incorporating key postures and positions) that can be mastered and then sequenced together to build the overall skill might be a reasonable strategy to teach the skill.

This process is illustrated in figure 7.2. The athlete gains competence in lifting the bar from the floor to above the knees (first-pull deadlift), moving the bar from the knees to the thigh (stiff-leg deadlift) and then pulling the bar from the thigh and recovering to standing from the point where the bar would be caught (not shown) in the catch of a full lift (front squat). Because each of these movements is a sound training movement in its own right,

the athlete is training while learning. As the athlete achieves mastery in each exercise, the movements are linked together and additional tasks are added to the movement repertoire.

The next progressions challenge the athlete to link the pull from thigh with a shrug and front squat to complete the clean from thigh, where the rapid and highly complex movement of rapidly descending under the bar to catch in the front squat position is practised. The stiff-leg deadlift and pull from thigh are linked into a pull from hang. The athlete also learns to lift from the floor, practising the first pull through first-pull deadlift (bar ending above the knees).

## Differentiation

Athletes will not follow a uniform rate of progression. Some athletes will quickly pick up the basic (level 1) movements but find clean from thigh much easier than pull from hang because

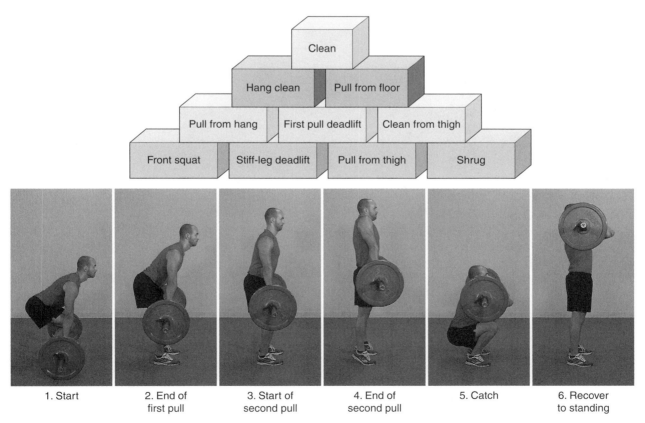

**Figure 7.2** Mastery in simple movements can progress towards learning more complex movements. A suggested strategy for learning the clean based on developed movement competency.

of the nature of the transition phase of the movement and rapid reflex of the knees under the bar as the hip extends in this lift. Other athletes may accelerate through levels 1 and 2 but struggle to link the pulling movements together to accelerate the bar from the floor to its highest position (pull from floor). The added movement range and coordination requirements may or may not slow their rate of progression.

The practitioner must be able to accommodate the athlete's rate of learning and level of competency within the overall curriculum progression, even within a group setting. This principle of physical education, known as differentiation, is fundamental. Although all individuals are doing the same practice, a number of individualized variations are appropriately applied to different people to enable all to receive the same level of challenge. As this chapter illustrates, and as chapters 8 through 10 describe in detail, every practice can be adapted in some way to make it more appropriately challenging for the athletes in the programme.

Differentiation can be illustrated in a number of ways and within different practical environments. Tables 7.2 and 7.3 demonstrate how this is possible within a strength-training

**Table 7.2**   Session 1: Basic Technique, Hip and Knee Extensors

**Team plan**

| Exercise | Sets | Reps | Notes | Load 1 | 2 | 3 | 4 | 5 |
|---|---|---|---|---|---|---|---|---|
| DB front foot raised split squat | 3 | 5 | Each leg | | | | ▨ | ▨ |
| Bungee-assisted razor curl | 3 | 8 | | | | | ▨ | ▨ |
| High-box DB step-up | 3 | 5 | Each leg | | | | ▨ | ▨ |
| Clean pull from thigh | 3 | 5 | | | | | ▨ | ▨ |
| Vertical leg shoot | 2 | 10 | | | | ▨ | ▨ | |

**Player 1:** Experienced player with good technical execution who is able to perform extensions of many of the exercises within the prescribed sessions

| Exercise | Sets | Reps | Notes | Load 1 | 2 | 3 | 4 | 5 |
|---|---|---|---|---|---|---|---|---|
| High-bar barbell front foot raised split squat | 3 | 5 | Each leg | | | | ▨ | ▨ |
| Razor curl | 3 | 8 | | | | | ▨ | ▨ |
| High-bar barbell step-up | 3 | 5 | Each leg | | | | ▨ | ▨ |
| Clean pull from hang | 3 | 5 | | | | | ▨ | ▨ |
| Candlestick | 2 | 10 | | | | ▨ | ▨ | |

**Player 2:** Less experienced player of young strength-training age who is developing basic technical competence and is being challenged by simplifications of the movements within the prescribed sessions

| Exercise | Sets | Reps | Notes | Load 1 | 2 | 3 | 4 | 5 |
|---|---|---|---|---|---|---|---|---|
| DB split squat | 3 | 5 | Each leg | | | | ▨ | ▨ |
| Bungee-assisted partial movement razor curl | 3 | 8 | Quality dictates reps and movement range | | | | ▨ | ▨ |
| Unloaded high-box step-up | 3 | 5 | Each leg | | | | ▨ | ▨ |
| Clean pull from thigh | 3 | 5 | | | | | ▨ | ▨ |
| Reverse curl | 2 | 10 | | | | ▨ | ▨ | |

context using the example of a weight-training programme for an elite female soccer squad. In many team situations, individualizing every player's programme may be impossible, perhaps because of time constraints (for example, when a squad is one of a number that passes through a facility in a week and only for specific training sessions). But the practitioner in charge can still establish a programme in which the training objectives can be achieved and individualized challenges can be provided across all exercises.

The objective for the female soccer team, which consisted of players of varying training ages and experience within a strength-training context, was to work on functional hip strength and postural control throughout the kinetic chain. Of particular concern to the coach and medical staff was the long-term development of players' ability to stabilize and maintain dynamic knee control in a range of sport-specific actions. For the 20 players, the presented programme (an example week from the start of a long-term programme) identifies the target exercises that form the core of the programme and includes exercise variations that can either reduce or increase the challenge to the athlete. Chapter 10 explores this

**Table 7.3**  Session 2: Basic Technique, Hip and Knee Extensors

**Team plan**

| Exercise | Sets | Reps | Notes | Load 1 | 2 | 3 | 4 | 5 |
|---|---|---|---|---|---|---|---|---|
| DB reverse lunge | 3 | 5 | Each leg | | | | ▓ | ▓ |
| Single-leg hop and hold | 3 | 4 | Each leg | | | | ▓ | ▓ |
| Behind-the-neck push press | 3 | 5 | | | | | ▓ | ▓ |
| Springbok | 3 | 8 | | | | | ▓ | ▓ |
| Rollout | 2 | 10 | | | | ▓ | ▓ | ▓ |

**Player 1:** Experienced player with good technical execution who is able to perform extensions of many of the exercises within the prescribed sessions

| Exercise | Sets | Reps | Notes | Load 1 | 2 | 3 | 4 | 5 |
|---|---|---|---|---|---|---|---|---|
| Barbell reverse lunge | 3 | 5 | Each leg | | | | ▓ | ▓ |
| Vertical drop single-leg land and hold | 3 | 4 | Each leg | | | | ▓ | ▓ |
| Behind-the-neck push press | 3 | 5 | | | | | ▓ | ▓ |
| Springbok with arms overhead | 3 | 8 | | | | | ▓ | ▓ |
| On-feet rollout | 2 | 10 | | | | ▓ | ▓ | ▓ |

**Player 2:** Less experienced player of young strength training age who is developing basic technical competence and is being challenged by simplifications of the movements within the prescribed sessions

| Exercise | Sets | Reps | Notes | Load 1 | 2 | 3 | 4 | 5 |
|---|---|---|---|---|---|---|---|---|
| Reverse lunge with arms overhead | 3 | 5 | Each leg | | | | ▓ | ▓ |
| Double-leg jump and hold | 3 | 4 | Each leg | | | | ▓ | ▓ |
| DB push press | 3 | 5 | | | | | ▓ | ▓ |
| Reverse springbok | 3 | 8 | | | | | ▓ | ▓ |
| Hip rollout | 2 | 10 | | | | ▓ | ▓ | ▓ |

concept in more detail and illustrates the idea that exercises can be regressed to a foundation movement or extended in terms of the challenge presented by increasing the movement complexity (position of bar relative to the centre of mass, speed of the movement, range of the movement, joints involved and so on). Further variation can be achieved at an individual level by increasing the resistive load to the movement.

The idea for foundation and extension movements is based on the notion of social competence. Players in group settings don't want to be given easier tasks and often want to go to the hardest tasks straight away. But practical delivery that has planned opportunity to 'go back a stage' often is not perceived in the same way. In the given team setting, in which everyone is working on the same exercise, differentiation based on movement competence and strength level can be delivered easily and quickly. Those who quickly progress beyond the extension exercises can be provided new movement challenges to suit their abilities as the programme develops. In this way, exercises that were once extension tasks quickly become foundation-level challenges.

Similar differentiation can occur in every range-of-movement and sport-specific skill setting. Consider a group coaching setting in which young children are practising the overarm throwing of a tennis ball. (Throwing is a fundamental movement skill; therefore, competence and confidence in the ability to throw well underpin a range of other sporting choices and abilities.) One practice challenge is for the practitioner to line up the children in front of a wall and see how many times in 1 minute they can throw a ball against the wall so that it comes back to them above head height. This practice encourages children to think about how they can adapt their throwing action to make it more forceful. In throwing and kicking tasks, in the early stages of skill learning with children, force is better to develop than accuracy because of the earlier neuromuscular development of the large-muscle groups compared with the muscles responsible for fine motor control, as explored in chapter 3.

The practitioner in charge follows good practice by lining up all athletes and having them throw the ball in the same direction against the same wall. The horizontal distance between them should be sufficient so that no one is hit by a thrown ball. Athlete A stands on the start line 6 metres from the wall, which provides a challenge suitable for his or her skill level, strength and coordination. Athlete B is more physically mature and has a mature skill action, in that he or she is able to step into the throw by turning the hips quickly and transferring weight from the back to the front as the arm comes forward. Athlete B also uses the non-throwing arm as a guide and rotational aid. For this reason, he or she stands farther from the wall, making the challenge appropriate to his or her level of competence in the task. Athlete C is limited not by his or her throwing competence (which is similar to that of athlete A) but by his or her inability to catch and retrieve the ball. If athlete C needs to spend time chasing and retrieving every ball that comes back over head height, he or she will need to spend much of the 60-second time off task and will not address the skill objective. Therefore, athlete C should be provided more tennis balls than the other participants so that he or she can have a similar opportunity to address the challenge of the task. Catching skills will not be ignored; the programme will offer other opportunities and relevant practices to address this skill.

To improve, all athletes need to be provided with an appropriate level of challenge that will stretch their ability to execute a particular technique or skill within a given situation. The excellent practitioner is able to provide the appropriate level of challenge to all participants so that they can experience sufficient success to reinforce developed movement patterns and experience the confidence that comes from achieving a successful outcome. This objective needs to be balanced with the need to provide variation to the challenge so that learning is reinforced and developed. Indeed, the need to experience failure (or noncompetence) is a recognized stimulus for learning and progression in many athletic (and nonathletic) situations.

The principles of individual need can be applied to aspects of physical stimulus, which depend on the athlete's training status. As with designing a learning programme, differentiating an imposed training load to an athlete within a group is important. Based on the supercompensation model for human adaptation to training stimuli,[5] figure 7.3 models the response of two athletes to the same training session. As can be seen, athlete 1 experiences little disruption to his or her homeostasis (habituated level), whereas athlete 2 is affected much differently by the same training load. Athlete 2 will need longer to recover between training episodes to avoid overtraining. This example explains why physical training loads need to be individualized. A training load (exercise complexity, exercise intensity, exercise volume) that stimulates one athlete may break (overreach) another yet not disrupt the physical capacities of a third person at all.

The training status of a person also changes over time as he or she adapts to the specifically imposed loads of the training programme. Therefore, what is considered a stimulating load at the start of a training block may well become a warm-up load later in the training progression. This transformation occurs because of the biological principle of accommodation, whereby the response of an athlete to a constant (or similar) environmental stimulus decreases over time. Hence, variations in the

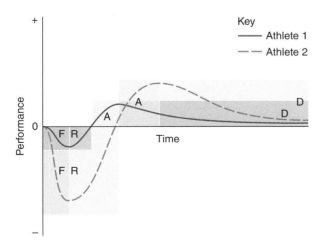

**Figure 7.3** The response to the same training event can be different between individuals depending on their training status. F = fatigue; R = recovery; A = adaptation; D = detraining.

training stimuli are needed to achieve overload that will cause performance improvement.

# Long-Term Approach to Motor Skill Development

The process of motor skill development starts with helping children develop a mature action for fundamental movement skills within themes such as agility, balance, coordination and speed. These actions involve the basic elements of a particular movement, but not the combination of these skills or the transition between one movement skill and the next. Typically, each fundamental skill is considered in relative isolation when programmes are being compiled to develop them.

The overriding strategy of the children's practitioner must be to develop the all-around athlete before focusing solely on sport-specific development and, if appropriate, the highest level of performance. Children not only need to develop the ability to undertake these basic movement skills but also must have a positive view of their abilities and be cognitively aware of their competence.

## Fundamental Motor Skills

Fundamental motor skills are part of a movement continuum that begins before birth and continues throughout life. With exposure to movement experiences, the young child begins to learn fundamental motor skills that will be refined over time through practice, instruction and modelling. Children who master fundamental motor skills in the early primary (elementary) school years will be more likely to be active and enjoy a range of recreational and sporting activities. Conversely, it has long been established that 'Children who possess inadequate motor skills are often relegated to a life of exclusion from organized and free play experiences of their peers, and subsequently to a lifetime of inactivity because of their frustrations in early movement behaviour.'[6]

Typically, fundamental actions are considered mature around the developmental ages of 5 to 7 years. Maturity means that the execution of the skill is observably distinct; for example, instead of toddling fast, the child is able to run and walk and the difference between the two actions is obvious and deliberate. The child has a sense that he or she can use distinct actions such as running, jumping, throwing and being balanced in a range of sporting tasks, even if these actions are not yet refined.

Effective movement skill programmes build on the competences and confidences achieved at fundamental stages and progress to high-level movement skills. Foundational stages of learning, however, do not apply only to children. Anyone who approaches a novel skill will go through this stage of learning. For example, an adult who wants to take up a new sport will be in the foundational stages of learning for all the skills related to that sport. Similarly, an experienced performer may be required to develop a new technique to continue his or her performance progression. The person doesn't become a foundation-level athlete, but for the new skill he or she will be considered at the foundation stage of learning. This concept is important, because the athlete's level of skill

learning typically informs the coaching methodologies and drill or session structures that should be employed to maximize learning.

In the foundational stages of skill learning, demonstration is particularly important. (See the sidebar Providing a High-Quality Demonstration.) At this stage, athletes first come across a new skill or technique[7] and therefore need a good picture of what skilled performance looks like so that they can begin to form their own movement interpretations.

When working with athletes at this stage, first teach movement techniques rather than skills and initially make these techniques as closed as possible. The distinction between a skill and a technique is important in this context. Techniques are the basic movements of any sport or event; for example, a block start in a 100-metre race and a volley at the net in tennis are techniques. Techniques can be combined into specific and recognizable movement patterns, such as a serve and volley in tennis or the run–hop–step–jump that constitutes a triple jump. A skill is an athlete's ability to choose and perform the right techniques at the

## Providing a High-Quality Demonstration

- Position the demonstration to provide an optimum view for all athletes.
- Present the demonstration from a range of angles so that the viewers can obtain a complete picture. With large groups, the demonstrator can often move more easily than the group can.
- If possible, position the athletes so that they have their backs to any potential interference with their concentration.
- Use verbal cues to direct the athletes' attention to the key aspects (one or two coaching points each time) of the technique they should focus on.
- Present a range of coaching cues to address the full range of learning styles that athletes may have. Use auditory cues; for example, in a plyometric action, say, 'Watch how Linda attacks the floor with the flat foot as she lands.'

Follow up with kinaesthetic cues such as saying, 'Imagine you are landing on hot coals' to help the athletes translate the picture into a feeling.

- The greater the athlete's experience is, the more precise and advanced the coaching points need to be. For example, to a beginner, you might say, 'Land on the ball of your foot and take off as quickly as possible. Imagine you are landing on hot coals.' To an intermediate athlete, you might say, 'Land so that the weight is through the middle of the foot but the heel is slightly off the floor. Feel as if you are using the stiff ankle as a spring that will rebound as quickly as possible.' To an advanced athlete, you might say, 'Be really active with the flat-foot contact and maintain a stiff ankle. You should be able to slide a credit card under the heels at ground contact. Really attack the floor just before you hit the ground.'

right time, successfully, regularly and with the appropriate amount of force. Skill is acquired and therefore has to be learned.

Most sport skills exist on a continuum between being open or closed. Two characteristics determine how open a skill is: the environment in which the skill is performed and the objective of the skill itself. Completely closed skills take place in an unchanging environment, and the movements that form the skill are the goal of skill execution. For example, gymnastic routines are closed skills, because they take place indoors on fixed equipment and the timing of skill executions is consistently rehearsed and completely within the athlete's control. How well the individual movements are executed determines the success of the performance. Contrast gymnastics with invasion sports such as soccer, American football, tennis, basketball and baseball, in which the environment is constantly changing as players (both teammates and opposition) interact with each other to shape the game. Similarly, the skilled movements that are executed within the performance are a means to an end; the outcome of the game (performance) is determined by an environmental outcome rather than the movements themselves.

In the early stages of learning, techniques should be progressed through practices that are as closed as possible. Athletes are building their movement patterns and learning the neuromuscular pathways that will develop into a motor programme and become the learned technique. Athletes must be given appropriate feedback and correction to address inappropriate technique before it becomes ingrained and learned behaviour. Making the practice as closed as possible enables the coach and athletes to focus on the technique itself rather than having it be influenced by environmental pressures.

This early stage of learning is characterized by inconsistency as well as large gains in skill performance. During this cognitive stage of learning, the learner must be provided with the necessary information, corrective guidance and time to establish sound movement patterns. Coaching emphasis should be placed on the quality of the performed movement rather than the speed or intensity of action. Early learners will make errors, and the environment needs to encourage this; without errors and constructive coaching, learning is often hindered.

## Sample Progressions to Develop Agility

The idea of manipulating the environment of a practice to induce a transition between learning techniques and expressing them as skills can be seen by looking at some specific aspects of developing agility. Table 7.4 introduces the range of techniques that a basketball point guard might need to be effective.

Each of these techniques can be developed through progressive practices that are gradually made more open as the athlete learns the technique. Table 7.5 provides a number of example practices to illustrate how this process can be achieved over time and how techniques can be gradually integrated into specific drills after the techniques are mastered to begin the development of the agility skills.

In level 1, techniques are performed at the lowest possible level of complexity. The drills are simple and entirely self-paced, and no transition occurs between techniques.

**Table 7.4**  Agility Techniques Required by a Basketball Point Guard

| Starting | Linear | Direction change | Transitional movements |
|---|---|---|---|
| Athletic position | Linear acceleration | Inside foot cut | Backpedal |
| Transition from running | Linear deceleration | Outside foot cut | Cross-step |
| Transition from jump landing | | Swerve | Side shuffle |
| | | 45- to 135-degree turn | |
| | | 180-degree turn | |

**Table 7.5**    Progressive Technique Drills to Develop Agility

|  | **Level 1** | **Level 2** | **Level 3** | **Level 4** | **Level 5** |
|---|---|---|---|---|---|
| Linear acceleration | Wall drills, uphill running | Advanced wall drills, partner-resisted march, 15-metre accelerations | Up tall and fall into 15-metre accelerations, face and chase | Transitional movement into linear acceleration (cone drill) | Transitional movement into directional change and linear acceleration (mirror drill with race) |
| Transitional movements | Backpedal, sidestep, cross-over step | Box drill | Mirror drill with partner | Mirror drill with partner | |
| Direction change | Cut drill to cone (slow) | Cut drill to static player (slow) | Cut drill to moving player (at tempo) | Linear acceleration into direction change (partner sprint and cut) | |

# LEVEL 1 DRILLS: LINEAR ACCELERATION

## Wall Drills

See chapter 8.

## Uphill Running

Sets of five or six accelerations up a 10- to 20-metre hill with a 3- to 8-degree gradient (with complete recovery between repetitions) can improve the athlete's ability to develop and direct propulsive forces.

# LEVEL 1 DRILLS: TRANSITIONAL MOVEMENTS

Practice backpedal, sidestep and cross-over step (figure 7.4) as individual techniques between two cones that are 6 to 10 metres apart.

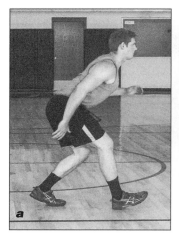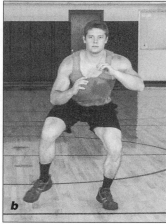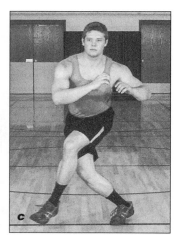

**Figure 7.4**    Level 1 transition drills: *(a)* backpedal; *(b)* sidestep; *(c)* cross-over step.

# LEVEL 1 DRILLS: DIRECTION CHANGE

## Cut Drill to Cone (Slow)

The athlete jogs (with increased pace as the technique becomes solidified) to the cone from 3 to 5 metres initially. At the cone he or she performs a cut (figure 7.5). The athlete should alternate the directions of the cut (following the technical specifications in chapter 8).

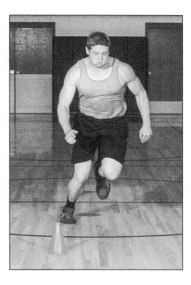

**Figure 7.5**   Cut drill to cone (slow).

The drills at level 2 are similar, although aspects are added to increase the complexity of the task. Techniques may be linked together so that the athlete is required to transition between different mechanical models, more people may be added, or movement velocity may be increased.

# LEVEL 2 DRILLS: LINEAR ACCELERATION

## Advanced Wall Drills

Wall drills and their progressions are described in chapter 8.

## Partner-Resisted March

Marching drills are described in chapter 8.

## 15-Metre Accelerations

The athlete performs maximal accelerations from a static or rolling start.

# LEVEL 2 DRILLS: TRANSITIONAL MOVEMENTS

## Box Drill

Working around a 10-by-10 metre square, the athlete sprints forward and transitions to a sidestep, a backpedal and then a sidestep back to the start (figure 7.6). The emphasis is on a rapid transition in movement each time the athlete reaches a cone.

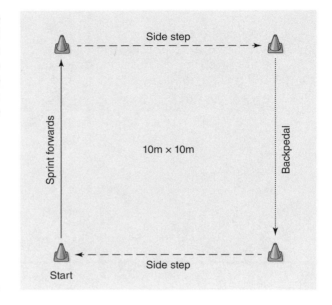

**Figure 7.6**   Box drill.

# LEVEL 2 DRILLS: DIRECTION CHANGE

## Cut Drill to Static Player (Slow)

The athlete jogs (with increased pace as the technique becomes solidified) to a passive opponent from 3 to 5 metres initially. The position of the static opponent enables judgement for the distance that the cut should be performed to be effective. The athlete should alternate the directions of the cut (following the technical specifications in chapter 8).

As athletes near the development or associative stages of learning, they need to find more challenging ways to practice techniques. The next level of progression adds reaction and decision making in response to the actions of others. The focus of the athletes at this stage often changes; for example, in mirror drills, the athlete's attention typically moves away from execution of sound mechanics to the need to lose the partner. The practitioner needs to use effective feedback and questioning techniques to focus the athlete's attention on how to move rather than the outcome of the practice. Gradually increasing the speed of movement in such practices decreases the athlete's thinking time, thereby developing decision making and reaction as well as mechanics.

Different levels of progressions might be needed, depending on the athlete's competency.

Table 7.5 also presents a simplified progression. Elements of the drills can be combined to provide different training stimuli at appropriate times. For example, linear acceleration (possibly initially taught from an up-tall-and-fall starting position) can be combined with a side shuffle between cones so that the athlete transitions from a lateral movement to a linear one. This drill can be built into an acceleration to a simple cut performed at a cone so that the athlete practices acceleration at higher levels and needs to cut at a higher velocity. Reducing the number of variables is useful for increasing the probability of success in the drill. Similar means of progression can be employed to link acceleration, deceleration, turning and single-foot pivot actions.

# LEVEL 3 DRILLS: LINEAR ACCELERATION

## Up Tall and Fall Into 15-Metre Accelerations

The drill is presented in chapter 8.

## Face and Chase

The drill is presented in chapter 8.

# LEVEL 3 DRILLS: TRANSITIONAL MOVEMENTS

## Mirror Drill With Partner

Two athletes stand 2 metres apart. Athlete A is the lead, and athlete B is the mirror. The job of the mirror is to stay exactly opposite the lead (figure 7.7). The lead can move side to side or forwards and backwards.

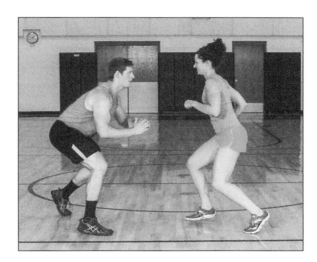

**Figure 7.7**   Mirror drill with partner.

# LEVEL 3 DRILLS: DIRECTION CHANGE

## Cut Drill to Moving Player (at tempo)

The athlete accelerates (with increased pace as the technique becomes solidified) to a moving opponent from 3 to 5 metres initially. The speed of opposed movement should be gradually increased to pressure the learner appropriately as he or she demonstrates competency.

As the practices in table 7.5 become more complex in terms of ability requirements, less equipment is typically required and the skills remain reasonably simple. At these introductory stages, change-of-direction techniques might be developed through practices that use cones or markers to guide movements and constrain the space that the athlete can use. But programmes need to progress beyond a process that relies on cones and drills. The objective has to be about finding the most effective ways for an athlete to learn and express movement mechanics whilst solving environmentally engineered challenges. This approach is different from simply applying ever more complex drills that require many cones laid out in ever decreasing circles.

## LEVEL 4 DRILLS: TRANSITIONAL MOVEMENT INTO LINEAR ACCELERATION

### Cone Drill

The athlete starts at cone 1. The athlete side shuffles to cone 2, turns and sprints across to cone 3 and then side shuffles back to cone 1 (figure 7.8). The coach calls out a cone number, and the athlete accelerates to that cone.

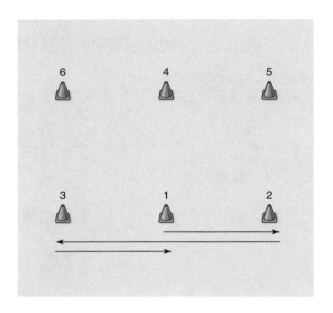

**Figure 7.8**   Cone drill.

## LEVEL 4 DRILLS: TRANSITIONAL MOVEMENTS

### Mirror Drill With Partner

The level 4 mirror drill is performed by having a third person decide which direction the athletes will move in by pointing an arm in one direction and changing arms as movement changes are required. One athlete responds to an external stimulus (rather than a self-made decision), and the other athlete responds to the movements of athlete 1.

# LEVEL 4 DRILLS: LINEAR ACCELERATION INTO DIRECTION CHANGE

## Partner Sprint and Cut

Two athletes face each other 20 metres apart. On the coach's command 'Go', they sprint to a line 10 metres in front of them, turn 180 degrees and sprint back. They cut past each other as they meet, going to the left or right as required (figure 7.9). Initially, the direction might be predetermined (using whichever technique they think is most appropriate), but with competency comes the need to perform this reactive, challenging decision making at high speed.

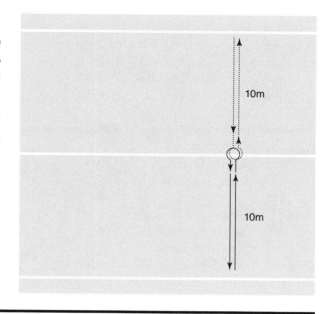

**Figure 7.9**    Partner sprint and cut.

By the time the programme reaches level 5, in which all techniques are integrated into an open agility drill, the athlete needs to have reached the autonomous or applied learning stage. The mechanics of the drill should be automatic, without conscious thought. Practices such as this can easily be made sport specific to develop agility within the sporting context as long as the practitioner has the imagination to do so without losing sight of the principles of effective mechanics and skill progression. Note here that although this section focuses on agility to guide the concept of progressions, similar and simultaneous progressions would be needed for strength and power development to maximize the physio-mechanical qualities that underpin agility skill execution.

# LEVEL 5 DRILL: TRANSITIONAL MOVEMENTS INTO DIRECTIONAL CHANGE AND LINEAR ACCELERATION

## Mirror Drill With Race

Two athletes face each other, 2 metres apart. Athlete A can move in any direction as long as he or she remains facing athlete B. Athlete B has to mirror athlete A, maintaining the 2-metre gap between them. If athlete A advances, athlete B retreats and so on. At any point, athlete B can call, 'Go'. At 'Go', athlete B changes direction past athlete A and accelerates to a finish point. Athlete A has to react to athlete B, change direction and race athlete B to the finish point.

# Repetition and Variation

The amount of repetition and variation provided in a learning programme is important in promoting the learning of specific techniques.[8] Indeed, the distribution of variation is an important consideration in how skilled learning is shaped over time. The balance between these two competing concepts is an interesting consideration for anyone designing a learning programme for athletes.

The central nervous system needs repetition to develop a motor programme for a coordinated sequencing of muscle actions that make up a skilled movement. Too much repetition, however, will cause the athlete's rate of learning (or indeed progression in any context) to stagnate. Similarly, the athlete will not be able to transfer learned movement patterns to a new situation or novel task. Too much variation will not allow an optimum rate of learning; too much repetition will not enable the technique learned to be transferred to a different context.

Typically, practices to develop movement technique can be structured as blocks or be more widely distributed over time (often referred to as random practice, although the pattern of distribution is planned rather than unpredictable or spontaneous). This means of structuring the amount of variation can apply both within sessions and between sessions, thus creating variation across time.[9]

Blocked practice has been shown to be more effective at short-term behavioural change, whereas random practice has been shown to result in better long-term learning (a more-or-less permanent change in behaviour). This differentiation is thought to result from the fact that during random practices, athletes must retrieve motor programmes from their long-term movement memory stores and apply those patterns to different contexts across time rather than repeat similar movement patterns in a block of time.[8] Practitioners may conclude that when introducing new techniques to complete beginners, a blocked approach to practice may be more effective, but beyond this, athletes may develop better with a more randomized approach to session structures.

This approach is illustrated in tables 7.6 and 7.7 for some elements of a movement programme development (and options for developing these aspects) for a young tennis player. Tennis requires a lot of movement across the baseline; players need to execute a number of 45- to 180-degree turns in rallies. Players are also required to maintain postural alignment and integrity whilst executing shots from a base provided by a single- or double-leg stance. The need to react to a moving ball and execute rapid three-step movements from a range of positions means that young players need to develop quickness within their tennis programmes. These specific athletic requirements can be isolated in the early stages of learning as individual techniques or movements to develop the physio-mechanical qualities associated with these techniques. At later stages of learning, these techniques can be refined into more sport-specific movement patterns that reflect specific on-court actions.

Each drill presented in tables 7.6 and 7.7 can have increased variability over time. Specific examples are presented in the following chapters about how this may be achieved for speed, power and strength drills. Trunk stability exercises can be added randomly to the end of sessions to develop postural strength in the lumbar–pelvic and abdominal areas. Some physical qualities such as strength in postural muscles are not suited to single sessions devoted entirely to one function, because the fatigue induced, particularly in novice athletes, will degrade skilled movement patterns and reinforce inappropriate movement patterns.

# Transition to the Practice Phase of Learning

As athletes begin to master the foundations of technique and develop an effective motor programme for isolated techniques, they move into what is regarded as the associative, or developmental, stage of learning.[8] This stage is also known as the practice phase of learning, when the athlete develops the ability to combine discreet movement skills into more sport-specific movement patterns.

**Table 7.6** Blocked Approach to Movement Skill Development Within a Tennis Programme

| SESSION 1: CHANGE OF DIRECTION | |
|---|---|
| **Drill** | **Description** |
| Z-pattern run | Cones are placed 2 metres apart in a zigzag pattern. Run between successive cones, alternating the cut-off foot inside each cone. |
| Pro-agility drill (20 metres) | Start midway between two cones that are 10 metres apart. Face forwards. Turn and sprint to one cone, touch the floor, turn, sprint to the other cone, touch the floor and return to start line. |
| Slide board with blocked direction change | Start in the middle of a slide board. Push laterally to slide the length of the board. Stop quickly without losing balance at the end. Reverse direction. |
| Overhead retrieves (tennis ball thrown overhead) | Stand in the ready position (see chapter 8) facing a server. The server throws a tennis ball over your head. When you hear the ball bounce just behind you, perform a hip turn (or other appropriate action) to turn and retrieve the ball. |
| **SESSION 2: QUICKNESS** | |
| Modified ultimate Frisbee | Play a small-sided game with two opposing teams. Players throw a Frisbee among themselves. The aim is to pass when static and move quickly into space to receive (or intercept) a pass to move down the pitch. |
| Crazy ball 21s | A crazy ball (or similar object with an unpredictable bounce) is thrown in the air. Track each bounce and score 1 point by catching the ball before it starts to roll. First player to 21 points wins. |
| Knee boxing | Stand in ready position an arm's length from a partner. Hit the inside of your opponent's knees with your hand whilst using footwork to avoid being struck yourself. |
| Compass race | Stand in the middle of a 10-metre circle with a partner. Eight points of the compass are marked by cones. Race with your partner to be the first to the correct cone when the direction is called. |
| **SESSION 3: SINGLE-LEG STANCE** | |
| Linear hop and hold | Hop as far as possible in a straight line. Land in a balanced static position before performing the next hop. Perform five to eight repetitions on each leg. |
| Single-leg shuffle on agility ladder | Start at the side of rung 1. Hop into the ladder, then diagonally forward to the far side, then laterally back into the ladder on rung 2 and so on down the length of the ladder. |
| Single-leg medicine ball rebound throw | Stand 1 to 3 metres from the wall in a single-leg stance with knee slightly bent. Throw the medicine ball as hard as possible against the wall. Catch it whilst maintaining a stable position. Change legs. |
| Cable supported single-leg squat | Using an appropriate resistance on the cable machine, perform a single-leg squat using the load to counterbalance the movement. |

Note that *phase* is a representative term. This process does not have defined landmarks that mark progression, but rather transitions. A novice athlete will become more developmental or exhibit fewer traits associated with the cognitive stages of learning as he or she becomes more confident and competent. In the same way that postural control can be assessed (see examples in chapter 6), so can movement skills, and practitioners should develop tools for evaluating athlete progressions in key movement and strength tasks based on the technical models presented in the following chapters.

During this phase, the focus remains on the core movement patterns for specific aspects of speed, agility, landing, jumping and functional

**Table 7.7** Random (Variable) Approach to Movement Skill Development Within a Tennis Programme

| SESSION 1 | |
|---|---|
| **Drill** | **Description** |
| Z-pattern run | Cones are placed 2 metres apart in a zigzag pattern. Run between successive cones, alternating the cut-off foot inside each cone. |
| Single-leg shuffle on agility ladder | Start at the side of rung 1. Hop into the ladder, then diagonally forward to the far side, then laterally back into the ladder on rung 2 and so on down the length of the ladder. |
| Crazy ball 21s | A crazy ball (or similar object with an unpredictable bounce) is thrown in the air. Track each bounce and score 1 point by catching the ball before it starts to roll. First player to 21 points wins. |
| Double foot bridge (chapter 10) | |
| **SESSION 2** | |
| Modified ultimate Frisbee | Play a small-sided game with two opposing teams. Players throw a Frisbee among themselves. The aim is to pass when static and move quickly into space to receive (or intercept) a pass to move down the pitch. |
| Pro-agility drill (20 metres) | Start midway between two cones that are 10 metres apart. Face forwards. Turn and sprint to one cone, touch the floor, turn, sprint to the other cone, touch the floor and return to start line. |
| Single-leg medicine ball rebound throw | Stand 1 to 3 metres from the wall in a single-leg stance, with knee slightly bent. Throw the medicine ball as hard as possible against the wall. Catch it whilst maintaining a stable position. Change legs. |
| Three-point Superman (chapter 10) | |
| **SESSION 3** | |
| Linear hop and hold | Hop as far as possible in a straight line. Land in a balanced static position before performing the next hop. Perform five to eight repetitions on each leg. |
| Knee boxing | Stand in ready position an arm's length from a partner. Hit the inside of your opponent's knees with your hand whilst using footwork to avoid being struck yourself. |
| Overhead retrieves (tennis ball thrown overhead) | Stand in the ready position (see chapter 8) facing a server. The server throws a tennis ball over your head. When you hear the ball bounce just behind you, perform a hip turn (or other appropriate action) to turn and retrieve the ball. |
| Stir the pot (chapter 10) | |
| **SESSION 4** | |
| Slide board with blocked direction change | Start in the middle of a slide board. Push laterally to slide the length of the board. Stop quickly without losing balance at the end. Reverse direction. |
| Compass race | Stand in the middle of a 10-metre circle with a partner. Eight points of the compass are marked by cones. Race with your partner to be the first to the correct cone when the direction is called. |
| Cable supported single-leg squat | Using an appropriate resistance on the cable machine, perform a single-leg squat using the load to counterbalance the movement. |
| Cable woodchopper (chapter 10) | |

strength. Where appropriate, however, the transitions and links between different aspects of movement can be explored and developed. For example, direction change may start from or lead into a jump after the specific take-off, landing and acceleration patterns are well developed in their own right.

Practices become more open as the athlete is subjected to variation in environmental pressures. Such variation may include considerations often not thought of in traditionally closed-skill environments such as the weight room. For example, in a unilateral stance, after the athlete is competent at the basic movement pattern of a split squat, variation in complexity can be achieved through adding a dynamic movement (e.g., a lunge pattern) or increasing the length of the kinetic chain by performing an overhead split squat or performing an overhead pressing action into the squat.

Examples of how planned variation can be achieved in the development of movement skills is further explored in table 7.8, which provides insight into the progressions outlined in more detail in the practical chapters that follow.

During the practice phase of learning, the athlete achieves success and familiarity with the basic techniques and is able to perform them automatically. Conscious thoughts for athletes now focus on what skills to use, when to execute them and how to link specific skills. When possible, practice structure should be made increasingly more open and more competitive to further learning.

## Games-Based Approach to Practice

The understanding of when to use specific techniques is often best developed not through drills but by a games-based approach that encourages decision making and provides a range of options from which an athlete has to choose. Since the early 1980s, much work has been undertaken in the coaching and educational fields about teaching games for understanding as a learning approach.[10] The games-based method originates from the idea that a technique may be successfully executed in more than one way and that skilled performances might better arise from individualized differences to the technical

**Table 7.8** Sample Methods for Achieving Variation in Movement Skill Practices

|  | Complexity of movement | Intensity of movement |
|---|---|---|
| Strength movement | Increase the number of joints involved in the action<br>Transition from a static base to a dynamic base<br>Increase the number of movement planes involved (e.g., use an uneven loading on a barbell) | Increase load<br>Increase lever arm in body-weight exercises<br>Increase velocity of the action (e.g., drop faster under the bar in a drop snatch) |
| Jumping action | Decrease ground contact time<br>Include multidirectional jumping action<br>Add equipment to coordinate with (e.g., hurdle) | Increase jump and drop height<br>Increase landing speed<br>Change from double-leg landing to single-leg landing |
| Speed and agility drills | Add transition between movements<br>Increase need for reaction speed or increase number of decisions to initiate movement<br>Increase pressure on movement time (decrease time, decrease space)<br>Increase movement options (e.g., available means to change direction around an opponent) | Increase movement velocity (best achieved through competition!) |

model. The other central tenant of this method is that drill-based approaches to technical development typically do not involve the decision making and problem solving required to execute a technique as a skill. In transferring movement skills to a sporting context, this applied ability is a central pillar of athletic success.

Using games to develop movement skills and understanding transfers the focus of the athlete away from asking, 'What is the skill and how is it performed?' to a more motivationally enhancing climate in which the activity (and probably increased fun!) can be emphasized rather than the correct movement pattern. This approach does not mean that technique coaching is ignored, only that athletes need to identify for themselves what techniques work and why and, equally important, which techniques don't work. To achieve this objective, athletes need to be placed in situations in which decision making is required to achieve a successful outcome.

The bull rush game (some cultures refer to it as sharks and minnows) is an example of a game that could be used with an athlete who is at the developmental stage of learning agility skills. Bull rush could be used to supplement the drill progressions provided in tables 7.6 and 7.7. In bull rush, a 'matador' stands in the centre of the ring. The matador has to identify and tempt an individual from a group of 'bulls' to run past him or her into a safe area without being caught. To catch the bull, the matador uses a single- or double-handed touch. Typically, bull rush is played in an area roughly 20 by 10 metres, but the size can be adjusted depending on the age and number of players involved. If the bull is successful, all the bulls cross the area and the matador has the chance to catch one of the bulls. Any bull who is caught becomes another matador; thus, over time the space available to the bulls decreases, increasing the need for spatial awareness and speed and agility skills to exploit the space. Note that with larger groups of athletes, having numerous small games is better than having one large game to increase the frequency of opportunity to participate.

This simple game can have conditions added to change the focus by emphasizing different aspects of chaotic speed. For example, inserting a scoring zone into the area to be crossed allows the bull to earn additional points (for example, a 'life') if he or she runs through this area. This condition focuses the athlete's attention on identifying target spaces within a playing area that can and should be targeted at every opportunity.

A similar emphasis can be placed on tactical awareness and decision making when the matador has to face away from the bulls and call a random number to determine which bull is attacking. When the matador faces away, the bulls can arrange themselves in any way in the safe zone so that when the matador turns, the matador is forced to scan and react to the starting positions of the bulls. If there is more than one matador, tactical awareness in terms of positioning and communication becomes important in achieving success. This practice can also be linked to sport-specific skills; for example, the matadors have a ball they throw among them. The bull has to be tagged by the ball held by a matador, but the ball can be passed only when a matador is stationary. This scenario emphasizes acceleration, deceleration, pass, catch and reacceleration aspects of sport-specific skill.

Another variation is to narrow the middle zone that the bull runs through. The athlete must encounter and evade a matador; in a wider space the bull may simply be able to outpace the matador depending on starting position and ability. The important concept is that the condition imposed on the game reflects the specific outcome that the programme requires. Each game should be stopped at regular intervals, and the athletes should be questioned so that they can reflect on their actions and thus enhance their learning.

Both the drill-led approach (which places the technique at the centre of the learning process) and the games-for-understanding approach (which places the context at the heart of the learning process) offer benefits. The reality for programme development is that both aspects have relative merits and should be included in the early stages of learning any skill. This mixed approach ensures that the athlete begins to shape individual variations of a technique whilst understanding how and when to best use it.

## Guided Discovery

A coaching method that goes somewhat towards combining aspects of both the drill and the games approaches is the guided discovery technique. Using this method, practitioners establish a drill or practice pattern and then use questions to guide or shape the athletes' learning and thus influence subsequent performance attempts. Effective questions are those that direct the athletes' focus to a particular aspect of the skilled performance, either the decision-making process or the technical aspects of a particular movement or skill execution.

During this stage of learning, the manner in which the practitioner delivers feedback to athletes also needs to change. As athletes develop competency, they typically need feedback less frequently. Similarly, the precision of both the instruction and feedback typically needs to increase. Questions are a particularly effective means of getting athletes to focus on their own performance. For example, when using games to develop jumping or agility skills, the practitioner delivering the session needs to use effective questioning to stimulate thinking about the game and the movements exhibited to progress the learning of the athletes and shape their skills.

## Autonomous Phase of Skill Learning

The apex of the learning pyramid is the autonomous phase of skill learning when skills are performed as automatic action, with little or no need for conscious thought from the athlete.[9] Indeed, many would argue that, in advanced performers, consciously thinking about how to execute an automatic skill during

---

# Asking Effective Questions

Ask questions that raise awareness and promote responsibility. Use *what* questions first:

- What did you do differently this time?
- Tell me what you felt in that movement.

Follow with questions that explore the following aspects:

- Where were you looking to help you decide where to move?
- When did you feel your heels coming off the floor as you descended?
- How much force do you think you used to push into the floor to jump upwards?

Or progress to asking for further explanation:

- Tell me more about how you felt the weight distribution change through your foot in the clean pull.
- Describe in more detail exactly where the bar was when you felt the weight shift forwards from your heels.

For less-experienced performers, you may direct their attention towards a specific focus. Relate feedback specifically to the coaching points on which you instructed the athlete to focus.

For experienced performers, you may want to focus on and follow the athlete's interest. Sometimes an experienced athlete will make you aware of something you could not see or had not focussed on; for example, the athlete may say, 'That didn't feel as powerful' or 'When I land on my left leg, I feel more unbalanced than on my right.'

Try a rating scale using the athlete's anchor words or images to keep the athlete from judging him- or herself. For example, ask, 'If 1 is no push at all and 10 is the most explosive push you can give, rate your push into the floor on that repetition.'

Really listen. Use your eyes as well as your ears. Listen to intent as well as content.

Give the athlete time to answer, especially when he or she is getting used to answering questions. Think about giving the athlete another skill attempt in which to come up with the answer to your question rather than providing the answer.

a performance might interfere with the fluent and efficient action already developed.

Nevertheless, many athletes can benefit from revisiting the practice phase and consciously readdressing certain techniques to refine them. For example, as the athlete progresses through a learning curriculum for plyometrics (see chapter 9), he or she may need to re-establish landing mechanics as drill complexity increases. As the following chapters illustrate, the autonomous stage doesn't pertain only to experienced athletes. With simple movement skills, learning can progress to this stage quickly. As technical complexity advances, the athlete will regress to a previous stage of the learning continuum until he or she achieves competency at that particular movement.

At this advanced stage of the learning process, the athlete typically requires little external feedback from the practitioner about how to execute a particular skill or technique. Therefore, the feedback has to be precise and directive to bring about meaningful change in the athlete's motor behaviour. In the weight room, for example, this feedback may relate to specific aspects of timing of joint actions that may be influenced by increasing loads on the bar for athletes who have undertaken a sound and progressive strength-training education.

Indeed, at this stage, the coach is helping the performer identify specific requirements for improvement. The coach needs to tap into the performer's knowledge of him- or herself to influence progress. Questioning athletes and discussing their answers at this stage of learning is an important part of the coaching process.

In terms of speed and agility movements, as table 7.9 illustrates for a soccer player, the nature of drills now has to be based on realizational movements, that is, the application of specific techniques to enhance performance in the game context. Athletes must automate some prerequisite techniques before they are subject to challenge and refinement in an open practice environment. Players will then be able to focus on how specific aspects of the environment might influence the skilled execution of the techniques rather than on the techniques themselves.

In particular, the athlete needs to contend with three environmental stimuli that will ultimately influence the decisions made relative to skilled execution:

1. Positional stimuli: the position of opponents, teammates, the ball
2. Velocity stimuli: the speed at which players or the ball is moving
3. Acceleration data: the rate of change in velocity and its influence on ball movement or the change in available space

The ability to develop and ultimately use such skills effectively can arguably be developed only through open and games-based practices.

To challenge the athlete's ability to perform skilful movements in the sport context, open practices need to be the focus of sport-specific practices. The technical staff can focus on what is being done as the athletic development professionals focus on how it is being done (i.e., how the athlete is moving). Practices can be highly integrated and sport specific. An appropriately high level of variation can be used in practices, requiring a wide and random distribution of drills.

Typically, this variation is achieved by moving technical practices that previously had been the focus of movement-specific skills training into a warm-up or preparation. For example, in a functional strength-training session, an overhead squat is an excellent exercise to develop functional postural control throughout the kinetic chain. After it is habitualized and executed easily, the overhead squat becomes an excellent potentiating exercise that involves full movement ranges and neuromuscular activation when used during a warm-up for other (loaded) exercises within a functional strength-training session. Similarly, full-range maximal velocity running technique drills can be used to activate and mobilize joint musculature in preparation for sessions that involve a lot of running activity.

## Training Principles

Much of this chapter has focused on the progressive learning of skills within a movement skill progression. Although these considerations

**Table 7.9**   Prerequisite Movement Patterns for the Development of Open Practices in Soccer

| Objective | Movement pattern | Specific prerequisite movement technique | Example practice format | Observational analysis and feedback |
|---|---|---|---|---|
| Initiation | Start to front<br>Start to side<br>Start to the rear<br>Change of direction | Acceleration pattern from these points:<br>Athletic position<br>Cross-step, hip turn<br>Drop step<br>45- to 180-degree turn<br>Cut | Lose the marker: The defender must keep in contact with an attacker in a marked zone from a static start. The attacker responds to a ball played into the zone. | Did either player select the appropriate technique to initiate the movement? Did the player execute the appropriate technique? |
| Transition | Jockeying<br>Move rearwards<br>Deceleration<br>Tracking diagonally | Side shuffle with hip turns<br>Backpedal<br>Decrease stride length with braking action to athletic position<br>Cross-step, diagonal backpedal | 3v2 and 2v1 games: Starting on the halfway line, attackers have to get the ball to the goal line to score, but the ball must be passed one, two or three times before a point can be scored. | Was the player positioned appropriately relative to the opponents? Did the player react to the correct cues in terms of where and when to move? Did the player execute the appropriate technique? |
| Actualization | Acceleration<br>Maximal velocity | Acceleration patterns from various initiation positions<br>Transition from acceleration | Attacking movement drill: The ball is played to the attacker, who comes off the defender to pass the ball back to another player before turning and accelerating onto a 20- to 30-metre diagonal ball into space. The attacker controls the ball, passes to a teammate on the wing, turns and reaccelerates into the penalty box for a cross. The defender has to react to the attacker's movement but cannot leave a defensive zone. | Did the player react correctly to the stimulus of the ball? Were the acceleration mechanics correct? Were the maximal velocity mechanics correct? |

are a major part of a curriculum, for the physio-mechanical qualities of skilled movement to progress, the programme needs to follow certain principles of training that allow the body to adapt to the training stimulus.

Training is based on a series of activities or exercises performed systematically to improve the physical abilities and skill acquisition connected to the performance of a sport.[5] All training effects are based on exercise-induced changes in the organism at a variety of levels, and each change specifically depends on type, intensity and duration of exercise.

This book has consistently focused on the idea that training equals learning, an important concept to remember when planning programmes. Every practice represents a learning opportunity for the athlete. The athlete's physiological capacities (as opposed to the neural networks of skill learning or cognitive functions associated with tactical development) need to be overloaded in some fashion to stimulate development. The nature of this overload depends on the nature of the training stimulus, which will be graded depending on the athlete for which it is targeted.

The neuromuscular system and the respective subcellular components adapt in highly specific ways but only to the demands (adaptive stress) imposed on them by the training load (the volume–intensity interaction). How each particular physiological mechanism responds specifically to a positive stressor is considered in the early chapters of this book. For a more comprehensive and detailed explanation of this process, see Stone, Stone and Sands (2007).[5]

# Summary

Earlier chapters focused on how the human body is engineered to produce athletic movement. The concept of measuring postural control to provide some baseline analysis for programme initiation was explored in chapter 6. The following chapters detail the training methodologies that can be progressively introduced to enhance or maximize the athletic movement of a sport performer. But the key to the success of an athletic movement programme is not just what is in the programme but also how the training methods are structured and sequenced within the programme to optimize the learning and adaptation processes.

This chapter explored several key features of programme design based on the need to individualize training prescription according to the athlete's stage of learning and training status. This concept is as important in a group setting as it is when working one on one with an athlete. Indeed, although the athletic development professional may work with a squad or team, he or she needs to remain focused on the idea that the athletes need to be treated as individuals if they are to progress physically.

The environmental manipulation of practices is important if a skill is to be progressed from a technique to a sport-specific application that can be used effectively under pressure. This manipulation can be achieved by making skills more open (subject to externally determined variables) or by introducing concepts related to games that can enhance tactical awareness or technical understanding.

Competency is a key determinant of when to progress or provide additional challenge to a technique. Competency is a key theme in the successful teaching of athletic movement control and the methods explored in the following chapters, whereby movements can be progressed or regressed in complexity or intensity depending on the capability of the individual athlete.

# CHAPTER 8

# Developing Running Speed and Agility Skills

In all arenas, sport performances have evolved continuously since competition became formalized and training modalities were developed to enable performers to push themselves to excel. Indeed, most sports have become more dynamic. The success of a play is often now determined by the intensity of action that the performers can achieve.

Running speed and movement agility are two performance characteristics that have been shown to correlate positively with game intensity[1] in team and invasion sports. Running is the principle form of locomotion in many sports and is thus regarded as a fundamental motor skill.* Running is a ballistic mode of locomotion consisting of alternating phases of single-leg support (foot in contact with the ground) and flight, which occurs from toe-off to the beginning of the support phase of the contralateral leg. (See the sidebar Running Gait Cycle.) By contrast, walking has no flight phase, and the support phase alternates between single- and double-foot contacts, depending on the stage of the cyclic action; therefore, walking can be considered a nonballistic action.

Technique and skill are functionally interrelated in the development of speed and agility. Indeed, an athlete's running speed, usually

regarded as a linear concept, can be determined by the technical skills and physio-mechanical abilities needed to achieve high movement velocities.[2] Agility can be understood as the skills and abilities needed to achieve explosive changes in movement direction, velocities or techniques in response to one or more stimuli.[3]

In basic terms, speed and agility are neuromuscular skills that rely on the athlete's ability to express (or resist) forces; that is, they are a movement manifestation of the athlete's functional strength. On the sport field or court, this strength is translated into sporting movements, and it can be improved in every athlete with correct coaching. Understanding movement and the way in which it changes with the performance context and the athlete's level of development is essential when developing a speed and agility programme.

This chapter has three progressive aims. First, it enables an understanding of the biomechanical principles of running speed and agility so that the practitioner knows the factors that need to be influenced to enhance an athlete's movement speed. Second, it introduces some basic technical models that can be used to analyse and develop the athlete's skill when executing movement. Third, it provides some examples of skill practices that can be used to develop the athlete towards the required technical model.

Many resources focus on the provision of drills for developing both speed[4] and agility.[5]

---

*As explored in chapter 3, mastery of fundamental motor skills is considered a precursor to their application in sport-specific contexts. Conversely, a lack of proficiency is recognized as a key reason for not participating in, or dropping out from, organized sport.

# Running Gait Cycle

In the running gait cycle, leg speed is influenced by arm action.

The cyclical and rhythmical movement includes three phases:

1. Drive phase: One foot pushes off the ground, and the other knee is forward.
2. Flight phase: Neither foot is in contact with the ground.
3. Ground contact phase: The lead foot is in contact with the ground.

The knee drives forwards as the opposite leg extends under and behind the body, bringing the ankle close to the buttocks as it moves forwards under the body. The ankles remain dorsiflexed (toes pulled towards the knees) in flight and through ground contact.

Stride length, the distance between toe-off on one foot and ground contact of the other foot, is determined by the force of the push into the ground. In sprinting (figure 8.1), the aim is to keep the centre of mass over or in front of the ground contact point.

The speed of running influences the running technique. Sprinting (figure 8.1) is different from slower running (figure 8.2). In sprinting, the heels don't contact the ground; the ball of the foot contacts the ground, and the toes are pulled up towards the knees. In slower-paced running, moving over the flat foot is generally considered an economical, energy-saving way to run, but individual styles vary. More of a heel–toe contact is evident in many runners.

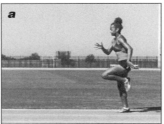
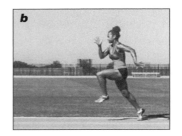
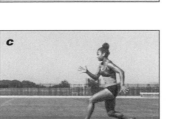
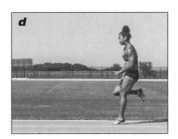

**Figure 8.1**  Gait cycle, sprinting: *(a)* stance; *(b)* toe-off; *(c)* flight; *(d)* ground contact.
Courtesy of Loren Seagrave.

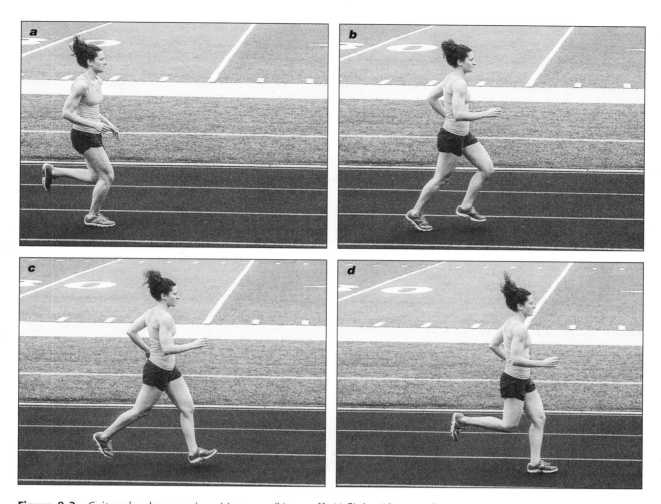

**Figure 8.2**  Gait cycle, slow running: *(a)* stance; *(b)* toe-off; *(c)* flight; *(d)* ground contact.

Without understanding and principles, these practices simply become drills to be followed; they cannot be progressed, regressed (as per the principle of differentiation based on competence) or usefully contextualized within an effective coaching programme. A holistic approach characterizes practitioners who will have the greatest success in enhancing the athletic qualities of their athletes.

# Biomechanics of Speed and Agility

To understand movement speed and agility, the practitioner must understand not only the athlete's technique but also the objectives of the skill being exhibited. These techniques and

objectives are underpinned by management of forces and therefore require an operational understanding of the concepts of impulse, momentum, velocity, acceleration and deceleration that were introduced in chapter 4. The athlete's control of posture (chapter 5) is also crucial in appropriately placing the centre of mass relative to the base of support and in optimizing the length, velocity and tension relationships in the musculature as a function of joint positioning.

Postural control helps the athlete maintain stability, making it easier to accelerate or decelerate while executing particular actions, such as when achieving full extension of the driving leg in the initial phases of acceleration mechanics. Indeed, the inverse relationship between stability and mobility is important to understand in the context of enabling accelerations from different positions.

Running is a cyclic activity that consists of a series of contralateral strides that launch the athlete's body as a projectile. Running speed is simply a relative concept relating to the distance that the athlete travels within a given period. Therefore, analysing sport-specific running-speed requirements is a concept of the relative intensity of the activity. The marathon runner who achieves the fastest speed over the 26 miles, 365 yards (42.2 km) of the course will win the event, in the same way that the baseball player who can beat the ball thrown to first base will be safe, whereas a slower player will be out.

The more intense the action requirements are, the greater the velocity of movement is required and the more explosively the athlete needs to be in applying forces to the ground to execute a movement. The intensity of running is usually differentiated into sprinting and submaximal activities. Sprinting requires the athlete to achieve maximal accelerations and maximal velocities, usually over brief distances and for brief durations. This chapter focuses on this specific running-skill requirement.

Outside track and field, sport-specific speed is largely determined by the variation in movement velocities and the direction of the movement required, giving rise to the concept of chaotic speed, the ability to sprint repeatedly and change direction efficiently without unnecessarily slowing down. Chaotic speed is a determinant of successful sport performance in field and court sports as shown by time and motion and coaching analysis and validation of testing batteries for elite and nonelite performers, and coaching analysis for sports such as rugby, field hockey, soccer and American football.[3]

Therefore, in most athletic contexts, chaotic movement, or agility, is as important an athletic quality as maximum velocity. Indeed, in court-based sports such as tennis and volleyball, agility is the key movement skill for a performer. The nature of required agility also changes with different sports (figure 8.3). For example, in invasion sports such as rugby, soccer or American football, the predominant requirement is the ability to accelerate into a space that either is occupied by an opponent (in a tackle context) or will create a territorial advantage (i.e., by moving into and attacking available space). Court sports such as tennis and volleyball are slightly different; the player needs to move into a position to intercept and return a ball and then decelerate to regain a position of stability from which to play a returning shot.

Many athletes also need to achieve optimal speed, the maximal velocity that the athlete can maintain, and still be able to control the execution of key sport-specific skills. For example, the critical speed variable for the long jumper isn't the maximal velocity he or she can attain during the run-up to the take-off board; it is the velocity at which the jumper can maintain control of the centre of mass and effectively apply force into the ground to change the trajectory of the centre of mass (i.e., jump) during the last three strides of the run-up. Spending lots of training time trying to achieve a maximum run-up velocity of 10 metres per second may be unproductive if the jumper's optimum take-off velocity is 7 metres per second. That doesn't mean maximum velocity should never be trained for, because by raising the maximum velocity threshold the range of optimal speeds that can be controlled may also increase. The point here is to consider how much emphasis to place on maximum velocity within the training programme and where it fits into the athlete's overall development plan.

Sprint coach Percy Duncan often described the difference between running and sprinting this way: 'You run on the ground; you sprint over it.' As the athlete accelerates by pushing the foot into the ground, the velocity of the centre of mass increases and the ground contact time decreases. A trained athlete typically requires 0.6 seconds to achieve maximal force production, but typical ground contact times in running are less than 0.2 seconds (submaximal running) and less than 0.1 seconds in maximal sprinting. Impulse and power are important training qualities for the athlete to develop; the resulting change in momentum is a product of the force produced and the time for which that force is applied.

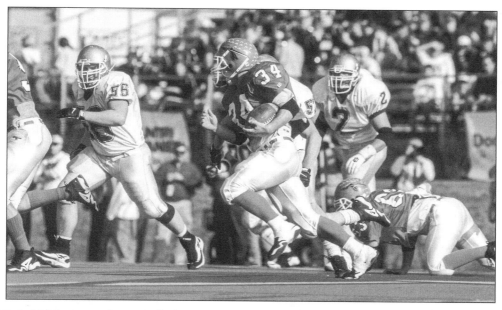

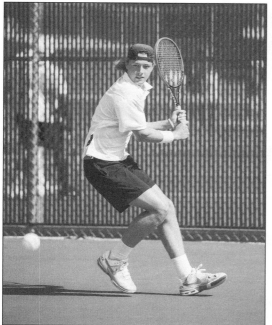

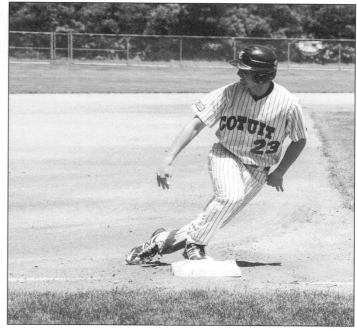

**Figure 8.3**  Sport-specific speed is a product of movement velocity and agility.

Plisk[2] illustrates that the mechanics of running should be analysed in light of how each of these variables influences performance. For example, more *force* is needed to accelerate and decelerate a predetermined mass (for example, the athlete's body) at a greater rate, more *impulse* is needed to achieve a greater momentum in a set period (for example, the time available to accelerate into space between opponents), and more *power* is needed achieve a higher maximum velocity with a set resistance (for example, the athlete's mass).

The ability to achieve high movement velocities requires skilful force application across a spectrum of power outputs and muscle actions that need to be developed within the overall context of the athlete development programme. High rates of force are developed predominantly through the stretch-shortening cycle that underpins explosive strength development (see chapter 9). In a running context, joint stiffness, particularly in the ankle, is essential to maximize the plyometric responses in the leg muscles, especially in the hip extensors of the rear kinetic chain (as explored in chapter 5). These forces, which may be many times body weight,[6] are transmitted through a single-leg stance. Therefore, the athlete's technical proficiency and functional strength need to be addressed simultaneously within the development programme to prevent injuries.

Developing positive, or acceleration, forces is not the only consideration in training for sport. For example, when decelerating, eccentric strength (especially in the knee extensor muscles in the thigh) is important in rapidly and effectively overcoming inertia to reduce the forward momentum in the athlete's body without injury (Newton's first law). The ability to produce high power outputs (high force, high velocity) is particularly important when collisions are a fundamental part of the movement problem, because the opponent's body mass has to be either decelerated (defensive move or tackle) or accelerated (offensive collision), depending on the context.

Movement efficiency is the result of the mechanical actions of the body in sparing metabolic activity that relies on the athlete's postural control, in particular the relationship between the centre of mass and the base of support. As shown in chapter 1, the stability of an object (i.e., its resistance to movement because of external forces) is inversely related to its mobility (i.e., its ability to move), a concept important to understand in the context of enabling accelerations from different positions.

To accelerate from a static position or to change direction when the body is moving, the athlete has to be able to move the centre of mass outside the base of support (i.e., move into a more unstable position). To decelerate, the opposite is true, and the athlete needs to bring the centre of mass back towards the base of support and create more stability. As shown in figure 8.4, deceleration is achieved by reducing stride length, increasing both stride frequency (number of times the foot is in contact with the ground) and the foot surface area in contact with the ground (increasing frictional braking force). Lowering the centre of mass as the trunk becomes more upright brings the centre of mass back inside the base of support.

Acceleration (figure 8.4a) requires instability. The centre of mass must be outside the base of support in the intended direction of motion. Deceleration (figure 8.4b) requires stability. The centre of mass must be brought within a wide base of support, and friction must be increased to retard forward momentum.

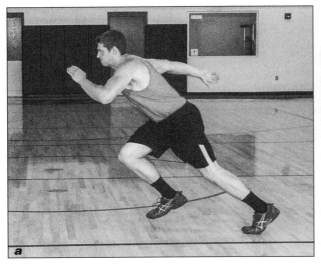
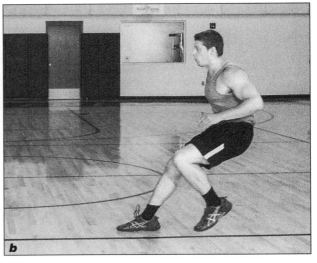

**Figure 8.4** The relationship between mobility, stability and the potential for changes in velocity: (a) Acceleration requires instability; (b) deceleration requires stability.

# Sport-Specific Running Requirements

Maximal velocity running is unsurprisingly best illustrated through the 100-metre sprint race, and the technical model for the various phases of a sprint performance in any sporting context is based on this. The application of speed within field sports, however, is typically quite different from the nature of speed in a linear track race. This consideration is important when developing programmes for athletes in a range of sporting contexts.

Those working within a particular sport should be familiar with activity analysis of a sport or event. In many cases, published papers provide this evidence for the coach, showing, for example, the number of accelerations, number of maximum sprints, number of transition movements as well as the sequencing, distances and patterns of such movements. Understanding such patterns is important, because the technique required for each activity will be different. Equally important, the transitions between activities should be smooth, effective and efficient.

Table 8.1 demonstrates the following phases to the movement pattern throughout the 100-metre sprint. This concept has been simplified to illustrate the phases of the race by relative distance, when in reality they should be looked at relative to time (for example, an athlete should have achieved maximal acceleration by 2 seconds). This makes analysis much more individualistic.

- **Reaction time (RT)**: This phase comprises the delay between the stimulus (i.e., the starter's gun being fired) and the first movement response (in this case derived from a sensor in the starting blocks) in the athlete. In a linear sprint activity such as the 100 metre, this phase is probably unrelated to the final time achieved. Practitioners should note that reaction time is not considered particularly trainable,[7] but it needs to be distinguished from reactive ability, which is a product of neuromuscular system excitability that can be improved through reactive and explosive

strength training (e.g., plyometrics, as explored chapter 9). As demonstrated later, in an agility context the training of reaction time is different and is an important part of 'skilful agility'.

- **Acceleration phase**: During this phase the athlete has to overcome inertia from a standing start to achieving the greatest rate of acceleration. This phase usually takes 8 to 10 strides, or 15 to 20 metres. Note that track athletes still accelerate (increase their velocity) after this point, but the rate of acceleration slows, as illustrated in table 8.1.

- **Transition phase**: This phase, which usually lasts for 2 to 2.5 seconds, represents the neuromuscular link between pure acceleration and maximum velocity running and the transitioning between the different technical requirements for each phase. The IAAF sprints editor and renowned coach Loren Seagrave often refers to this as the most difficult phase to coach, because the athlete often retains acceleration mechanics too long or, equally inappropriately, incorporates maximum velocity mechanics into the action too early.

- **Maximum velocity phase**: Typically, sprint coaches analyse this phase of the race in two sections. In phase 1, quality sprinters usually achieve maximum velocity around 40 to 60 metres and maintain it for around 20 metres. In the second maximum velocity phase, usually around 60 to 80 metres, the athlete slows very slightly as he or she tries to maintain maximal velocity. (Note that female sprinters are usually less able to hold this speed than males are.[7]) Sprinters can achieve maximum velocity earlier than this (and do so for specialist sprint races, such as the indoor world championships run over 60 metres), but those who achieve their maximum velocity too early through the 100 metres struggle to achieve a good overall time because they cannot maintain this velocity long enough. Table 8.1 shows that Usain Bolt achieved his highest velocity between 60 and 80 metres in achieving the then world record (12.42 metres per second).

- **Speed endurance phase**: Although commentators in a 100-metre event talk about athletes 'pulling away from others' in the last 20 metres of the race, this doesn't actually occur because of active acceleration. During this phase of the race, athletes decelerate because they cannot maintain maximum velocity. The athletes who are seen to be pulling ahead are actually just decelerating less than their opponents are, as shown in table 8.1. In contrast, the activity analysis of field sport athletes shows different patterns of acceleration, deceleration and maximum velocity that are determined both by the positions the players play and the opportunities available for movement on the field at any one time. As figure 8.5 illustrates, technological advances in athlete tracking enable individual player activity profiles to be established. Such analysis typically shows that field sport athletes sprint 10 to 30 metres, or for 2 to 3 seconds, which means that to be effective, they need to be able to achieve maximum velocity much quicker than the track athlete (even though maximum velocity will ultimately not be as quick, or held for so long).

Therefore, high-speed movements in sport often can be characterized by an activity sequence that enables the athlete to manipulate the temporal and spatial situations encountered in a game. Such sequences are typified by transitions from acceleration to deceleration and corresponding changes in movement direction to exploit space, manipulate opponents or achieve technical advantage (i.e., be better placed to execute a desired action). In this context sport-specific speed might be described as the following:

- **Acceleration**: The initial movement response is acceleration, often from an already moving position, such as a walk, submaximal run or landing from a jump.
- **Deceleration**: In many movement sequences in field sports, space is initially limited, so periods of rapid acceleration are often followed, after a couple of metres or a second, by a (rapid) deceleration. Deceleration may enable the athlete to achieve a more advantageous body position to execute another movement skill (for example, to change direction) or to initiate a movement response in an opposition player to create some space or uncertainty in the defender's mind and therefore improve relative positioning.

**Table 8.1** Analysis of the 2009 100-Metre Men's World Championship Final, Berlin

| Start | Acceleration phase | | Transition phase | | Maximum velocity phase | | | | Speed endurance phase | | |
|---|---|---|---|---|---|---|---|---|---|---|---|
| | | | **TYPICALLY 20 TO 40 M** | | **PHASE 1: TYPICALLY 40 TO 60 M** | | **PHASE 2: TYPICALLY 60 TO 80 M** | | **TYPICALLY 80 TO 100 M** | | |
| | Reaction time (s) | 20 m (s) | Velocity 0 to 20 m (m/s) | 40 m (s) | Velocity 20 to 40 m (m/s) | 60 m (s) | Velocity 40 to 60 m (m/s) | 80 m (s) | Velocity 60 to 80 m (m/s) | 100 m | Velocity 80 to 100 m (m/s) |
| Bolt | 0.146 | 2.88 | 6.94 | 4.64 | 11.36 | 6.31 | 11.98 | 7.92 | 12.42 | 9.58 | 12.05 |
| Gay | 0.144 | 2.92 | 6.85 | 4.70 | 11.24 | 6.39 | 11.83 | 8.02 | 12.27 | 9.71 | 11.83 |
| Powell | 0.134 | 2.91 | 6.87 | 4.71 | 11.11 | 6.42 | 11.70 | 8.10 | 11.90 | 9.84 | 11.49 |
| Bailey | 0.129 | 2.92 | 6.85 | 4.73 | 11.05 | 6.48 | 11.43 | 8.18 | 11.76 | 9.93 | 11.43 |
| Thompson | 0.119 | 2.90 | 6.90 | 4.71 | 11.05 | 6.45 | 11.49 | 8.17 | 11.63 | 9.93 | 11.36 |
| Chambers | 0.123 | 2.93 | 6.83 | 4.75 | 10.99 | 6.50 | 11.43 | 8.22 | 11.63 | 10.00 | 11.24 |
| Burns | 0.165 | 2.94 | 6.80 | 4.76 | 10.99 | 6.52 | 11.36 | 8.24 | 11.63 | 10.00 | 11.36 |
| Patton | 0.149 | 2.93 | 6.76 | 4.85 | 10.58 | 6.65 | 11.11 | 8.42 | 11.30 | 10.34 | 10.42 |

The durations provided for each phase of the race are illustrative as described in the text. At an individual level, these would be analysed according to time, not relative distance.

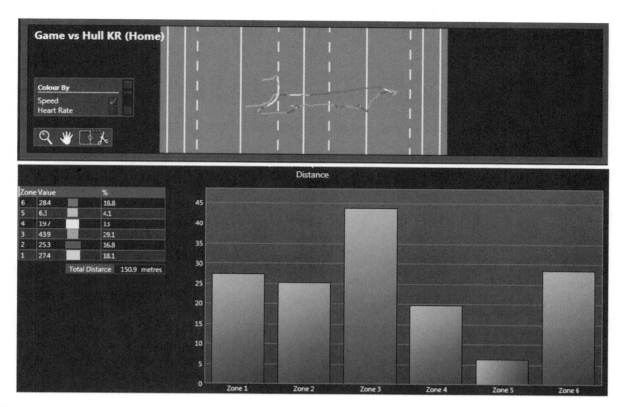

**Figure 8.5**    A movement speed profile for an elite rugby league player during one passage of game play.

- **Direction change**: The player may change direction to exploit or create space in response to an opponent's body position or a change in the direction of play.

- **Reacceleration**: The greater the rate of acceleration that the player is able to achieve, the more he or she is able to exploit the space or time available.

- **Maximum velocity**: Field players can typically attain their maximum velocity within 10 to 30 metres. After a space has been created (for example, a defensive line breached), athletes usually run in a straight line, because it is the quickest way to cover the ground between where they are and their objective (goal, scoring zone).

Understand such sequencing is a necessary generalization, because the nature of agility movements is determined by the specific athletic situations at a particular time in the sport context. Athletes need to have the movement tools in their toolboxes so that they are prepared to solve any problem. (Specific techniques to consider when developing this toolbox are explored later in this chapter.) Practitioners should be prepared to incorporate reactionary responses into the start of movement sequences as practices become increasingly sport specific.

The initiation of sporting movements is important to consider, because the effectiveness of a starting movement often determines how successful the successive stages of the movement are. Therefore, linking decision making to starting positions and mechanics is important. The situational nature of skilful agility movement responses is so idiosyncratic that the perceptual and cognitive components that initiate the skill cannot be ignored. A number of possible reaction and decision-making situations can be incorporated into skill development practices depending on the context being trained.[8]

Simple conditions (no spatial or temporal uncertainly) apply to closed-skill situations in which the performer entirely determines the execution of the skill. Examples include the execution of a particular skill during a routine, such as a walkover sequence on the balance beam.

In temporal situations (no spatial uncertainty, but temporal uncertainty) the athlete knows where to go but not when to react. The easiest example is the sprint start, in which the performer responds to a single stimulus with a set response.

In spatial situations (no temporal uncertainty, but spatial uncertainty) the athlete knows when to go, but not where to go. An example is a soccer goalkeeper reacting to a set-piece move such as a penalty kick. The goalkeeper knows when to dive but is trying to determine in which direction and at what height to dive as the penalty taker approaches the ball. In tennis the player waiting to receive the serve knows when the ball will arrive, but the attacking player may vary the speed, direction and height of the serve.

Universal situations (temporal and spatial uncertainty) are the most common in field sports. The positioning of the opposition and the emerging play determine where and when the athlete moves. The relative movement of attacking and defending players alike depends on the decisions made by those in possession as the play unfolds. The relative positioning of other players influences the space available and the relative timing of particular actions.

# Technical Models for Specific Running Skills

Whether accelerations are from a static start or a transition from submaximal running, or maximum velocities are achieved over 50 to 60 metres or 10 to 30 metres, the technical model on which these skills are applied is the same for athletes in both track and invasion game contexts. Remember that 'correct technique' does not necessarily look the same for every athlete, and experienced practitioners need to adapt the technical model (the description of the ideal technique) to suit the individual anthropometrical and physio-mechanical qualities of each athlete to achieve the desired efficient motion.

Sound technique is a prerequisite for an athlete to begin to run well and develop optimum speed. The technical model is based on putting the posture in the optimum position to achieve the objectives according to the laws of physics and the mechanical properties of the human motor system. Skill is not just reliant on technique; it is also intrinsically linked with the athlete's motor capacity, in particular the neuromuscular qualities related to rate of force development. The athlete's programme should develop technique in tandem with these qualities to ensure optimal development.

# Running: Important Features of the Skill

Running is not just a fundamental movement skill. Observation of children in free play shows that it is normally a child's preferred method of moving between two points.

A fundamental movement skill can be characterized as mature when all the component parts of a motor pattern are integrated into a well-coordinated, mechanically correct and efficient act.[9] An effective athlete development programme facilitates refinement and advancement of the basic movement pattern.

The running action is not typically considered mature until a child is approximately 7 years old (biological age). At this stage the neuromuscular system (and hence motor coordination) is undergoing intensive development. Despite this, the basic running action of children at this stage is natural and does not differ from the critical features of the technical model for experienced athletes.

This running action is one that we might see in an adult jogging, a marathon runner racing or a games player moving around a field when not involved in the immediate action.

This section introduces the mature action of running (i.e., the basic technical features). This action is typified by the late childhood stages, and therefore many of the basic errors described here are often seen in children as they progress. Later in the chapter, specific technical detail will be presented for technique considerations in relation to acceleration and maximum velocity phases of the advanced, high-speed running model.

## Mature Running Action

In the drive phase of a child's mature running action (figure 8.6), the posture is upright and has a slight forward lean. The forward lean is achieved through the entire posture; it does not result from the child bending forward at the waist. In the initial stages of movement, greater acceleration results in a further forward lean. The head remains up, and the eyes face forward, which enables the child to scan the environment while moving and keep the posture optimally positioned. Head movement, especially side to side, detracts from both the ability to see in the direction of travel and the forward momentum of the body as a whole.

Arms are surprisingly important in running. A contralateral action (opposite arm and leg forward at the same time) prevents rotations

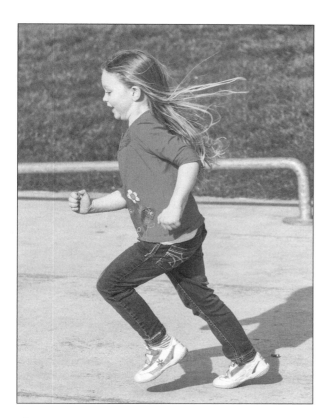

**Figure 8.6** The drive phase in a mature running action of a 7-year-old in a playground game.

about the hips and trunk. Therefore leg speed is influenced by arm speed. This relationship can be illustrated to the sceptical athlete by taking him or her through the following activity sequence:

1. The athlete jogs on the spot, keeping the arms by the sides.
2. In response to the 'Go' command, the athlete moves the feet as fast as possible whilst keeping the arms by the sides.
3. After 3 to 5 seconds, a second 'Go' command is given, at which point the athlete moves the arms as well as the feet. The athlete will feel the rate of leg turnover increase as the arms are engaged in the action.

The elbows are bent to approximately 90 degrees and move through a path that keeps them close to the sides of the body. The arms drive from the shoulders in a backwards direction with no accompanying trunk rotation. A slight extension of the elbows may occur with the backwards momentum of the arm. At the extent of the rearward drive, the stretch reflex in the biceps and anterior shoulders causes the arm to drive forcibly forwards without an active or voluntary movement on the part of the child. The athlete develops this movement as the arm action becomes more forceful, and it is not something that necessarily needs to be 'coached into' the child. A common error seen in the arm action is for the arms to swing forwards across the body, causing unwanted rotations in the transverse plane through the trunk. Similarly, a child who does not drive the arms backwards from the shoulders may develop an action in which the arms bend and straighten from the elbows only, an action that is much less forceful and therefore not beneficial.

## Running Gait Cycle

The running movement is cyclical and rhythmical. In the drive phase, one foot pushes off the ground as the knee is forward on the other leg. The knee drives forward as the driving leg extends under and behind the

# Common Errors in Children Developing a Mature Running Action

Slumped posture (rounded back), 'sit in a bucket' posture.

Arm action is not coordinated with the legs.

Arms swing across the body, causing rotation.

Arm drive is from the elbows (arms bend and straighten), not from the shoulders.

Knee is driven high, not forward.

Ankle does not come under the buttocks in a straight line but comes out to the side as it passes under the body.

The leg reaches as it comes into the ground so that overstriding occurs (ground is contacted too far in front of the centre of mass).

Toes are pointed in flight so that the child contacts the ground with the toes first.

---

body. As the knee drives forward, the ankle remains dorsiflexed and is brought as close to the buttocks as possible as it moves forward under the body. This positioning reduces the moment arm between the pivot (the hip) and the ankle, conserving angular momentum and increasing the speed at which the leg can rotate. This positioning also reduces the energy involved, making the action more efficient. In the flight phase, neither foot is in contact with the ground. The ground contact phase is entered as the lead leg comes into contact with the ground and lasts until the drive phase commences in that foot.

The length of the stride—the distance between toe-off on one foot and ground contact of the other foot—is determined by the force of the push into the ground. Typically, stride length is the product of both the athlete's strength and the length of the limbs. Limb length changes relative to trunk length as the child grows, meaning that changes in stride pattern are evident as the child progresses through the various stages of growth. The length of the legs relative to the trunk determines the optimal running position for the athlete. For example, the multiple world and Olympic 200-metre and 400-metre champion Michael Johnson ran with a technique different from the conventional technical model because of the length of his torso relative to his legs.

## Developing Running Technique in an Athlete Development Programme

The running component of athlete development programmes typically does not attempt to develop stride length as a function of technique because such attempts often lead to overstriding, a common error in which the athlete reaches forward with the leg coming into the ground. Ground contact then occurs a long way in front of the centre of mass, which decelerates the athlete's forward movement. Indeed, in efficient maximal velocity running, the horizontal distance between the centre of mass and the contact point of the foot during impact should be as short as possible.

Instead, a focus on the ability to develop and use neuromuscular strength through technique will enable the athlete to develop an optimal stride length for his or her physique. The practitioner should find a range of practice activities that encourage the athlete to run whilst contacting the ground with the foot under the body, examples of which will be introduced later in this chapter.

The speed at which the athlete runs influences the optimal technique that the athlete will exhibit. In acceleration, for example, the athlete needs to have a forward body lean to keep the centre of mass in front of the base of support (i.e., the feet). The resultant force vector accelerates the body forward. In high-speed running or sprinting, maintaining this position isn't possible, but the aim is to keep the centre of mass over the ground contact point as much as possible. In distance running, in which the velocity of movement is much less, this forward lean isn't necessarily a consideration until the athlete needs to accelerate for a sprint finish. At more energy-sparing paces, the athlete tends to adopt a more upright running posture.

The speed of movement also typically influences the nature of the ground contact. In sprinting, much of the foot surface should contact the ground (enabling a large surface area through which to generate ground reaction force) without the athlete's heel making contact. The practitioner leading the technical development programme should be conscious of the coaching cues provided to the young athlete. 'On your toes', for example, is a commonly used coaching term, as is 'on the balls of your feet'. In reality, both of these cues encourage the child to use a part of the foot with small surface areas to contact the ground, reducing the potential for forceful ground contact. Analogies such as the credit card rule—'I always want to be able to get just a credit card between your heels and the ground when you run'—may be more appropriate for developing the foot contact into the ground.

At slower running speeds, when the efforts are submaximal in terms of speeds, not cardiovascular effort, ground contact is usually different and similar to the walking action. The athlete typically contacts the ground with the heel first, rotates through a flat-foot position at midstance phase and then onto the forefoot for toe-off. This heel-to-toe action is considered more energy sparing and absorbs more ground reaction forces, which is important when multiple foot contacts occur in longer-distance running.

In adults, for example, the transition from walking to running generally occurs at a speed of 2.3 metres per second to make locomotion more efficient. At 2.5 metres per second, the stride rate increases by 44 per cent over that seen in walking, and the stride length increases by 15 per cent as the flight phase becomes more pronounced. Increased flexion occurs at the knees and hip joints, and flexion continues to increase with the velocity of movement.[10]

A common error is 'sitting in a bucket' (i.e., sticking the hips backwards and leaning forward from the trunk). This posture is usually most evident as an inefficient athlete changes speed. Ground reaction forces aren't optimized because hip drive is limited, and forces are not effectively transferred through an object or structure that isn't straight. Similarly, a rounded shoulder position in the forward lean is often seen in younger athletes. This posture detracts from the optimum sagittal plane shoulder drive and should therefore be discouraged. Activities such as overhead medicine ball marching or overhead stick running (figure 8.7) are excellent postural activities for correcting this practice.

The opposite arm and leg forward action, with a fast, short arm movement throughout, should be maintained. A leg action that is not coordinated with the arms will result in a clumsy, nonfluid movement that will have visible rotations in the transverse plane. As the lead leg moves forwards, the knee should drive forwards as the foot leaves the ground. Simultaneously, the ankle dorsiflexes, so that the knees are pulled towards the toes in flight. The greater the running speed is, the closer the ankle should be towards the buttocks to enable a rapid rotation underneath the body. This transition from rear-side mechanics (from midstance through push-off to the drive leg passing underneath the body) to front-side mechanics (the lead leg accelerates towards the floor to ground contact) should be smooth, and an active transfer of weight should occur between the legs through an unsupported flight phase. The ankle should remain dorsiflexed during the flight, ground preparation and ground contact phases.

The knee and ankle movements during this action are common sources of error in young athletes. For example, as the athlete prepares for ground contact, the toe may be pointed towards the floor (the ankle is plantarflexed). The toe then makes ground contact, meaning that the movement is inefficient. Subsequently, the muscle actions of the gluteus maximus and calf muscle complex are liable to be inhibited.

The forward movement of the knee is also important. The knee should be driven forward

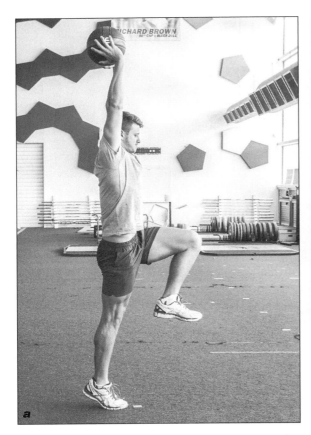 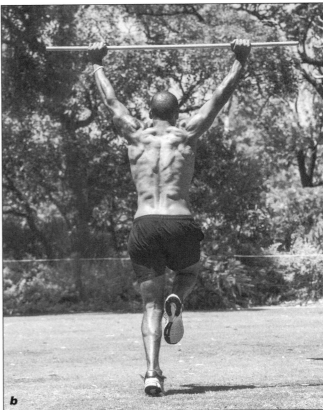

**Figure 8.7**    Postural running drills such as *(a)* the overhead medicine ball march and *(b)* overhead stick runs are excellent means to encouraging sound postural mechanics.

with the ankle pulled towards the buttocks rather than driven high. Typically, the high knee action changes the athlete's body lean from one slightly forward to upright or even rearwards, especially with athletes who have tight hamstrings and overactive hip flexor muscles. Some traditional coaching drills, such as butt kicks and high knees, develop inappropriate knee positions that do not benefit the athlete in high-velocity running. Although these drills are often touted as useful dynamic stretching activities, practitioners can use alternative means of achieving these stretches without developing inappropriate running responses in athletes.

# Running Activities to Develop a Mature Action

As children develop towards a mature action, they move through several stages of progression as the flight phase becomes more evident,

stride lengths become more even, and the extension of the driving leg following push-off becomes more complete. These characteristics can be aided by fun activities that encourage the child to explore different ways of running and then progress towards exploring how to run efficiently and effectively at various speeds and in different directions. Such practices can incorporate running within many game contexts and specific sporting situations.

The small, tall, high, low, fast, slow game is such a developmental activity that is appropriate for a medium-sized group of young children who might be at different stages of running skill development. The objective of this practice is for children to identify how running technique is influenced by changes in the running action and speed. This practice also develops spatial awareness and stamina.

In getting children to relate their actions to technique outcomes, practitioners need to

---

# SMALL, TALL, HIGH, LOW, FAST, SLOW

## Coaching Points

- The speed at which you move will influence your technique.
- Keep your head level and still.
- Keep a straight body position.
- Maintain a fast, short arm movement and hold the elbows bent at 90 degrees and close to the sides of the body.
- Drive the leg downwards and backwards as if striking and pushing the ground.

## Equipment

Place dish markers to define the boundary of the playing area. The specific size of the playing area depends on the number of players, but an area of 15 by 6 metres is typically suitable for 8 to 10 children.

## Organization

The children spread out around the playing area, which should be big enough so that the children can run around without bumping into each other and without limiting the speed they can achieve. The instructor tells the children to jog around the space while remaining aware of where the others are; they need to run with their heads up. The children are told to run towards space and avoid other children throughout the activity.

As the children run about, the instructor shouts instructions to them every 5 to 6 seconds, telling them to run in different ways, such as the following:

- 'Run tall': Children try to maintain a tall and upright body posture as they run.
- 'Run small': Children bend their bodies and assume a crouched position while running.
- 'Run fast': Children run as fast as they can within the area.
- 'Run slow': Children run slowly but don't walk.
- 'Run with big steps': Children try to run with as long a stride as possible.
- 'Run with short steps': Children try to run with as short a stride and as many foot contacts as possible.

The instructor should alternate between more demanding and less demanding running actions. After 30 to 45 seconds, children get a short rest break during which they are encouraged to think about and reflect on how they moved.

---

encourage pupils to think about (perhaps by calling out) the different parts of their bodies that contribute to a high or low posture, including balls of their feet, torso, head and arms. Asking questions ('Tell me' or 'Show me') is useful in getting children to identify what body parts change when they change pace and to consider whether the change is effective or ineffective in making them better runners.

Although running is the primary focus of the activity, spatial awareness can be developed by altering the space available. The children

need to have sufficient space to run at full pace but not so much space that they don't have to avoid others as they move. Visually impaired children can be integrated into drills of this nature if they can partner with a sighted child who is bound to them with a ribbon or cord.

To develop high-quality, high-speed actions and benefit endurance, many short sprints are better than a few long sprints, and children will recover quickly between efforts.

Simple playground games are highly effective means of developing context-specific speed and agility in children who have more mature actions. Multidirectional running in sport involves making a decision about where to move, accelerating towards that space and then maybe decelerating, changing direction and accelerating again. Games such as rats and rabbits develop these skills in a fun and interactive manner that encourages children to want to execute these skills at maximal intensities. After all, if someone is racing or chasing them, children are motivated to move faster and change direction more quickly.

Such games commonly lead the practitioner to focus on the outcomes of the game (who scored points, how many, who won) and cause the children to focus on the strategies they used to achieve the points. But the focus should be on how the children move rather than where and when. The coach will have to use effective questioning strategies to get the children to identify how they moved to accelerate or decelerate effectively.

A variation on this structure is to organize the group into two parallel lines and set up

---

# RATS AND RABBITS

### Coaching Points
- Keep your head up so that you can see what is going on around you.
- Accelerate into space by leaning forward but keep your posture straight; don't lean forward just from the upper body. Keep your tummy tight.
- Accelerate by taking small strides that get longer and pushing into the ground with the balls of the feet.
- Decelerate by leaning backwards and taking smaller strides, pushing into the ground with a flat foot or heel.

### Equipment
- Cones to mark boundary areas
- Mats or other equipment to mark safe areas
- Bibs or shirts to distinguish between two teams

### Organization
Set up a playing area that has defined boundaries. Players must stay within the playing area. The area should be large enough to allow players to run around without restraint but small enough that players have to dodge other children while moving. Within the player area, mark safe areas for players. The size and number depends on the space available and the number of children playing. These safe areas form a warren for the rabbits and a nest for the rats. Divide the group into two teams, the rats and the rabbits.

Children spread out evenly in the playing area. The instructor starts the game by telling the children to move around wherever they want. Children can be made to run, walk, skip, hop, and so on as part of the game if variations are desired.

The instructor calls out either rats or rabbits. When 'Rats' is called, the rabbits have to run to the safe areas (or warrens) and the rats have to try to catch them by tagging them. When 'Rabbits' is called, the rats have to run to their nests before the rabbits tag them. The number of rabbits or rats that are able to go into one safe zone should be limited to make it more challenging (i.e., maximum of one or two per safe area, depending on equipment and numbers). This rule forces the children to identify their options and move to those areas quickly.

For every player who makes it to the safe area without being tagged, the escaping team scores 1 point. For every player who is caught, the chasing team gets 1 point. The first team to score 20 points wins. (This figure can be adjusted depending on the number of players.)

five evenly spaced cones approximately 20 metres away from the rabbits and five cones approximately 20 metres away from the rats; these areas act as a warren and a nest. This setup encourages more linear speed and less reactive decision making, but it is an option for practitioners who wish to focus a practice more on developing running speed and mechanics and less on dodging, multidirectional speed and decision making.

# Advancing a Specialized Running Action

Running speed can be seen as a product of power and neuromuscular coordination. As described in chapters 1 and 2, the interaction of the neuromuscular and musculoskeletal systems to put the posture into the correct position to exert and transmit forces can be thought of as technique. Within the athlete's movement development programme, speed, therefore, isn't simply about developing good running mechanics. Technique has to be coupled with developing the athlete's ability to produce great forces and apply them in the proper direction within a very short period. Therefore, technical development must be considered in parallel with the progression in the rate of force development that the athlete is able to achieve.

As with all forms of training, a long-term planned process must be in place to enable the child to progress from a mature skill to the more advanced levels of technical development that characterize high-level athletic performance. The programme must have structured progressions that move from structured play to deliberate practice and involve the progressive development of biomotor abilities linked with technical competencies to develop specific movement competencies.

## Developing Acceleration Technique

As with any advanced skill, the look and feel of the athlete's acceleration action can progress from the basic skill (outlined in the technical model for a mature action) to an automatic presentation of excellent technical characteristics of an advanced model. To accomplish this progression, the learning conditions must be right, the athlete must have the appropriate physical capacities to execute the powerful skilled action, and the athlete must have the motivation to practise towards excellence. Typical progressions that might be observed as the athlete becomes more competent at acceleration mechanics (and indeed accelerating) can be seen in table 8.2.

Analysis of any world class 100-metre race will demonstrate that elite sprinters achieve more than 80 per cent of their maximum speed by the time that they have sprinted 20 metres. As noted earlier, many team-sport athletes need to be able to reach maximal velocities within very short durations or distances.

Acceleration mechanics are best understood by the realization that, regardless of the context in which he or she is moving, the athlete needs to increase the magnitude of horizontal propulsive force to overcome inertia and increase power output and then speed (figure 8.8). The athlete needs to adopt a posture that will enable him or her to push hard, and often, into the ground, so that ground reaction forces can propel the athlete forward. This action means longer ground contact times and a high stride frequency. Indeed, one of the most effective prompts that can be given to an athlete in the first few steps of accelerating is to focus on nothing other than 'push, push, push' into the ground.

In chapter 4 the physics of good acceleration technique were explored. The athlete looking to overcome inertia and create horizontal momentum needs to exert equal amounts of horizontal and vertical force into the ground. For this reason, accelerations typically require the athlete to have a marked forward lean and to begin to accelerate from a low body position that will rise to a higher one as the athlete achieves maximal velocity. Many sports require athletes to accelerate from different start positions, whether upright or from a crouched position (such as the three-point stance of the linebacker in American football or the sprinter exploding from the blocks). The key focus for practices looking to develop speed from either

**Table 8.2**  Progression Towards Advanced Acceleration Competence: Athlete Development Model

| PROGRESSIVE DEVELOPMENTAL MARKERS | | | | | | | |
| --- | --- | --- | --- | --- | --- | --- | --- |
| Maturing | | | Developing | | | Refining | |
| Ready active position: staggered feet, low centre of gravity, forward body lean | Ability to push off (downwards and backwards action) with feet | Effective falling start technique with straight-line body position maintained as gravity assists acceleration | Quick reactions and rapid acceleration from a variety of starting signals | Posturally able to hold and accelerate from a crouch start; front knee bent to 90 degrees and rear leg at 120- to 140-degree angle | Balance and control from sprint start, with short, powerful and progressively lengthening strides | Rear foot brought through and down quickly and forcefully (with a forefoot contact) to commence second stride | Push off with both front and rear foot |
| Strongest foot forward, rear foot about shoulder-width behind, opposite foot and arm pattern | Accelerate quickly from a variety of static positions (standing, lying down, kneeling and so on) | Bring rear foot through low to drive | Posturally able to hold and accelerate from an effective three-point start | Rapid forward movement of the rear leg in the drive phase as the body maintains an effective forward lean | Low body angle maintained while driving out of the start position | Feet kept low and driven back with a down-and-back piston-like action in the first 5 to 8 strides | Fluid start into drive phase with the transition and then the full flight running phases |
| Response to a simple starting stimulus ('Go') | Demonstrate basic (shallow angle) falling start with balance and control | | | | | Gradual rise of body from stride 7 or 8 to full height by stride 14 to 17 with smooth transition | |

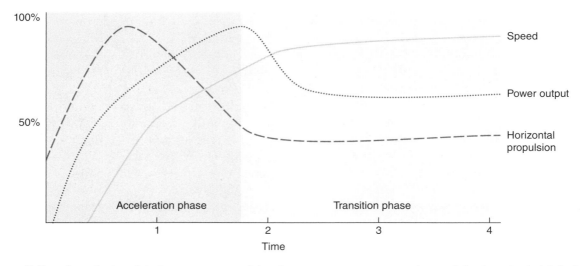

**Figure 8.8**  The relationship between propulsive force, power output and speed during the initial phases of a sprint.

position is to place the athlete into the optimal position to take the first three strides.

The starting and initial driving mechanics should place the athlete in a position where two definitive consequences must occur. First, the athlete's centre of mass must be in front of the base of support. Second, the hips must be placed in a position from whence one leg can powerfully move forward whilst the other leg can forcibly extend, thus providing the initial impulse into the ground or the start blocks.

As can be seen in both figures 8.9 and 8.10, the shoulders of the athlete are directly above or in front of the hands in the different stances. In the three-point stance, this setup is facilitated by hips rising to a level above the shoulders, inclining the trunk forward. In this position,

the weight is fully on the athlete's hands, and the athlete will feel as if he or she is ready to go forward. The athlete's centre of mass is outside the base of support, making him or her unstable. As the athlete begins to drive forward, the rear leg pushes hard into the ground but moves rapidly forward, with a short stride, so that it is quickly repositioned in front of the body where the ball of the foot can contact the ground. Simultaneously, the front leg pushes for a longer period so that maximum extension in the leg is achieved before the next foot contact.

Games players typically accelerate from an upright position, such as the athletic ready stance (figure 8.11), which may or may not be static. The athletic ready position is a standing start position that is taught across many sports

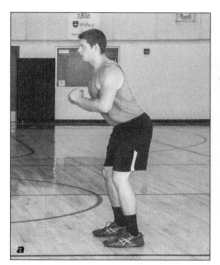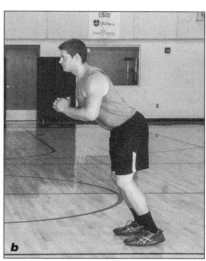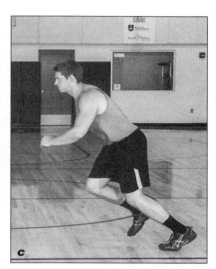

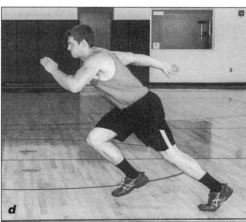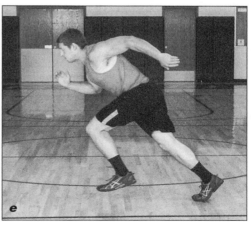

**Figure 8.9** Starting mechanics from a crouched position: *(a)* position of optimal preparatory support; *(b)* optimal starting position with weight moving forward; *(c)* hands and shoulders rise in preparation for the first stride; *(d)* rear leg push is hard and fast; *(e)* rear leg pushed to full hip extension.

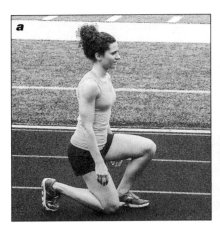
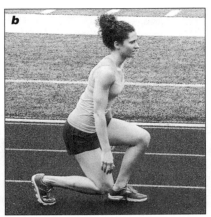
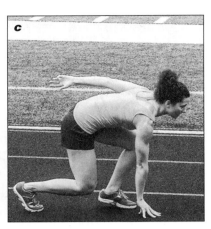

**Figure 8.10** Positioning the athlete for a three-point stance: *(a)* kneel upright with the knee of one leg level with the instep of the other foot; *(b)* raise the hips vertically; *(c)* fall forward so that the weight is on the fingers and the shoulders are in front of the hands.

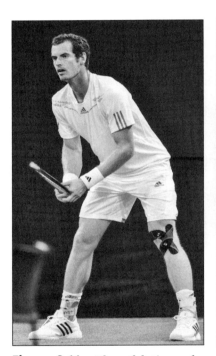
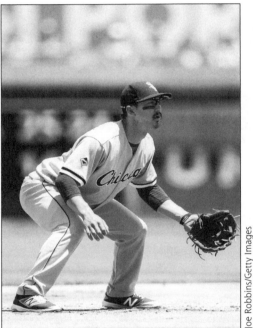
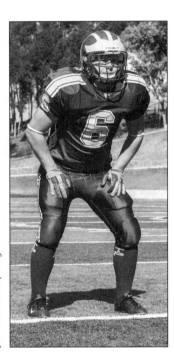

Joe Robbins/Getty Images

**Figure 8.11** The athletic ready position.

as a preparatory stance for movement in any direction. With the weight evenly distributed between left and right feet, and the hips and shoulders level, the athlete should be ready to move in any direction. In such a position, achieving instability in the direction of travel (i.e., the forward lean that places the centre of mass in front of the base of support) is harder. The temptation may be to achieve this by leaning forward from the waist, but this approach disrupts the straight-line body position that is most effective for transmitting ground reaction forces (figure 8.12). The athlete cannot wait for the trunk to lean forward before applying the propulsive effort from the hips; thus, the principles of the movement remain the same but the resultant action may look slightly different depending on how the athlete is able to prepare for the movement. But to accelerate forwards, the ground contact must always occur behind the centre of mass. The closer the contact is to the line of vertical action of the centre of mass, the greater is the resultant vertical force that a step will produce.

The athlete is looking to produce high propulsive forces in a short time to produce a high impulse that overcomes inertia in the centre of mass. To do this, the large hip extensor muscles in the gluteal and hamstring groups need to contract concentrically, followed by the powerful knee extensors in the quadriceps. The length of the athlete's stride is determined at this stage by the magnitude of the force provided with each foot contact, the direction of the force and the duration of the force. As chapter 4 detailed, if the athlete's shin angles aren't the same in the

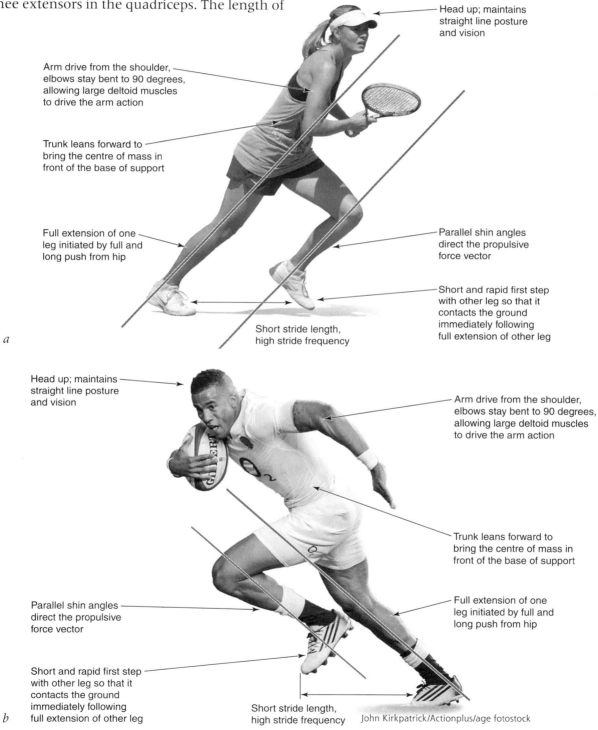

Head up; maintains straight line posture and vision

Arm drive from the shoulder, elbows stay bent to 90 degrees, allowing large deltoid muscles to drive the arm action

Trunk leans forward to bring the centre of mass in front of the base of support

Full extension of one leg initiated by full and long push from hip

Parallel shin angles direct the propulsive force vector

Short and rapid first step with other leg so that it contacts the ground immediately following full extension of other leg

Short stride length, high stride frequency

*a*

Head up; maintains straight line posture and vision

Arm drive from the shoulder, elbows stay bent to 90 degrees, allowing large deltoid muscles to drive the arm action

Trunk leans forward to bring the centre of mass in front of the base of support

Full extension of one leg initiated by full and long push from hip

Parallel shin angles direct the propulsive force vector

Short and rapid first step with other leg so that it contacts the ground immediately following full extension of other leg

Short stride length, high stride frequency

John Kirkpatrick/Actionplus/age fotostock

*b*

**Figure 8.12** Drive mechanics: *(a)* from a standing position with both feet equal; *(b)* from a jogging start.

first few steps, the resultant forces on ground contact will have a greater vertical component than desired, the result of Newton's law of equal and opposite reaction. The positioning of the athlete's body determines the resultant line of action of force. If the athlete's body position is too upright, the push into the ground will result in a more vertical reactive force and less horizontal propulsion. Conversely, if the athlete overbalances and falls too far forward, foot contact with the ground will be insufficient to generate large forces. So achieving a forward-leaning posture with as straight a line as possible between the flat foot at the end of the leg drive and the knee, hip and shoulder joints creates a powerline through the body that maximizes horizontal propulsion. Typically, during the first couple of strides, the athlete's forward lean may be as much as 45 degrees, but by the time the athlete reaches 20 metres, he or she will be in an upright position as stride length increases.

Ground contact time during acceleration is longer than that seen in maximal velocity running, but the foot contact time is still short (for example, in elite sprinters it may be 0.2 seconds for the first stride) because of the need to achieve a greater impulse at this stage of the movement. The athlete's legs should extend backwards effectively, forcefully and rapidly. The ground reaction forces cause a triple-flexion response in the hip, knee and ankle, thus repositioning the foot to attack the ground again. The ankle must be dorsiflexed in the recovery phase to position the foot optimally to contact the ground with an active flat foot (a concept fully explored in chapter 9). If the athlete contacts the ground with a plantarflexed ankle, then little surface area can be used to contact the ground and the resultant ground reaction will be ineffective in accelerating the body.

The propulsive force from the hip through the knee to the ankle and into the ground results in a triple extension of the driving leg through ground contact. Because the athlete is leaning forward, the leg action largely occurs behind the athlete, and there is little front-side mechanics to consider. Generally, as long as the duration of ground contact time isn't compromised, the higher the frequency is of foot contacts in acceleration, the more opportunities the athlete has to generate impulse. The leg action requires a piston (triple flexion, triple extension) behind the athlete; the recovery of the heel in the drive leg occurs below the level of the knee in the lead leg.

Assuming that the athlete is able to extend the hip and knee optimally through full range and the propulsive forces are appropriately channelled, stride length will increase incrementally during the acceleration phase. As the athlete's stride length increases, the shins gradually become more vertical, leading the transition into a more upright stance and maximum velocity running mechanics.

## Developing Acceleration Mechanics

Debate continues about whether acceleration mechanics are best developed through technique drills or by modifying the performance conditions under which the acceleration is performed. As with many questions relating to training methodologies, there is no definitive answer. The best programme embraces both concepts and combines them with functional strength and power development to ensure a balanced approach to acceleration development. The importance of combining speed drills to enhance technical ability with the development of athletic qualities through plyometrics and multimuscle, multijoint, high-force exercises (such as squats and cleans) cannot be underestimated in terms of developing an explosive athlete.

Resistance accelerations can be achieved either using gravity (for example, running up hills or steps) or an external resistance. Various forms of speed work can be used depending on whether the athlete is working on acceleration mechanics or maximum velocity mechanics, which is considered in the next section. Although a more conservative approach to resistance may be required for maximum velocity mechanics, the benefits for acceleration mechanics should not be overestimated.

For example, 10- to 20-metre hill accelerations up a slope that has a gradient of approximately 3 to 8 degrees can improve the athlete's ability to develop and direct propulsive forces. Because each step requires the athlete to contact the ground at a higher relative height than the last ground contact, the athlete must exert high forces into the ground. The task can really encourage the athlete to feel the need to drive backwards and apply forces into the ground to move forward.

The gradient of the slope tends to reinforce the athlete's force direction through the appropriate shin angles so that the environment itself positions the athlete, not the coach or the drill. The slope also encourages the athlete to drive the knee forward fast, with a low heel recovery, which may also have a beneficial training benefit to stride length and stride frequency when the athlete returns to running on the flat or in the normal performance environment.

A typical session for hill sprints might look something like 5 × 20 metres falling start, 5 × 25 metres falling start and 5 × 20 metres press-up start, so the total session distance is 325 metres, all at maximal intensity with complete recovery.

External resistances can be provided from sleds or cords attached to a harness or by a partner when working in group situations. A heavy external load can be used to support the athlete as he or she leans forward to initiate the movement. Indeed, for athletes who need to be encouraged to adopt a greater forward lean in the early phases of acceleration, this strategy helps them learn to accelerate from a low to high posture.

Some athletes know they can initiate forward movement simply by leaning forward. Although the forward lean is part of the required motor programme, it will not result in an explosive forward movement unless it is accompanied by the driving action from the legs. Using an external load means that simply moving the centre of mass in front of the body will not result in forward movement, so the athlete needs to focus on a highly explosive leg drive to overcome the inertia of the system mass (athlete plus resistive load). In contrast to maximum velocity mechanics, acceleration may benefit from relatively higher levels of resistance (e.g., 25 per cent of body mass) for this reason. The athlete needs to start the action consistently from the appropriate starting position to reinforce the need for sound mechanics through the driving action.

Wall sprints were introduced as an effective tool for developing acceleration mechanics in chapter 4. This series of drills is easy to introduce and can be progressed or regressed in difficulty based on the athlete's competence. The first thing to develop is the athlete's ability to create and maintain an effective ready position. The athlete stands with feet flat on the floor, ankle dorsiflexed, arms straight and the trunk leaning to approximately a 45-degree angle.

The ankle position is important, because a plantarflexed ankle will take the athlete high onto the balls of the feet (or the toes), reducing the area of the foot available for ground surface contact and therefore reducing ground reaction force. Coaches should cue the athlete to maintain the credit card rule at all times during the drill. A straight line should run from the shoulder through the pelvis (which is in neutral with the trunk braced), knee and ankle. When the athlete can hold this position, he or she is ready to progress to the ready position (figure 8.13). The front knee is punched forward (a common mistake is to take the knee high rather than forward) and the toe is dorsiflexed so that the sole of the foot is parallel with the floor. The toe should now be behind the knee so that the shin angle is the same as the body lean, and this angle should be the same in both legs (i.e., the shins are parallel). The foot in contact with the floor should remain flat, and the toes should remain dorsiflexed.

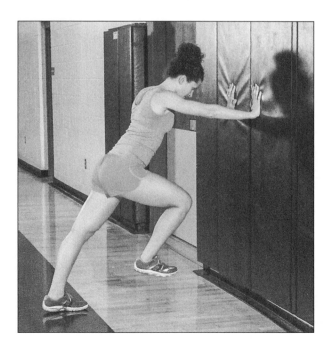

**Figure 8.13**   Wall sprint power position.

The practitioner may need to correct the athlete until the athlete feels it; an athlete who is told to get the shins at the same angle may need to look down, which will change the position of the head and the trunk. Although shin angle is a technical requirement, it is not necessarily a good coaching cue.

After the athlete can establish and statically maintain the start and ready positions, movement is introduced to the drill and then progressively increased in speed and complexity. Wall drills progress by varying the sequences between single- and double-leg support positions and by alternating between the left and right foot driving backwards to the floor. Initially, the speed of movement is not important; the maintenance of correct body position and the mechanical actions need to be consistently executed before the drills are increased in complexity or speed. Progression through this drill series is based on competency and the athlete's ability to maintain extension mechanics consistently with both legs through increasing speeds and complexities.

Postural mechanics need to be consistently reinforced during the transitions from hip and knee extension to flexion. An athlete practising this movement may lose the neutral lumbar–pelvic alignment as the knee is driven forward, especially if he or she relies too much on the hip flexor muscles. A posterior pelvic tilt in the ready position will become evident if this happens. It needs to be corrected by slowing down the movement or adjusting the temporal patterning between repetitions to enable the athlete to maintain consistent mechanics. As described in chapter 5, observing the distance between the sternum and belly button (and ensuring that this distance remains constant) might be an observational aid when delivering this drill to an athlete.

The driving leg in each progression must contact the ground with full extension. As the drill complexity increases, the athlete often loses focus on the need to drive the foot forcefully into the ground with full extension through the leg. Therefore, the ground contact occurs closer to the wall than desirable, changing the line of action of the ground reaction force (as evidenced by a change in shin angle at ground contact) and causing the athlete to lose the forward-leaning position.

# Wall Drill Progressions

### Wall Sprint Single-Leg March

From the ready position, keeping the standing foot flat (heel slightly off) and the body angle and straight-line position the same, extend the bent leg fully. Contact the floor right next to the other foot, and have the ankle in a dorsiflexed position. Initially, speed is not important; speed will come as technique becomes proficient. The key is being able to maintain the correct body position. Reset the position and repeat for repetitions on each leg.

### Wall Sprint Single-Leg Drive

From the straight-line body position, drive one knee forward (towards the wall) into the ready position with the toes dorsiflexed, positive shin and body angle, knee forward and toe behind the knee. At the top of the knee drive, the glutes fire to drive the leg towards the ground, returning the foot (ankle still dorsiflexed) to the start position. Speed can be added as the technique becomes proficient.

### Wall Sprint Two-Step

Start with one leg forward in the ready position. From here, drive the raised leg backwards to the floor and at the same time fire the knee of the opposite leg forward. Maintain all the technique points throughout this sequence. After proficiency is achieved, sequences of three or more repetitions can be added together.

When the athlete is proficient at these drills, sequences of two or more repetitions can be put together so that the athlete is forced to focus on both the forceful drive into the ground and a powerful reflex action in driving the knee forward whilst maintaining postural integrity and without altering the trunk lean.

Encouraging the games player to adopt a forward lean to start the acceleration pattern can be achieved through use of the up tall and fall drill. This practice also emphasizes the importance of the relationship between the centre of mass and the base of support in promoting accelerations or decelerations. All the technique points emphasized in the power position for the wall drills also apply to the athlete in this context. If the athlete takes a big step forward with one foot when released by the partner, this action will widen the base of support and bring the centre of mass into the middle of it, making the athlete's position very stable.

# UP TALL AND FALL

### Coaching Points

- A straight line should be maintained from the head (which should face forwards), through the shoulders, hips, knees and ankles as the athlete leans forward. Most of the foot should be in contact with the floor (the credit card rule applies to the heels).
- If the straight body position is lost (coaches should check that the head is looking forward and the straight-line body position is maintained), gravity will probably cause the athlete to stumble as he or she overbalances.
- The first acceleration steps should be short and forceful, and the athlete should achieve full and rapid extension of the driving leg with each stride.

### Equipment

No equipment is required.

### Organization

Stand with feet together and lean forward into a partner (if available), who takes the weight of the body as you lean forward. This straight-line position, with the ankles remaining in the dorsiflexed position and a credit-card-width distance between the ground and the heel, is referred to as the drive position (figure 8.14a). After the partner has your full body weight, the partner steps to one side, causing you to fall forward (figure 8.14b). (If no partner is available, maintain the correct body position and fall forward until the point at which you overbalance.) As soon as the support is removed and you fall forward, immediately accelerate away (figure 8.14c).

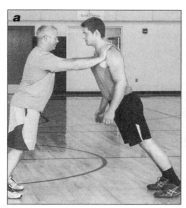 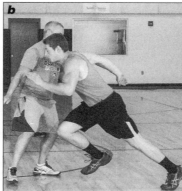 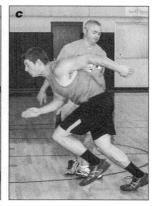

**Figure 8.14** Up tall and fall drill: *(a)* starting position; *(b)* release to drive mechanics; *(c)* release to stable position.

To accelerate during the first few strides, the centre of mass needs to be kept in front of the base of support. Therefore, the initial stride length needs to be short and powerful to assist in forward propulsion as the athlete is released. Without the feet action, the athlete will still accelerate because the motion is gravity assisted, but this acceleration will be towards the floor, meaning that the athlete will stumble and potentially fall over. This also will occur if the postural integrity of the straight-line body position is lost (for example, by the athlete looking down or 'breaking' at the hip) so that forces cannot be directed appropriately.

Using gravity to force the athlete into effective acceleration mechanics, with the emphasis on the driving action back into the floor ('Push, push, push'), is a good means of encouraging the athlete to develop technique. The partner who is spotting the starting technique doesn't push the athlete backwards when stepping sideways; the partner simply removes the support without applying a decelerating force. The athlete can also do this drill by working alone; the athlete simply leans forward, maintaining a straight-line posture, until he or she overbalances and moves the feet rapidly and forcefully to achieve an effective acceleration. Emphasize that the arm action is essential, because the arms are not constrained as they are in a wall drill. A forward leg swing requires a forceful backward arm countermovement that may be exaggerated in some instances during the first few strides.

The starting position for the up tall and fall drill can also be used to develop a resisted high-force marching drill during which each backward leg drive into the ground drives the resistive mass (the partner) backwards. The partner can provide face-to-face resistance or use a harness resistance behind the athlete, which allows the athlete greater freedom to generate a more rhythmical, if not necessarily forceful, action. Combining these approaches is effective in emphasizing force and rhythm in an athlete's technique.

These drills can be performed using a contrast technique by initially resisting the march or run and then midway through the drill removing the resistance (the partner lets go or releases the harness). Note that these drills should not be done with bungee cords if they are providing the resistive load, because the recoil from a bungee under tension can cause serious injury. Specialist release cords are available that can release tension on the harness without any undue recoil effect.

These drills work exceptionally well in an athlete who has good mechanics. Working against a resistive load encourages the central nervous system to activate (potentiate) more motor units, increasing the neuromuscular force of each leg drive and creating more force into the ground. As the resistive mass is suddenly removed, the same motor units work to exert the same forces, thus generating greater impulse and momentum with each subsequent foot strike.

Many athletes may need additional incentive to be motivated to exert maximal forces through the floor in acceleration practices. Try making the drills competitive. This approach is covered in more detail when agility and directional change are being considered (because acceleration typically follows a directional change), but introducing the concept here is helpful whilst linear acceleration drills are being discussed. The obvious means of introducing direct competition is to make a drill into a race. In doing this, practitioners must ensure that they do not emphasize performance intensity at the expense of good movement mechanics. Ultimately, athletes cannot get quicker without bringing maximal intent to acceleration drills, but they must learn good mechanics before attempting maximal efforts.

How competition is introduced is important. For example, if two athletes were supported in the start position of the up tall and fall drill and the support was removed from each on a 'Go' command, the athletes would receive a prompt that would cue them to the release instead of using gravity to trick the body into sound mechanics. But drills such as face and chase encourage colleagues to race each other over short distances following a starting practice that is designed to reinforce sound mechanical principles.

# FACE AND CHASE

## Coaching Points

- A straight line should be maintained from the head (which should face forwards) through the shoulders, hips, knees and ankles as the athlete leans forward. Most of the foot is in contact with the floor (the credit card rule applies to the heels).
- If the straight body position is lost (coaches should check that the head is looking forward and the straight-line body position is maintained), gravity will probably cause the athlete to stumble as he or she overbalances.
- The first acceleration steps should be short and forceful, and the athlete should achieve full and rapid extension of the driving leg with each stride.
- Forceful steps in the drive and acceleration phases will lengthen the athlete's stride length.
- Turning mechanics are introduced and focused on in later drills.

## Equipment

No equipment required.

## Organization

Two athletes start 5 metres apart, facing each other. Target lines are 15 metres behind each athlete. On the appropriate command or visual signal, one athlete runs to the line he or she is facing. The other has a 5-metre buffer zone in which to turn and accelerate to the same line so that the athletes are racing each other.

As the athlete's direction changes mechanics become more proficient, chase me drills can easily entertain and challenge groups of athletes in equal measure. For example, having two athletes starting 5 metres apart and facing each other with target lines that are 15 metres behind each athlete makes such drills very simple. On the appropriate command, one athlete runs to the line he or she is facing. The other has a 5-metre buffer zone in which to turn and accelerate to the same line so that they are racing each other.

Acceleration efforts (as opposed to drills that focus on acceleration mechanics) need to reflect aspects of both the starting positions from which an athlete might accelerate in a given sport and the various distances over which an athlete might be expected to accelerate (noting that anything over 20 metres is typically not going to be focused on acceleration only). Repetitions need to be done with maximum intensity and have maximal recovery between them so that fatigue does not influence movement quality.

A typical acceleration session for a team-sport athlete might be 2 or 3 × (4+1 unresisted) × 25 metres with a resisted sled followed by 1 or 2 × 4 × 15 metres with active recovery between repetitions (total session volume = 310 to 495 metres).

Besides considering how the sprints may start, the sport performer (as opposed to the track athlete) must learn to transition between movements at different speeds. For example, in sports such as soccer, the players may walk and run relatively large distances but perform only a small number of sprints (table 8.3, where a sprint is defined as exceeding 25.2 kilometres per hour). Although tactical and positional demands determine much of this contribution to the game, the player needs to be able to transition efficiently and effectively between movement speeds (i.e., accelerate and decelerate) to maximize the space available or gain an advantage over an opponent.

Drills such as hollow sprints are designed to enable the player to transition between acceleration and lower-intensity running, focusing

**Table 8.3**    Distances Covered in a 2014 Premiership Soccer Game

| Player | Total distance covered in km (miles) | Total number of sprints* | Maximal sprint velocity (m/s) |
|---|---|---|---|
| Midfield 1 | 12.62 (7.84) | 39 | 8.8 |
| Midfield 2 | 12.19 (7.57) | 55 | 8.9 |
| Winger | 11.79 (7.33) | 45 | 9.1 |
| Winger | 11.61 (7.21) | 53 | 8.8 |
| Midfield 3 | 9.81 (6.10) | 26 | 9.0 |
| Fullback | 9.69 (6.02) | 41 | 9.4 |
| Central defender 1 | 9.44 (5.87) | 25 | 8.5 |
| Central defender 2 | 9.24 (5.74) | 12 | 7.4 |

*In soccer, a sprint is regarded as faster than 7 m/s.

the player on changing body positioning and stride pattern. For each change in pace, the athlete should observably change body position to achieve a lower centre of mass and a forward lean. After each acceleration period, the posture becomes more upright as the athlete reaches maximal velocity, and this high centre of mass can be maintained comfortably for the cruising phase of the drill. But the athlete must prepare for, and execute, sound acceleration mechanics as he or she reaches each acceleration marker.

These drills are based on the athlete working over a 100-metre course that has been marked into 20-metre intervals. From the starting position, the athlete sprints for the first 20 metres, cruises or jogs for 20 metres (deceleration is passive rather than active), sprints for 20 metres, cruises for 20 metres and sprints for the final 20 metres. Recovery should be active and complete. A 4- to 6-minute walk back to the starting position might be necessary if the exertions have been truly maximal. This effort can be repeated for one or two sets of four to eight repetitions depending on the planned training volume.

Similar drills can be achieved with less residual fatigue within efforts by marking out a 30-metre course into two sections that are either 10 metres and 20 metres in length or each 15 metres in length. The athlete should transition from 50 per cent speed to maximal acceleration at the designated point of the course (at either the 10- or 15-metre mark) and sprint until the end of the 30-metre distance. Performing one or two sets of six to eight repetitions of maximal intensity (i.e., maximal quality) is appropriate for working on the development of acceleration from submaximal linear running.

Much debate has occurred among the athletic development community about how appropriate it is for the sport performer to use a drop step to initiate forward acceleration. This technique involves the performer moving from the athletic ready position through a split position to accelerate forward.

Although sending one foot backwards to accelerate forwards may seem counterintuitive, this observation is often a misinterpretation of what may be an instinctive motor response for an athlete. Performed incorrectly, the backwards movement widens the base of support and moves the centre of mass rearwards, hindering forward acceleration and making the athlete slower. But the drop, or split, step should be very short and rapid and be accompanied by a forward postural lean that initiates the forward movement of the centre of mass, placing it in front of the base of support. If performed correctly, this countermovement action can initiate a stretch-shortening cycle in the lower limb, especially with the ankle stiff and dorsiflexed, which enables a more forceful triple extensor effort in both legs. The rear leg pushes into the ground to accelerate forward rapidly, whilst the front leg pushes hard into the ground for a longer time to full extension.

Professionals have not reached a consensus about the efficacy of this technique in promoting positive acceleration. A reasonable premise is that in those athletes who do this naturally, coaching can aid and improve the effectiveness of the movement, which needs to be done very rapidly and forcefully. But the drop step isn't a technique to teach to an athlete who doesn't naturally perform it, and in those who attempt a drop step but who do not manage to execute it well, it might be discouraged.

# Maximum Velocity Running

Maximal sprinting speed is important to most sports that occur outside a court or aquatic environment. Invasion games such as soccer, American football, rugby and baseball require players to reach maximal sprinting speeds quickly and maintain those speeds for short durations to achieve a competitive advantage. The quicker an athlete can achieve maximal velocity, the more effective he or she will be in a sporting situation because of the ability to evade an opponent or create and exploit space.

Lower-leg acceleration mechanics are best related to the actions of a piston driving the body forward. Maximum velocity lower-limb mechanics are much more cyclical in nature, because contralateral activity occurs both in front of and behind the body. As with most sporting actions, correct technique is a prerequisite for an athlete to begin to run well and for optimal technical development to occur.

Maximal velocity is determined by the nature of the sport. An elite track sprinter is required to achieve speeds of up to 12 metres per second in single maximal efforts that are unconstrained by spatial considerations and the demands of any external variable that would influence a team-sport player. In sports such as rugby or soccer, sprints may be recorded as speeds that are greater than 6 or 7 metres per second, respectively. Maximal velocities in such sports may reach up to 10.5 metres per second for short durations

as dictated by game play. The sprinter is not required to undertake the additional mileage outside of sprinting that game play demands, so they will understandably be much faster and more technically proficient. But they are not as durable, or indeed as robust, as the repeat-sprint athlete needs to be.

In achieving maximal velocities, the trunk is upright and the shoulders are on top of the hips. As explained in chapter 4, the ground reaction forces are now predominantly vertical, and the athlete's posture needs to be erect and stable to transfer the vertical ground reaction forces to overcome the downward force of gravity. Therefore, the natural lumbar–pelvic curve should be evident, and the athlete's torso should be braced.

The goal of maximal velocity sprinting mechanics is to achieve a high stride frequency in conjunction with an optimal stride length. The aim is to produce an athlete who is able to produce large horizontal propulsive efforts with minimal vertical impulse, which requires specific neuromuscular qualities for the hip, knee and ankle musculature. The main concern for the athlete is to use a stride pattern that prevents negative (i.e., downward) vertical displacement of the centre of mass in flight.

Athletic development professionals need to consider this concept carefully. If the goal of acceleration mechanics is to maximize horizontal propulsion, why should this not be the same with the physio-mechanical qualities of maximal velocity running? Isn't horizontal speed still the desired outcome? The answer can be found in understanding the biomechanics of sprinting, which underpin the technical model of maximal velocity mechanics and therefore the drills that can be employed to develop such qualities.

After maximum velocity has been achieved (i.e., the athlete is no longer accelerating), the athlete's centre of mass has a lot of horizontal momentum propelling the body forwards. When running at maximum velocity, the body position is much more upright, which enables optimal mobility at the hip joint and therefore maximizes the range of movement at the thigh. Because of this upright position, the ground reaction forces are predominantly vertical. The athlete has to apply higher peak forces during a shorter contact period (i.e., the same total impulse is generated, but in less time, typically less than 0.09 seconds in an elite sprinter), and all force production is used to overcome the downward force of gravity. The athlete can keep the centre of mass high and therefore maximize stride length, the distance between the centre of mass at the point of touchdown on one foot to the position of the centre of mass at the point of touchdown on the other foot.

As shown in figure 8.15, at ground contact the ankle should be dorsiflexed so that the athlete can achieve active ground contact and maintain it throughout the ground contact phase. The supporting leg should be stiff, and no flexion should occur at the hips, knees or ankles throughout the support (ground contact) phase. The athlete needs to be able to recruit high levels of single-leg strength in sprinting, because ankle stiffness is essential if the athlete is to explode through the ground with an active ground contact.

The leg contacts the ground below the body's centre of mass. The ankle is dorsiflexed, yet the ground contact is active, a concept explored in more depth in chapter 9. For this reason, the leg should not reach in front of the body, because this will project the foot too far forward of the centre of mass (overstriding), which will effectively decelerate the body on ground contact. Indeed, all the active ground contact should take place slightly in front of the midline of the body, as the athlete is encouraged to 'tear

back the track' (a favourite cue of coach Loren Seagrave). As the foot contacts the ground, the shin should be nearly vertical as the other leg (which is in the recovery phase) is brought rapidly forward. The knees of both legs should be together as the lead leg makes ground contact.

During the propulsion phase of ground contact, the ankle joint should not push off actively. The athlete pushes through the ground following midstance, but the drive is from the hip extensors and forces transferred through the stiff leg. In particular, the gluteal and hamstring muscle groups, with their mechanically advantageous leverage around the hip joint, are essential in this action. Therefore, a sport performer needs to be functionally strong throughout this muscle group (as explored in detail in chapters 9 and 10).

If a high force is applied early in the ground contact phase, the athlete does not need to stay on the ground and attempt to apply more force into the ground through toe-off. The leg must remain stiff throughout ground contact, and, unlike in acceleration mechanics, it does not fully extend after the toe leaves the ground at the end of the propulsive phase. Indeed, as evident in figure 8.15, at toe-off the horizontal distance between the ankle and the hip is not as significant as it is during acceleration. Trying to push actively through the ankle will cause problems further up the kinetic chain that will inevitably cause overstriding and increase the likelihood of soft-tissue injuries. Stride length is effectively determined by the athlete's ability

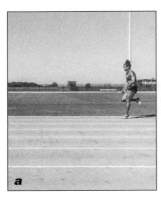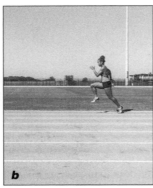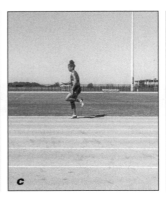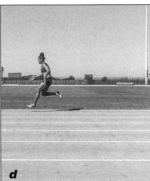

**Figure 8.15**    Sprinting technique at maximal velocity: *(a)* ground contact; *(b)* propulsion; *(c)* recovery phase; *(d)* ground preparation.

Courtesy of Loren Seagrave.

to generate vertical impulse (practical application of Newton's second and third laws) and the athlete's limb length, and is not something that typically needs to be coached.

Indeed, although faster athletes typically have longer stride lengths than slower athletes, the longer stride length is achieved with less time spent with each foot in contact with the ground. The more effective a person becomes at maximal speed running, the more power he or she is able to generate in a shorter time. Therefore, maximal velocity is principally governed by the ability to express large muscle forces using the stretch-shortening properties of the neuromuscular system whilst minimizing ground contact time. This rule suggests that the goal of an athlete development programme with respect to maximum velocity running is to improve the power output capacities of the athlete whilst reducing ground contact times.

Following toe-off, the thigh of the trailing leg immediately begins to accelerate forward as the heel begins to rise. The ankle remains dorsiflexed, and the toe is pulled up towards the knee. Ensuring that the trunk remains upright and the pelvis stays neutral maximizes the range of movement about the hip as the knee accelerates forward (not high) and the ankle steps over or crosses above the opposite knee just as the athlete approaches toe-off on the other leg. The closer the ankle can get to the butt during this movement, the more effective the forward acceleration of the thigh by the hip flexors is, because this positioning presents a shorter lever arm that conserves the angular momentum of the thigh around the hip joint.

As the knee moves to a point in front of the body and the thigh approaches horizontal, the eccentric actions of the hip and knee extensors (principally the hamstrings) block the forward movement of the thigh and begin to accelerate it negatively towards the floor in preparation for ground contact. As this happens, the lower limb moves forward of the knee joint with the ankle dorsiflexed. An active action of powerfully bringing the thigh back to generate negative footspeed now occurs (i.e., accelerating the foot down and back into the ground). Immediately before ground contact, the knee should be stabilized with an active cocontraction in the quadriceps and hamstrings as the athlete 'grabs grass' by accelerating the flat foot actively into the ground.

During this time, a weak or inefficient hamstring muscle is typically most vulnerable to injury. For this reason, as illustrated in chapter 10, eccentric and isometric hamstring-strengthening exercises, with the knee bent to approximately 140 degrees, may be beneficial in preventing hamstring injury and benefitting performance as part of the athlete's overall programme.

As table 8.4 illustrates, athletes pass through a number of progressive landmarks as their technical competence at maximal velocity mechanics improves with practice and the development of the prerequisite physical capacities.

# Developing Maximal Velocity Mechanics

A range of drills can be used to develop the cyclical action of upright running. These drills typify the three key phases of the movement: ground preparation, ground contact and efficient recovery. Developing recovery mechanics is about efficiency in the movement, not reducing the time for the recovery phase of the action. A more forceful and rapid ground contact, aided by correct ground preparation, is where time is reduced in maximal velocity sprinting.

These drills should not be limited to athletes who require maximal velocity running mechanics; they are equally important for middle- and long-distance runners who want to make their upright running posture more efficient. As the athlete becomes more proficient at these individual practices, they can be combined to provide a highly demanding neuromuscular and coordinative challenge, regardless of the mechanical benefits for running technique.

The aim of this book isn't to provide an exhaustive range of drills or practices that can be incorporated into athlete development

**Progressive developmental markers**

| MATURING | | | | DEVELOPING | | REFINING | |
|---|---|---|---|---|---|---|---|
| Walk tall with head up, shoulders relaxed and high hips | Jog and skip tall with relaxed shoulders, arm movement hip to lip, high hips, good upright posture and balance | Run tall with relaxed shoulders, sound arm action, high hips and good upright posture | Run tall at increasing pace with balanced action, relaxed shoulders, sound arm action, high hips and good upright posture. Fast and powerful (yet relaxed) arm action emphasizing the drive backwards | Maintain relaxed running technique with no visual tension at increasing velocities | Maintain technical quality at increased velocities and under increasing pressure through varied competitive demands | Transition effectively from acceleration phase into maximum velocity running | Smooth transition from explosive drive to acceleration phase, gradually rising to maximum velocity mechanics with efficient and powerful action |
| | Walk or march with knee up, heel coming underneath butt and dorsiflexed ankle action | Jog and skip with knee up, heel coming underneath butt and dorsiflexed ankle action | Run with knee up, heel coming underneath butt and dorsiflexed ankle action | High knee (thigh parallel) enabling effective swing phase during front-side mechanics | Active flat-foot strike following a powerful down-and-back motion into ground contact | Maintain postural integrity and upright, linear action (no rotational components to detract from forward momentum) | No evidence of rotational movements or postural collapse that would detract from linear velocity at higher speeds and distances |
| | | Jog and skip with good technique maintaining upright posture and no backwards lean to accommodate leg actions | Run with good technique maintaining upright posture | Active and quick down-and-back motion into touchdown during front-side mechanics | | | |
| | | | Demonstrate active strike on front of foot with no heel contact | Strong support leg (no sinking at the hip or knee) through support phase into rear-side mechanics | Execute technique drills for both single-side (left or right side) and alternating (left and right side) actions | Execute advanced technique drills including complex actions | Ability to maintain maximum velocity and mechanics for longer distances up to 150 metres |
| | | Start, stop and change pace with control in response to verbal or visual cues | Incorporate curved or bent running on top of pace change ability with no loss of control or coordination | Smooth and controlled transitions from change of pace and change of angle in running | | | High levels of self-awareness of technical execution |

progressions. Professionals, however, can use their understanding of the physio-mechanical benefits of core drills and progress them according to the principles of learning and science to develop a series of beneficial progressions.

As with many drill progressions, the best initial drills are those that can be practiced statically but can be progressed through intensities in terms of complexity and speed (e.g., skips into bounds).

## Ground Preparation Drills

Ground preparation drills emphasize the key features of upright action during which the leg is accelerated towards the ground; the emphasis is on accelerating the leg back towards the ground to contact the ground slightly in front of the centre of mass. The knee should be stiff (the coactivation of the knee flexors and extensors stabilizes the joint), and the ankle needs to be stiff and dorsiflexed.

# FAST GRAB

### Coaching Points

- Start with the knee punched forward so that the thigh is horizontal.
- The ankle remains dorsiflexed throughout the movement.
- The thigh is accelerated towards the floor, and contact is under the centre of mass without the centre of mass moving.
- The standing leg remains stiff.

### Organization

This static drill enables the athlete to reinforce ground preparation mechanics, and it emphasizes the importance of grabbing the ground with a stiff and dorsiflexed ankle. The athlete stands on one (stiff) leg next to a wall for support, with the trunk upright (figure 8.16a). The heel of the standing foot is slightly off the floor. The working leg is positioned so that the thigh is horizontal with the toe of the dorsiflexed ankle just below the raised knee. From here, the thigh is accelerated towards the floor so that the ball of the foot contacts the ground just in front of the centre of mass (figure 8.16b). The foot scrapes the floor and returns to the start position, where the movement is paused and then repeated.

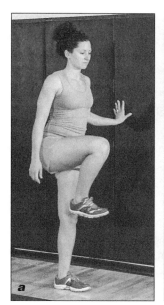 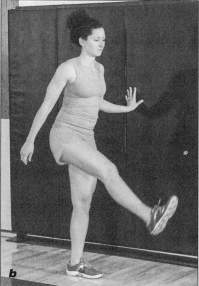 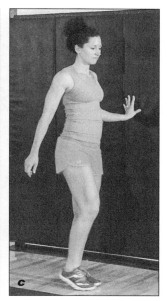

**Figure 8.16** Fast grab.

# STRAIGHT-LEG SKIP

### Coaching Points

- The drill is performed with straight legs and maintaining the opposite arm, opposite leg pattern.
- The ankles remain dorsiflexed throughout the drill.
- The ground contact is through an active flat foot.
- The athlete accelerates the leg towards the floor using the hamstrings, causing a rhythmical forward skipping movement.

### Organization

This drill is performed over a straight 30 to 60 metres. The athlete stands tall, brings a straight leg forward (with the toe pulled back towards the knee) with an opposite arm, opposite leg action (figure 8.17) and then uses the hip extensor muscles to accelerate the foot back towards the floor. Straight-leg skips reproduce the technical model of the active foot contact; the leg accelerates back towards the ground mechanically. Active flat-foot contact with the ground is below the centre of mass, and the credit card rule is applied to the foot (i.e., the heel is raised just slightly off the floor). This action accelerates the athlete forward in a rhythmical left, right skipping action.

After the athlete is strong enough in the hamstrings, the drill can progress to the more dynamic, forceful and plyometric straight-leg bound (see chapter 9) in which each successive foot contact accelerates the athlete forward.

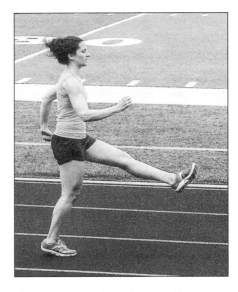

**Figure 8.17**   Straight-leg skip.

# REACH AND GRAB GRASS

### Coaching Points

- Accelerate the foot towards the floor.
- Contact the ground with an active flat foot (heel slightly off, ankle dorsiflexed) slightly in front of the centre of mass.
- The trunk should remain upright, and the athlete uses an opposite arm, opposite leg action.
- Think 'knee up, leg reach, grab the grass' during the drill to coordinate the sequence.

### Organization

This marching drill takes place over a 40- to 60-metre course. From a standing start, one knee is lifted forward. When the knee reaches its most forward point (the trunk is kept upright), the lower leg is extended forward (figure 8.18). The hamstring muscles decelerate this action as the knee reaches extension, and the athlete then 'paws' the foot down into the ground so that the active flat foot contacts the floor directly under the centre of mass ('Grab the ground'). The emphasis is on contacting the ground actively and forcefully beneath the centre of mass with each successive foot contact so that the athlete marches forward. An alternating arm and leg action is used for the duration of the drill.

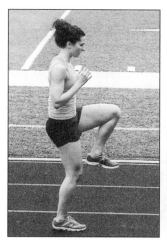
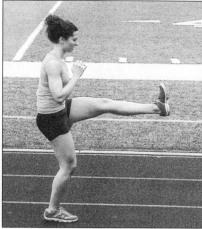
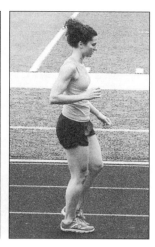

**Figure 8.18** Reach and grab grass.

## Ground Contact

Drills that emphasize ground contact mechanics are based on the need to maintain a stiff ankle through active ground contact, using the elastic properties of the neuromuscular system in the ankle joint to transfer forces from the hip extensor muscles into a ground reaction. Drills typically are based on (or progressed from) low-intensity and complex plyometric drills as explored in chapter 9.

In executing these drills, the athlete is looking to have an active and extremely rapid flat-foot contact with the ground (heels should not contact the ground; a credit card should be able to be slid under them at all times).

# DOUBLE-FOOT ANKLE JUMP

### Coaching Points
- The athlete should stay tall and not flex at the hip or knee joint at ground contact.
- The athlete should attack the floor with an active foot contact. The ankle should remain dorsiflexed in preparation for ground contact.
- The aim is to spend as little time on the floor as possible. 'Imagine you are landing on hot coals' is a good coaching cue.

### Organization
Bouncing repeatedly (without emphasizing height or distance) on an active flat foot encourages the correct landing technique to promote high vertical impulse with each foot contact. The greater the frequency that can be achieved in a small distance, the better. The athlete should stay tall and not flex at the hip or knee to generate momentum (figure 8.19). All work should be done through the elastic properties of the gastrocsoleus–Achilles complex around the ankle joint. This drill can be progressed to bounces over a 10- to 20-metre distance (encouraging many rapid foot contacts over the distance).

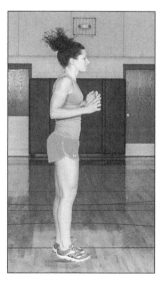

**Figure 8.19** Double-foot ankle jump.

# DEADLEGS

### Coaching Points

- The athlete should stay tall and not flex at the hip or knee joint at ground contact.
- The athlete should attack the floor with an active foot contact. The ankle should remain dorsiflexed in preparation for ground contact.
- The athlete should have a rhythmical opposing arm and leg action
- The aim is to spend as little time on the floor as possible. 'Imagine you are landing on hot coals' is a good coaching cue.

## Single-Foot Deadlegs

This drill is an alternating-leg (skipping) version of the double-foot ankle jump. In deadleg drills, the athlete stays tall with hips and knees stiff and toes pointing forward. The ground contact is rhythmically up and down with a stiff ankle and with an opposite arm and leg action (figure 8.20). The greater the frequency of foot contacts that can be achieved in a small distance, the better. Athletes, especially those with tight hip flexors, are often tempted to turn the hips outwards in this drill, which takes the foot contact out in front of the centre of mass rather than below it. This drill can be progressed to a course over a 20-metre distance (encouraging many rapid foot contacts over the distance).

Deadleg drills can also be performed by having one leg serve as the deadleg (hips and knees stiff, ankles dorsiflexed, active ground contact with the foot and the heel adhering to the credit card rule) and having the opposite leg perform other drills, such as A-skips, B-skips or straight-leg skips.

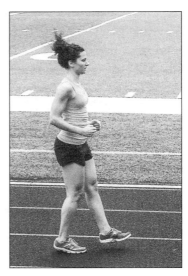

**Figure 8.20** Single-foot deadlegs.

## Single-Foot Deadlegs With High Ankle

The athlete brings the ankle of one leg up over the height of the other knee following ground contact (figure 8.21). The aim is to use ground reaction force to bring the ankle high, simultaneously driving the knee forward. The contralateral leg remains in a single-leg deadleg action (i.e., it is stiff at the knee and ankle with an active flat-foot contact).

This drill can be performed as a single-leg drill (i.e., one leg is a deadleg, while the other does a high ankle action every foot strike) for a distance, or the legs can be alternated in sequence (three high ankles with the left foot, then three right). A more complex variant is to perform a sequence in which the ankle action is performed this way: left leg, right leg, right leg, left leg, left leg, right leg and so on.

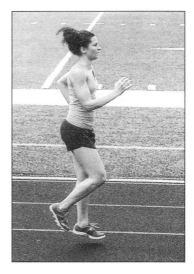

**Figure 8.21** Single-foot deadlegs with high ankle.

## Single-Foot Deadlegs With Hurdles

This drill is performed over a 10- to 20-metre course that has microhurdles set up at three foot lengths apart (marked by placing the first hurdle and then measuring the heel-to-toe length of the athlete's shoe) for the length of the course. The athlete performs the drill laterally to the hurdles, using the outside foot as the deadleg and making contact with the ground after every hurdle (figure 8.22). The inside leg is driven high over each hurdle in succession. The introduction of a microhurdle provides a sensory cue (the athlete should not look down because doing so will alter the postural mechanics) that encourages the ankle to rise high following a rapid ground contact. Using a hurdle also encourages rapid ground contact. If the athlete is too long in ground contact on the lifted leg, the foot will make contact with the next hurdle.

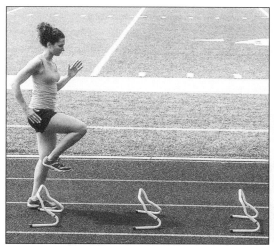 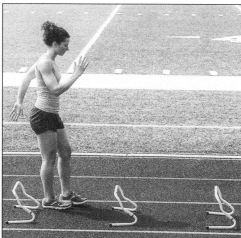

**Figure 8.22** Single-foot deadlegs with hurdles.

## Recovery Mechanics

The focus of these drills is for the athlete to establish a pattern in which the thigh is able to accelerate forward from behind the body to in front of the body, ready to transition into ground preparation and accelerate towards the ground. The ankle recovery above the opposite knee and the dorsiflexed ankle position are key features of this movement. These points should be continually cued and corrected, especially during the early stages of learning.

Advanced athletes can perform these drills by having one leg perform the recovery drill action and the other perform a deadleg action (i.e., modelling ground preparation mechanics).

Mechanical drills are not the only means of enhancing maximal velocity running, and they are not exclusively the preserve of sports that require maximal velocity running. The level of neuromuscular coordination required to perform variations of these drills makes them ideal for motor skill development in sports such as tennis or basketball, in which acceleration and chaotic speed movements predominate over high-speed running. Because these drills elicit high mobility and muscle activation requirements, these and other variations of upright running are also ideal for incorporation into extended warm-ups for any practice sessions (or competitive performances) that will involve running.

Although drills can be useful in developing technique, an athlete will never achieve efficient top-speed mechanics if he or she is not subjected to maximal velocity running sessions in which the techniques become skills. Such sessions vary with the experience of the athletes and the context in which they are working. (For example, 200-metre runners typically require much more speed endurance than 100-metre runners do, and team-sport athletes typically do not reach the velocities or sprint the distances that track athletes do, so session structures will differ.) An example session for maximal speed running might be structured around the following examples; the distances can be manipulated to suit the specific needs of the athlete's sport or position. Each maximal effort has to be done with maximal intensity (and therefore intent), so maximal recovery is required between efforts. As a guideline, recovery may take up to a minute for every 10 metres sprinted.

Example 1: 4 × (4 × 30 metres) maximal sprints with different starting positions for each set (total session volume = 480 metres)

Example 2: 4 × 40 metres, 3 × 50 metres, 2 × 60 metres, 1 × 70 metres (total session volume = 500 metres)

Example 3: Mark out a 50-metre course into 2 × 25-metre sections. The athlete starts by running at 50 per cent speed and increases the pace with each stride until reaching full pace by the end of the 25 metres. The athlete should maintain maximal speed for the final 25 metres. Repeat for three sets of four repetitions (total session volume = 600 metres).

# LONG BACKWARD STRIDES

## Coaching Points

- The heel passes close to the butt as the athlete stretches the recovery leg out behind him- or herself.
- The athlete makes a toe-first contact with the ground because the ankle remains dorsiflexed.
- The trunk remains upright, the shoulders and hips are square, and the trunk is braced.

## Organization

This drill emphasizes both recovery mechanics and ground contact. The aim is to reproduce optimal sprint mechanics whilst moving backwards (figure 8.23). The ground contact pattern, coupled with the need for a rearward propulsive force, emphasizes the importance of using the explosive strength characteristics of the hip flexors to produce force against the ground.

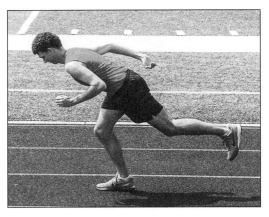

**Figure 8.23**   Long backward strides.

# SIDE-LYING AND STANDING RECOVERY

## Coaching Points

- Replicate the sprint recovery action in a lying position. The ankle in recovery moves rearward of the centre of mass, and then the knee drives forward.
- The ankle of the working leg remains dorsiflexed throughout the drill.
- The trunk should be straight, and the lumbar–pelvic area should be stabilized in a neutral position to enable the leg action to occur effectively.

## Organization

Side-lying and standing recovery drills allow the athlete to practice the motion of recovering the leg using the triple-flexor actions at the hip, knee and ankle, with the joints working in synchronization. The athlete begins lying on the side in a straight-line body position with the ankle dorsiflexed (figure 8.24). Introducing the model in lying removes the resistance of gravity and enables the athlete to focus on rapid leg recovery mechanics. From this starting position, the ankle of the top leg is brought forcefully rearwards. Then the knee is driven forward, and the ankle is moved as close to the butt as possible to mimic the cyclical pattern of leg recovery. The drill ends with the knee as far forward as it goes with the ankle cocked and close to the athlete's butt. After the pattern is established, the action should be explosive from and to a static start position and repeated for sets of 10 repetitions on each leg.

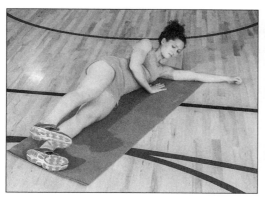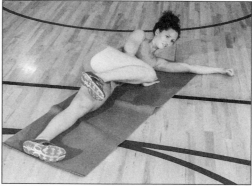

**Figure 8.24**    Side-lying recovery.

Performing the drill while standing obviously is more realistic to skilled performance because it is gravity resisted and requires postural control. The athlete stands on the support leg (a wall can be used to aid stability in the upper trunk during the drill), and the recovery leg action does not change from the side-lying version of the drill.

# A-SKIP AND ALTERNATING A-SKIP

**Coaching Points**

- The athlete displays a fluid and rhythmical action.
- The thigh drives forward, the ankle is high and close to the butt, and the ankle is dorsiflexed.
- The recovery action should be rapid.
- The support foot should perform a small skip as the other leg accelerates towards the ground.
- The trunk should remain upright throughout the action, and an opposing arm and leg action should be used to overcome rotations.

**Organization**

The A-skip drills (figure 8.25) are similar in appearance to the high-ankle drills, but as a maximum velocity technique drill, the emphasis changes from ground contact to the triple-flexor action in the hip, knee and ankle in the recovery mechanics. This means that the knee comes forward as the ankle comes high and as close as possible

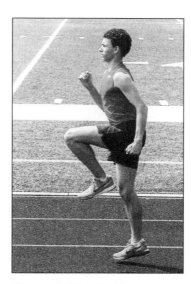

**Figure 8.25**    A-skip.

*(continued)*

## A-Skip and Alternating A-Skip *(continued)*

to the butt and through towards the ground. The trunk should remain upright throughout. The A-skip drill also can be done with a contralateral action; the athlete changes legs whilst one leg performs the deadleg drill to emphasize ground contact.

Athletes who are advanced enough can combine this drill with a straight-leg skip; one leg works on ground preparation, and the other works on recovery mechanics. The sequencing for this action can be adapted to suit the level of challenge required by the individual athlete. Take care not to introduce such complex drills before the athlete is competent enough.

# B-SKIP

### Coaching Points

- Accelerate the foot towards the floor.
- Contact the ground with an active flat foot (heel slightly off, ankle dorsiflexed) slightly in front of the centre of mass.
- The trunk should remain upright, and the athlete uses an opposite arm and leg action.
- Think 'knee up, leg reach, grab the grass' during the drill to coordinate the sequence.

### Organization

The rhythmical and cyclical action of a B-skip (figure 8.26) is designed to emphasize recovery and transition mechanics into ground preparation. Earlier, the reach and grab grass drill presented the B-skip movement as a marching drill; the B-skip extends it by having the athlete performing a slight bounce in the standing leg as the knee is lifted forward. The pattern reinforces the basic recovery movement patterns of knee high and forward by extending the knee and cycling the thigh forward following toe-off whilst moving forwards (the role of the contralateral skip). When the knee reaches its most forward point (the trunk is kept upright), the lower leg is extended forward. The hamstring muscles decelerate this action as the knee reaches extension, and the athlete should now 'paw' the foot down into the ground so that the active flat foot contacts the floor directly under the centre of mass.

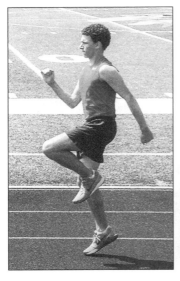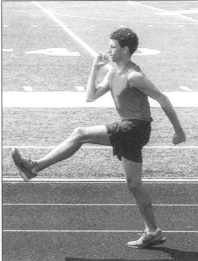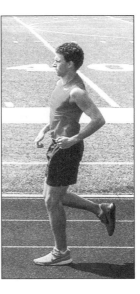

**Figure 8.26**   B-skip.

The emphasis is on the athlete actively and forcefully contacting the ground beneath the centre of mass with each successive foot contact so that the athlete continually accelerates forward in a rhythmical skipping manner. An alternating arm and leg action is used for the duration of the drill.

---

# STEP-OVER RUN

## Coaching Points

- The ankle passes as close to the butt as possible whilst the athlete maintains an upright posture.
- The athlete contacts the floor with an active ground contact, with the heel slightly raised, below the centre of mass.
- The action is fluid and rhythmical as the athlete transitions into the run.

## Organization

Step-over runs encourage appropriate recovery mechanics whilst maintaining postural control. The athlete can transition into a step-over run from any number of drills (for example, straight-leg skips, or alternate single-leg B-skips). The step-over run itself is an exaggerated running action, in which the athlete visualizes the ankle picking up and stepping over a small hurdle (to achieve the knee forward, high-ankle action) as he or she runs down the track for 20 to 40 metres.

Step-over runs can be performed in a variety of conditions (for example, while holding a medicine ball, with arms overhead or while using the arms) to require the athlete to maintain an upright and forward-facing trunk without the arms to counter the rotations generated in the legs.

---

## Assisted Running

Assisted running drills often have been considered beneficial for athletes looking to improve their high-speed running. A number of techniques have been introduced to assist in the development and maintenance of high velocities by focusing on the neuromuscular system. These techniques cause the athlete to run at supramaximal speeds by increasing the stride frequency that the athlete is able to achieve within a given distance.

Downhill running, for example, often has been considered particularly favourable. It is inexpensive because it uses gravity to speed up the athlete's descent down a slope. The key determinant of the success of this type of training is the gradient that the athlete descends. Experts cannot agree whether a slope should have a negligible incline or be slightly steeper; recommendations vary between 2 and 7 degrees.[2]

The mitigating factor that determines the efficacy of this type of training appears to be the athlete's ability to maintain foot speed with sufficient cadence that the athlete doesn't overstride (with little or no change in stride frequency). If overstriding ensues, as usually happens when slopes are too steep, the reverse of the desired training effect occurs, in that the athlete will be trained in eccentric braking actions that enhance deceleration rather than high-speed running.

Some practitioners overcome the controversy of the slope incline by using supramaximal speeds on motorized treadmills, so that the athlete is forced to increase leg cadence to maintain position on the treadmill. Although this type of training may have the desired effect with regards to the running action, the benefits in terms of running economy and neuromuscular potential are questionable because the movements elicited from passive foot contact (i.e., the ground moves under the athlete, as opposed to the athlete moving over the ground) are very different in terms of both quality and muscular recruitment. The athlete has little need for the high-velocity backwards-clawing action from ground preparation through ground contact, and therefore the recruitment patterns and active demands for the hip extensor and knee flexor muscles in the posterior chain (particularly the hamstring muscle group) are reduced significantly.

Towing by a partner or bungee cord may be more practical and beneficial in introducing overspeed training to an athletic development programme. The intention of this type of work is to cause the athlete to accelerate from a standing start and transition into supramaximal speeds without a change in the required running technique. For the athlete to achieve this and maintain an upright running position without overbalancing forward, the stride frequency must be increased with sound ground contact.

These techniques enable the athlete to follow the natural transitional process from acceleration mechanics into maximal velocity running; thus, a natural progressive action is achieved. But maintaining such drills for longer than 30 to 40 metres is not advisable, because the physio-mechanical demands of supramaximal running typically force the athlete into a fatigued action that results in overstriding and braking. A similar result will occur if the task demand is too great (i.e., if the overspeed requirements exceed the athletic qualities of the athlete). Towing partners (or bungee tensions) need to be carefully selected so that only a 2 to 5 per cent increase in speed demand is required from the athlete in training.

## Resisted Maximal Velocity Running

As with many training methodologies, the use of resistances in maximal velocity running is a topic for lively discussion amongst professionals. As with many such debates, definitive answers have never been found, but if the practitioner understands the full benefits of the activity and the potential consequences of inappropriate prescription, then he or she can make an informed decision about when or if and how to include such drills in the programme.

The use of external loads challenges the neuromuscular system to recruit more motor units to execute a task than would normally be required under volitional neural drive. But this potential benefit needs to be balanced against the realization that the easiest way to hinder maximal speed running is to retard the athlete's upright posture or interfere with natural stride lengths.

The key to the success of this technique is to ensure that an optimal resistive load is selected to overload the athlete. The outcome is for the athlete to attain (and for a short period sustain) maximal velocity with an external load. Therefore, the resistive load cannot be so great that it slows down the athlete. Unlike in acceleration mechanics, in which drag may encourage the athlete to adopt a forward-leaning posture, the resistive load must not cause the athlete to adopt a forward lean (or even more inappropriately bend forward from the trunk) to move the load. Both of these maladaptations are seen by practitioners who use loads that are too heavy for their athletes' capabilities.

Therefore, loads that typically provide a 2 to 5 per cent increase in resistive load (i.e., body weight) might be considered appropriate in such practices, although this amount depends on the reactive strength properties of the athlete and the frictional drag of the surface (for example, on turf a sled may slide far more efficiently than it does on a hard court). Practitioners should also remember that in any form of resisted or assisted running, to achieve maximum benefit from the increased motor unit activation as applied to normal running technique, some form of contrast must be incorporated; loaded repetitions should be followed by unloaded repetitions so that the athlete learns to incorporate the increased motor unit activity into his or her performance. Therefore, a session might comprise four sets of three resisted (assisted) runs and one unresisted run over 40 to 50 metres with complete recovery between repetitions and longer recovery between sets.

# Agility

Agility is a unique physical attribute that encompasses every aspect of an athlete's motor and cognitive ability. In a sporting context, agility represents the athlete's perceptual and decision-making qualities as well as his or her coordinative and forceful movement speed qualities. Developing agility is a more sport specific yet a more interdisciplinary practice than many other aspects of movement skills. For example, direction change mechanics can be taught in many drills, but if the athlete does not have the physio-mechanical qualities of reaction strength to reaccelerate from a directional change, or the eccentric strength qualities to decelerate momentum as a precursor to directional change, then technique cannot be functionally applied as a skill. Similarly, high-level sport is full of examples of athletes who were able to read the play so well that regardless of their physical qualities, they were always a metre in front of their opponents or always in position to return the ball with force.

Change-of-direction speed involves preplanned actions to alter the direction of movement, whereas agility takes into account the perceptual and decision-making skills of the athlete, the technique required for direction change and the physical qualities needed to turn a reaction to a stimulus into an effective movement response.[11]

Sport-specific speed typically is defined by the athlete's ability to generate high speeds over multiple short distances accompanied by directional changes. The changes in body position and body direction, as well as changes in movement speed that an athlete needs to achieve in a sport-specific context (figure 8.27), are grounded within the movement demands of the sport.

These varying requirements don't mean that agility can, or should, be taught only within sport-specific contexts. The athlete is a generalist who has to be able to use a range of tools well before being able to decide which one best fits the task. The role of the athletic development programme is to provide the athlete with the movement tools, underpinned by the physical qualities to use those tools effectively, that he or she can apply to any movement context. This idea was introduced in chapter 1, which explained the concept of generic movement techniques that are progressed to movement skills that become sport-specific applications.

This chapter looks at various movement tasks that relate to directional change mechanics, analysing what skilful execution of these tasks looks like and how this can be developed with specific practices and drills, building on

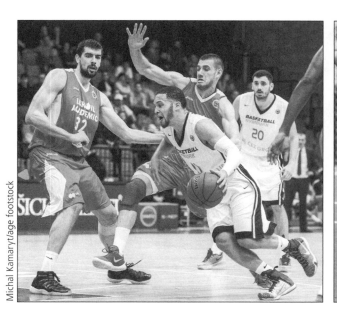 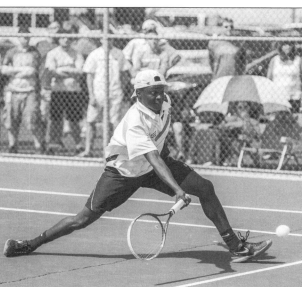

**Figure 8.27** Agility demands are very different between sports.

the example progression principles outlined in chapter 7. The aim is to communicate the principles of teaching agility mechanics, rather than focus on specific agility drills. Practitioners must be able to analyse and develop mechanics by applying principles to their own drills rather than copy a range of drills without understanding how they can be differentiated to progress the movement competence of an athlete.

Indeed, many books[5] provide a wide range of drills and sport-specific movement practices for informed coaches to dissect and develop to their own ends after they understand the movement outcomes required in their athletes.

Recent research[3] indicates that, although most sport performers need the ability to accelerate to maximal speeds in a range of time frames, linear speed and directional change ability are not highly correlated. Therefore, training for change-of-direction speed and agility must involve highly specific training that develops directional change skills that can be incorporated into the specific demands of the sport. A deterministic model for agility illustrates the factors that need to be considered when designing an agility development programme for an athlete.

As figure 8.28 illustrates, perceptual and decision-making skills, as well as physical qualities, play a large role, and technique is one building block that can be developed. Fitting with the philosophical and practical considerations for curriculum development (chapter 7), the athletic development professional is advised to focus on the range of technical and physical characteristics associated with change-of-direction speed before progressing to the open and reactive (sport-specific) practices that will enhance perceptual and decision-making skills. These qualities aren't being ignored, because they are being simultaneously developed in the sport-specific aspects of the athlete's educational programming.

That recognized, many agility games with young children should incorporate aspects of decision making and environmental adaptation. Games that are fun and competitive and require children to change direction and understand how to improve direction changes (strategically and physically) are important foundation activities for an athlete education programme that begins in the early years. The rats and rabbits game covered earlier in

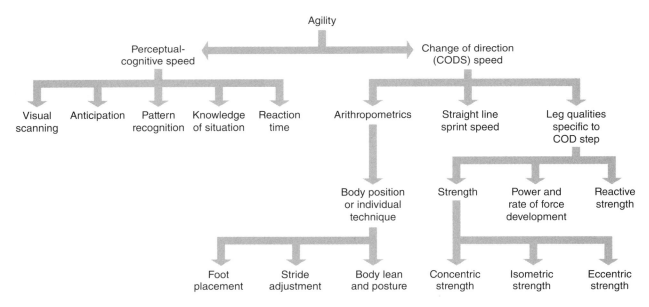

**Figure 8.28** Deterministic model of agility.

Reprinted, by permission, from S. Nimphius, 2014, Increasing agility. In *High-performance training for sports*, edited by D. Joyce and D. Lewindon (Champaign, IL: Human Kinetics), 187. Adapted from W.B. Young, R. James, and I. Montgomery, 2002, "Is muscle power related to running speed with changes of direction?" *Journal of Sports Medicine and Physical Fitness*, 42(3): 282–288; and J.M. Sheppard and W.B. Young, 2006, "Agility literature review: Classifications, training and testing", *Journal of Sports Sciences*, 24(9): 919–932.

# CAT AND MOUSE TAG

## Coaching Points

- Make quick, firm decisions.
- Change direction with a low body position.
- Plant one foot and quickly change direction. Push through the foot in the direction opposite where you want to move.
- Accelerate after changing direction.

## Equipment

- Coloured bibs
- Marker cones or appropriate equipment to define a movement area that enables free movement with the numbers participating but also constrains and forces directional changes

## Organization

Choose an appropriate number of cats (ideally a 1:4 ratio of cats to mice) and give each cat a distinguishing coloured bib. The rest of the group are mice. Position the cats in the middle of the playing space and the rest of the group around the outside. On your command, the mice should be encouraged to escape from the cats, whose aim is to tag them. After being tagged, the mice should stand still. Other free mice should try to release their captured classmates by circling them once (basic level) or twice (more advanced) without being caught. The object of the activity is for the cats to capture all the mice. The coach should allow the game to progress for 1 to 3 minutes before providing a rest period.

---

the chapter and cat and mouse tag are two examples.

A movement vocabulary (chapters 1 and 2) based on a range of skilful agility movements for a sport-specific context needs to be based on certain principles that relate to changes in velocity (acceleration or deceleration), transitions between movement directions (backwards, sideways, forwards) and specific directional change skills (for example, cuts, swerves and turns through varying degrees of motion).

As identified in chapter 1, an inverse relationship between the concepts of mobility and stability can be established by the relationship between the athlete's posture, the position of the centre of mass and the relationship of the centre of mass to the base of support (and the width of the base of support). The positioning of the joints and the trunk is also important because it determines the ability of the trunk to optimize force transmission from the ground through the posture. In particular,

joint and trunk positioning dictates the muscular involvement in producing optimal forces (from the hip, then the knee, then the ankle, to the ground).

This concept is well illustrated in figure 8.29. Movement starts from a relatively static position that is not stable. (The photo on the left illustrates that the athlete is performing slight jumping actions from the athletic position before settling onto both feet to receive the opponent's serve.) The player is remaining on the balls of the feet with the heels not in contact with the ground. The greater the surface area in contact with the ground is, the higher the stability is.

Before movement is initiated, the feet are hip-width apart, the trunk is upright, and the flexion in the knees and hips places the athlete at an optimal angle for maximizing the stretch reflex in the hip and knee extensors. The centre of mass is relatively high (which decreases stability), but it is over the midline of the base of support (meaning that it will

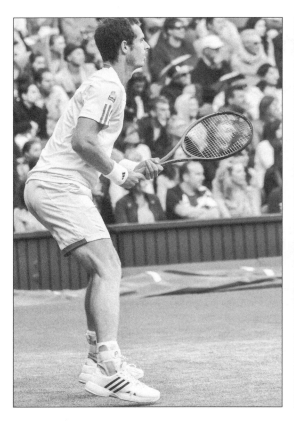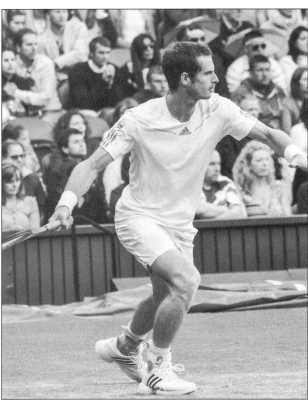

**Figure 8.29**  Applying the physio-mechanical principles of agility.

require an external force to move the centre of mass). The wider the base of support is, the lower the centre of mass is, and the more stable (and less reactive) the athlete becomes.

As the player reacts to the opponent's shot, several things occur that promote the direction of travel and the optimization of propulsive forces in that direction. The hip of the lead leg externally rotates, so that the lead leg and foot point in the direction of intended movement. The athlete also rotates the head and shoulders with the hips and moves them until they are in front of the hips, immediately moving the centre of mass laterally to the base of support, enabling the force vector to move in the intended direction of travel. This movement enables the hips of the driving leg to generate propulsive power and the leg to extend fully, optimizing force transference through the hip, then the knee, then the ankle and foot, into the ground. The straight-line body position enables efficient transfer of ground reaction forces through the posture in the direction of travel.

Agility movements typically achieve four broad objectives related to initiation of the movement, directional change and evasion, or transition between movement skills, and finally the important link to linear acceleration and maximal velocity that should follow a directional change. Exploring these aspects of the athlete's movement capability can identify specific baseline movement skills that can be developed through specific practices. Agility is a reactive quality; therefore, exhibiting change-of-direction skills at pace requires the athlete to have high levels of reactive strength and plyometric qualities (chapter 9) to control eccentric forces and create reactive concentric forces to achieve explosive and effective changes in body positioning.

## Deceleration

Athletes decelerate in the sporting arena for a number of reasons—sometimes to come to a dead stop, often to enable them to change direction and many times simply to transition efficiently from one moving velocity to another (for example, from a sprint to a jog or walk in soccer). Any deceleration that involves a directional change also involves asymmetrical actions through the legs and hips, therefore requiring the management of rotational forces through the athlete's posture.

Logically enough, the mechanics of linear deceleration to a stop are opposite those for linear acceleration. The key is ensuring that the posture is aligned to apply forces into the ground to retard forward momentum of the athlete's centre of mass. In essence, the athlete is trying to bring the centre of mass back within the base of support to achieve a stable position. Besides having a good technique, stopping efficiently involves high ground reaction forces and eccentric muscle actions through the posterior chain, especially if the athlete is travelling at high speeds (required force equals athlete's mass times acceleration). Therefore, the athlete needs to be physically strong to produce effective actions and minimize the potential for an acute overreaching injury.

As soon as the athlete begins to slow down (figure 8.30), the ankle is dorsiflexed to provide pretension through the lower leg in preparation for a ground contact with the heel. Ground contact takes place in front of the centre of mass to retard forward momentum and bring the centre of mass closer towards the base of support. This foot position enables a horizontal braking force to be applied through the heel.

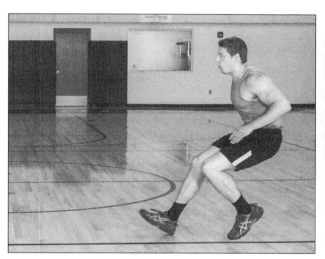
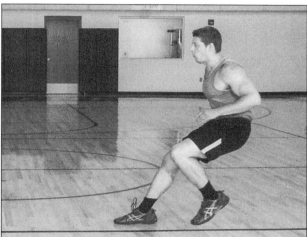
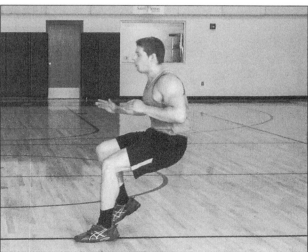
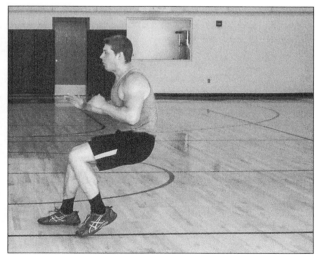

**Figure 8.30**  Deceleration.

The braking force is absorbed through the knees and hips as the athlete rapidly rolls onto the forefoot to create a frictional drag that aids the braking action.

Depending on the athlete's velocity, a number of shortened gait cycles are typically needed to decelerate safely while maintaining a balanced body position. The athlete lowers the centre of mass and widens the base of support throughout the action sequence. As with accelerating, a high frequency of foot contacts provides greater interaction between the body and the ground, in this case to absorb the high eccentric forces needed to decelerate the athlete's momentum.

If the skill is to be effectively transferred to a sporting context, the athlete needs to be able to undertake this action whilst maintaining a level hip and shoulder and keeping the head and trunk upright. The athlete will then be able to transition quickly to any other movement pattern in any direction. If an athlete cannot maintain a position in which the hips and shoulders are level as deceleration occurs, any subsequent reacceleration in any given direction is limited.

Linear decelerations can be practised using the typical progression from closed (limited number of decisions to be made by the athlete) to increasingly open (difficult decision making determined by external environmental factors) practices. Such a progression is illustrated in figure 8.31. The athlete must accelerate from a static starting position as hard as possible past the 10- to 20-metre stop line. This distance can be manipulated depending on the athlete's ability to accelerate and his or her eccentric strength. The higher the athlete's velocity is at the stop line, the greater the eccentric must be to brake forward momentum.

Immediately after crossing the stop line, the athlete needs to hit the brakes as quickly as possible. Typically, during early attempts at this drill the athlete will not accelerate as hard as possible so that the stopping action is easier. Although this approach may encourage familiarity with the practice, it will not promote the technical model required! The practitioner needs to ensure that the athlete is running as hard as possible at the stop line and starts to slow only after crossing that line. Speed gates or competitions to see who can cross the line first may encourage maximum effort, as long as they do not detract from the overall purpose of the drill (i.e., stopping as quickly as possible, from high speeds, after crossing the line).

To progress the drill, the athlete can be challenged to decrease the stopping distance. Place a marker at the point where the athlete comes to a dead stop (figure 8.31*b*) and tell the athlete he or she must beat this mark without slowing down the acceleration. Provide feedback on the outcome (i.e., whether the athlete slowed before the respective marker) as well as the technique that the athlete uses. After the athlete has demonstrated a general level of movement competence and can stop effectively, a number of options for progression are available.

One option is to remove the stop line and introduce a verbal or visual cue that the athlete needs to respond to in order to stop. This method externalizes the athlete's decision about when to stop but makes it difficult to challenge or objectively measure progress in terms of subsequent actions. Alternatively, the athlete can be challenged to reaccelerate as soon as he or she achieves a dead stop (figure 8.31*c*). This option removes the reactive element of the drill but focuses the athlete on the need to maintain technique and stop with a good body position before reaccelerating.

Just as maximal acceleration should be emphasized in the first part of the drill, the athlete must achieve a dead stop (rather than simply slow down) before reaccelerating. Those who are not able to control their posture effectively and stop in a stable position will not be able to reaccelerate effectively. Observers may see athletes overbalance as they transition from a high to low body position and then move the centre of mass back inside the base of support before taking it forward again during the first steps of acceleration.

These drills typically progress to an open practice in which the athlete is required to accelerate, decelerate to stop and reaccelerate entirely in response to an opponent's actions (figure 8.31*d*). Include evasion skills to get past

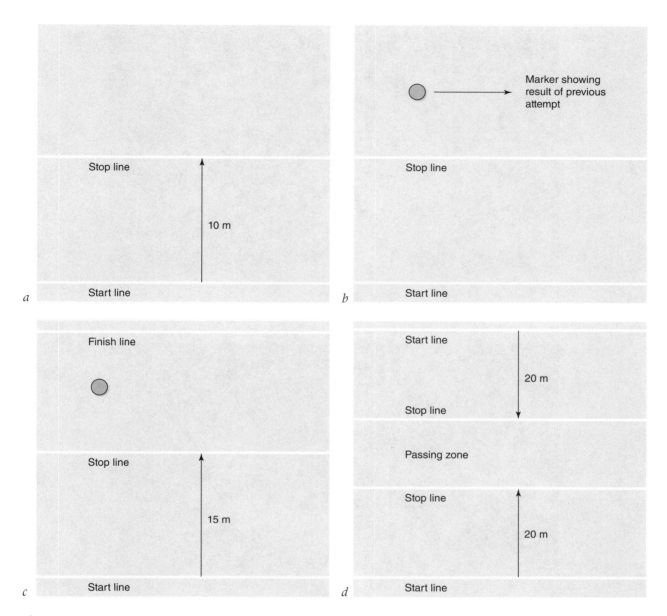

**Figure 8.31**  Sample progression of linear deceleration practice linked with transitional reacceleration: *(a)* linear deceleration; *(b)* linear deceleration with a target; *(c)* reacceleration after dead stop; *(d)* reacceleration in response to an opponent's actions.

the opponent in the subsequent reacceleration attempts if the athlete is competent in the execution of all the prerequisite skills. Note that not all decelerations in sport require the athlete to come to a dead stop, but when the athlete masters coming to a dead stop, variations of slowing to a reduced speed before reaccelerating can be incorporated into practices.

Nonlinear decelerations are highly common in all sports that involve an element of

invasion. Indeed, such movements are typically more common than linear decelerations. These movements are highly complex and situationally specific (figure 8.32). Many such actions require high eccentric muscle forces to be generated through a single-leg stance, and the upper-body actions are often not related to the lower-body requirements. For example, in tennis, the leg may be decelerating whilst the upper body is playing a shot.

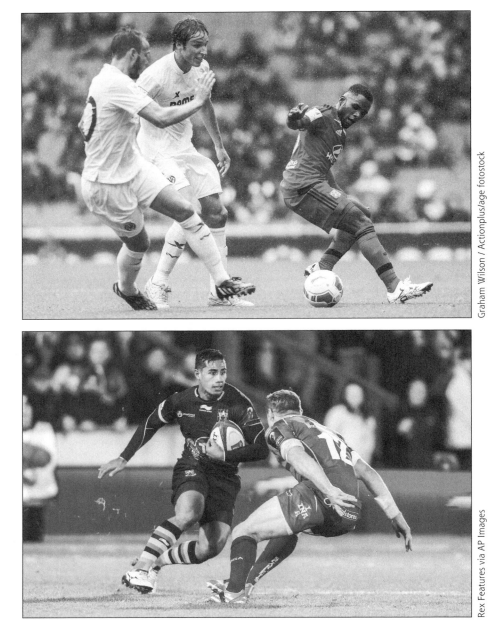

**Figure 8.32**   Nonlinear decelerations are highly situation specific.

Thus, the pattern of rotational force control and multidirectional force absorption is not uniform across sports. Indeed, as the pictures in figure 8.32 show, many deceleration actions and positions are determined by the movements that follow the deceleration, as will become evident in the following sections of this chapter. That said, the principles of decelerating remain the same. The athlete needs to be low to the ground, have the base of support as wide as possible and have the centre of mass as central to the base of support as practical. The greater the surface area of the foot in contact with the ground is, the greater the frictional force needed to decelerate forward momentum is. The athlete needs to be strong through the posterior chain to produce high eccentric forces through a single- or double-leg stance whilst controlling rotational (or maybe even collision) forces through the trunk and upper body.

# Transitional Movements

Often in sport, athletes need to initiate movements to enable an efficient and effective transition between distinct movement patterns. For example, a defender in soccer may sprint towards an opponent he or she is marking, decelerate when an anticipated pass isn't made and move laterally a couple of steps into space before accelerating forward to make a clearing header. The ability to link forwards, sideways and backwards movements provides the athlete with a clear competitive advantage over opponents and an efficient and energy-saving means of moving around the playing area whilst viewing play.

The starting point for any transitional movement is the athlete's preparedness to move. The athlete must have a stimulus to react to or make a decision to move. Similarly, the athlete must be in the best physical position to move in any direction. For this reason, the athletic ready position is essential for athletes from all sports.

The backpedal (figure 8.33) is the most familiar skill for backwards movement. The backpedal can be performed either as a linear or an angled movement. The key to performing this skill successfully is to keep the hips and shoulders square at all times, ensuring that the hips can be directed in any required movement direction in the subsequent seconds. The athlete keeps the ankle dorsiflexed and reaches back to contact the floor with the toe. This technique enables the athlete to push backwards through the whole of the foot as the weight moves onto the heel. As the weight transfers onto the planted foot behind the body, the momentum causes the front foot to rise from the floor if the toes remain dorsiflexed. Therefore, the athlete should be encouraged to show the bottom of the shoes to the front as the weight transfers backwards.

The backpedal can be adapted to an angled movement by manipulating the forces exerted into the floor through the base of the feet. By adding a lateral force through the inside or outside of the feet, depending on the desired direction of movement, the resultant force sends the athlete laterally as well as rearwards. Through this skill adaptation, the athlete can respond effectively to any necessary change in direction of the movement as long as the hips and shoulders remain square. If the hips orientate in any direction other than forward, the athlete will not be able to respond rapidly to any required directional change, which opens up opportunities for an opponent to pass the athlete on the side the body has turned away from.

Lateral movement is also important in many sports. The simplest skill for travelling a short distance laterally but maintaining a readiness to react in any direction is the lateral shuffle (figure 8.34), a lateral pushing action in which the athlete pushes from the inside of one foot and the outside of the other foot to achieve sideways movement. The push-to-move

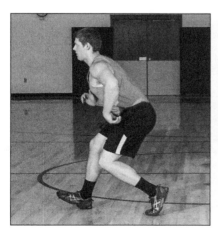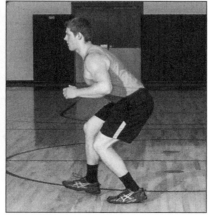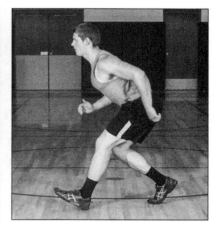

**Figure 8.33**   Backpedal.

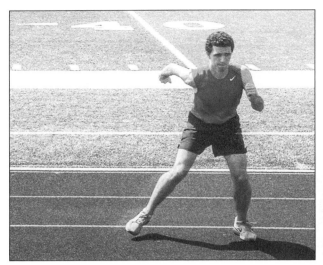 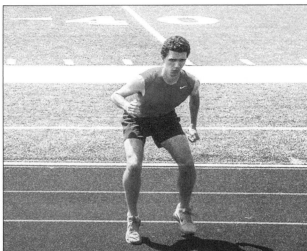

**Figure 8.34** Lateral shuffle.

concept is much more effective than the reach-and-pull approach to achieve lateral movement; the athlete initiates movement by reaching the foot laterally in the direction of travel and then uses the groin muscles to pull the body across whilst pushing off the other foot. Typically, the reach-and-pull action not only is slower and less forceful but also decreases the athlete's mobility because the initial movement widens the base of support. The pushing action enables the athlete's feet to remain close to the ground and under the hips so that he or she is able to transition into something approximating the athletic ready position.

To develop these movement skills, simple closed practices can be established that can then be developed into more open and dynamic situations that require the athlete to react to externally contrived situations (the context of which can be sport specific) whilst not losing body position. Although many would correctly propose that, for example, the quickest way to move laterally through 10 metres isn't to side shuffle but to turn and sprint, remember that these progressive approaches to developing movements are not about sport-specific contexts, but about developing the movement tools for the athletes to use in their performances. In the specific sporting situation, the athlete may need to shuffle or backpedal for only one or two steps but will have developed the ability to do this.

The key requirement in planning such drills is to ensure that the work remains high quality and that rest is adequate to ensure that the drill does not become a conditioning task. For example, if the drill shown in figure 8.35 was performed on a 10-by-10 metre grid, the athlete would need to do 70 metres of multidirectional work, which is highly fatiguing. Alternatively, this sequence could be limited to a three-cone movement drill, halving the volume to maintain the quality of the work. The directions of movement can then be varied to ensure bilateral skill development.

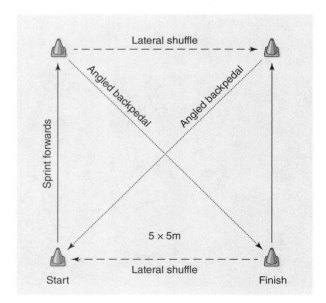

**Figure 8.35** Transitional movement skill drill.

Readers will note the point where a change-of-direction practice becomes more of an agility drill, because reactions and decision making become involved in the progression and are highly involved in mirror drills (see chapter 7). Drills should be kept to 5- to 6-second activities of high quality with complete rest between efforts. The more chaotic or reactive the drill becomes, the greater the requirement is for the athlete to maintain the hips-square position during movement transitions. This condition can be really exploited by requiring the athletes to sprint forwards in response to an externally provided 'Now' shout during the mirror sequence. Alternatively, if athlete A sees that athlete B is in a disadvantageous position, he or she may be tasked with trying to sprint and evade athlete B (or vice versa) to end the mirror drill. The tasks become very competitive and demanding in terms of reaction and decision making.

## Changing Direction

Throughout this chapter, the managed application of forces into the ground has been emphasized as the key to optimizing acceleration, maximal velocity and movement transition. The same principles apply to direction change mechanics; the athlete simply needs to provide sufficient forces in the appropriate direction to enable acceleration. These movement tasks are highly specific to the situational context of the sport, and they rely on the athlete being able to undertake technically correct actions whilst exerting large forces rapidly into the ground from the hips and knees.

Athletes are required to change direction from both static and moving situations, and the skills can be used either in evasion tasks, to exploit or create space or in moving to intercept an object (for example, a player moving from the ready position into a forehand or backhand in tennis or an outfielder retrieving a hit in baseball). The very movement of the athlete through the transverse plane creates torque that the athlete needs to be able to control throughout the kinetic chain. This links with the concept of developing functional strength and rate of force development examined

further in chapters 9 and 10. If force production is developed (and trained) only in the sagittal plane, athletes can have movement inefficiencies and possibly develop injuries when required to exert forces through the transverse or frontal planes.

Direction changes from a static position are typified by a turn and acceleration through a range of possible angles. The shallower the angle is, the greater the range of techniques available to the athlete is. All these techniques, when successfully executed, are characterized by some commonalities. First, the centre of mass is lowered and moved towards the direction of travel. This movement is led by the head and shoulders, and rotation is aided by a forceful and rapid driving of the arms in the intended direction of travel. As the athlete is moving into a position of acceleration, as described previously in terms of linear acceleration, the centre of mass needs to be in front of the lead foot at the point of toe-off, the rear leg needs to extend fully and the line of force must be through a straight-line driving position throughout the posture at the point of toe-off.

For example, the pivot step (figure 8.36) is characterized by the external rotation of the lead leg in the direction of travel as the athlete sinks low and loads the extensors in the other leg. Simultaneously, the contralateral arm is driven across the body, rotating the torso towards the direction of travel. As the trail leg extends completely, the body is rotated through the full range of movement ready to accelerate into the straight sprint.

Similarly, the cross-over step (figure 8.37) uses the weight transfer from both legs into the lead leg, although the torso remains more upright without the forward-sinking movement of the pivot step. The rapid arm drive, close to the body, rotates the torso (rather than simply the lower body) with simultaneous external rotation in the lead leg (which acts as the pivot). Unlike with the pivot step, the trail leg is also internally rotated slightly before take-off. As the lead leg remains in contact with the ground, the other leg crosses in front of the body as the contralateral arm drives forcefully backwards, putting the athlete into the driving position to accelerate forwards. The different

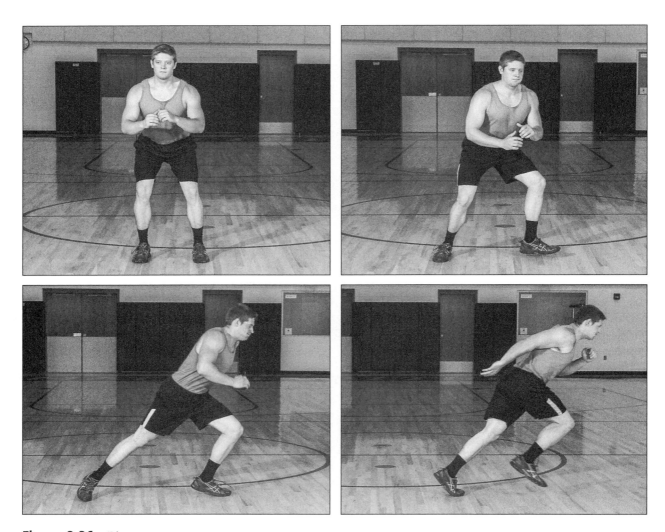

**Figure 8.36** Pivot step.

hip actions between these two illustrative (but not exhaustive) techniques also result in a shorter initial first step into linear acceleration in the cross-over movement, enabling a high stride frequency in the initial stages of the subsequent sprinting action.

Changing direction through angles greater than 90 degrees is relatively common in sporting situations. For example, in soccer the ball may have been cleared over an athlete's head, or in basketball a defence may be turned into attack. Such manoeuvres may need to be executed from a static or dynamic context; regardless, the principles are the same and can be equally applied.

The first requirement is to initiate movement in the desired direction of travel. The athlete uses the stretch-shortening properties of the muscle by loading the hip and hip extensors to produce forceful reflex contractions that increase the velocity of the turn. From a static start (figure 8.38), this loading might be done by performing a rapid and shallow squat to precede the movement. The squat movement also helps to move the centre of mass rearwards of the base of support, so that it is already moving in the intended direction of travel. As with linear acceleration, this movement optimizes the horizontal propulsive force that can be applied through the floor and in the intended direction of travel.

To perform this turn effectively from a forward acceleration (figure 8.39), the athlete first needs to perform several adjustment steps to

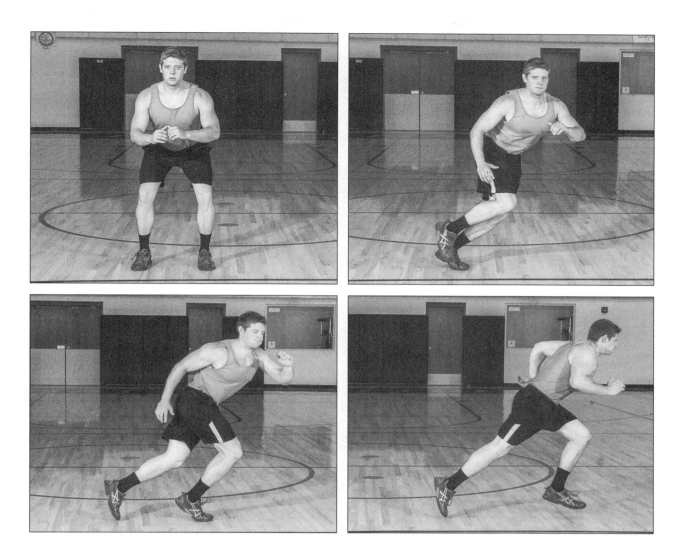

**Figure 8.37**    Cross-over step.

decelerate forward momentum into the turn. The steps are shortened and ground contact times become longer through a heel–toe foot action. At this point the athlete is also relying on large forces produced through eccentric muscle actions to overcome the forward momentum of the centre of mass. Note that the athlete lowers the centre of mass when approaching the turn and leans back towards the direction of the turn. This action helps reduce forward momentum by placing the ground contact in front of the centre of mass.

Early initiation of the turn also helps the successful completion of a rapid turning action. This action is achieved through the rotation of the hips and legs into the new direction during the final adjustment steps of the approach. The athlete requires less rotation during the subsequent phases of the movement because of this preparation. Indeed, executing the full turn during the plant may take additional time and even require additional steps to be taken before accelerating in the new direction.

Overcoming rotational inertia (i.e., the resistance to change in the orientation of the body) is a major consideration in the effectiveness of turning actions, especially when the athlete is beginning from a static start. To make this action more efficient (reduce the effect of inertia), the arms and legs should rotate close to the body (thus reducing the radius of the body's turning circle). This action is aided

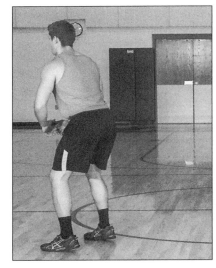
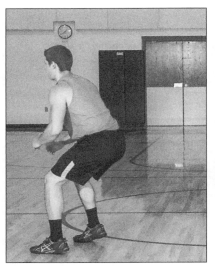
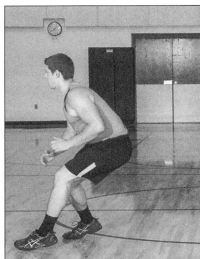
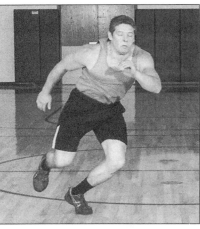
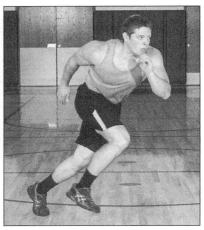

**Figure 8.38**   Turning through 180 degrees from a static start.

by an early head turn during the action that precedes the turning of the shoulders and then the hips, which by this point are optimally placed for power generation. Turning the head early is advantageous to most sports because it enables visual scanning that can buy additional time for the athlete to observe and react to the changing environment.

In dynamic actions, during the deceleration movement the plant foot is positioned away from the rotational axis (other foot) for the final ground contact before the directional change to produce a large torque (turning force) in opposition to the intended direction of travel. This action rapidly produces a stretch-shortening action in the muscles that will enhance the acceleration steps that occur immediately after the directional change.

Assuming that the player is required to accelerate away from the turning point following the change of direction, it follows that the next steps will see a marked forward lean that maximizes horizontal distance between the take-off foot and the centre of mass. This enables the driving leg to extend fully, thus achieving maximum horizontal propulsion.

Depending on the sporting scenario, the player may also be required to turn and jump or turn and side step or even backpedal to catch a ball (for example, a wide receiver cutting back to catch a quarterback's pass thrown short of a defender). Such movements require different positions following a turn. For example, if more vertical propulsion is needed (e.g., into a jump), then the powerline of the body needs to be more vertical and the distance between

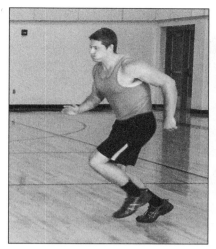
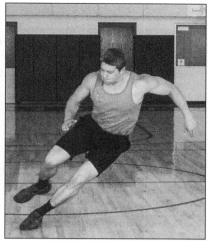
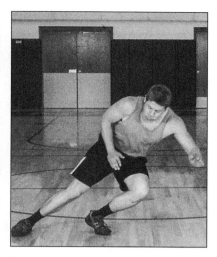
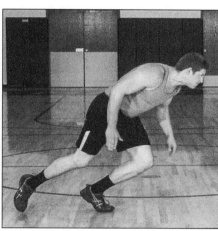
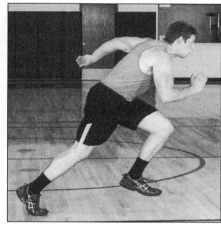

**Figure 8.39**    Turning through 180 degrees from a dynamic start.

the take-off foot and the centre of mass needs to be reduced. A similar position is needed for a backpedal or lateral shuffle step. Therefore, practicing a range of scenario-based outcomes for the skill will enable the athlete to develop a movement vocabulary about how to exit the turning action.

## Evasion Skills

Throughout the evolution of sport performance, many methods have been described that can be used to change direction and accelerate past, or exploit space around, opposition players. These methods have typically included sport-specific skills designed to throw the opposition off balance by feinting in one direction and then moving in another. Other related strategies include deliberate deceleration in the approach to a defender to get the defender to adjust body position relative to the attacker's velocity and then, as the defender becomes more stable, rapid acceleration past the defender. The ability to maintain velocity and running mechanics whilst accelerating into or past an opponent is important, because without this ability, competitive advantage is significantly reduced.

Although a range of evasion techniques might be explored, most of these techniques have a basis in a small number of skills that involve powerful changes of direction with either the inside or outside leg. These actions are typified by variations of the inside foot cut or the outside foot cut.

Cutting actions highlight the importance of the athlete being able to plant the foot and then reaccelerate effectively, involving deceleration, direction change and reacceleration in approximately 0.2 seconds, depending on the nature of the action.

### Outside Foot Cut

The outside foot cut (figure 8.40), or power cut, is considered the optimal technique for achieving powerful directional change through an acute angle. The athlete has to decelerate slightly to optimize the foot placement and preloading of the neuromuscular system before accelerating out of the direction change. In the approach to executing the action, the planted foot contacts the ground laterally to the centre of mass. The knee of the planted foot is located medially (i.e., inside) the foot. If the shin is vertical (i.e. the knee tracks the line of the toes), the athlete will not be able to exert the required lateral force to execute the movement.

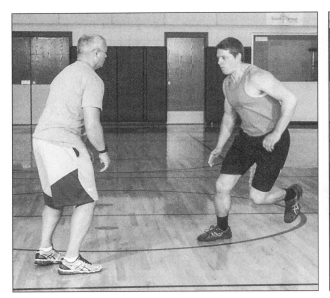
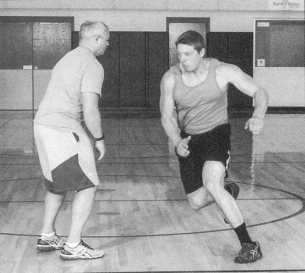
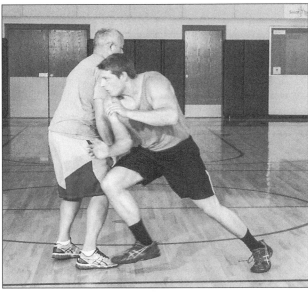

**Figure 8.40**   The outside foot, or power, cut.

# Outside Foot, or Power, Cut

Spatial awareness is crucial. Getting too close will cause a collision to occur; being too far away gives the opponent time to adjust.

The optimal position for executing the outside foot cut is to put the planted foot in line with the middle of the opponent's body, the centre of mass out to the side of travel and the knee of the planted leg medial to the foot. If the foot is planted too far towards the defender's shoulders, the athlete will accelerate into the opponent. Approaching the defender too far towards his or her right side will cue the defender to shut down that space.

As the centre of mass begins to accelerate with hip and knee extension, the outside foot externally rotates in the direction of travel and is positioned so that it can contact the ground behind the centre of mass and forcefully continue to accelerate the body forward in the new direction. If space is to be created and exploited by a change in direction, the athlete must use the created forces and accelerate away from the change-of-direction step.

The full foot is in contact with the ground, and the ground contact time is relatively long. Combined with the lowering of the centre of mass into the turn, this full, relatively long contact ensures that the extensor muscles of the hip and knee joint are optimally preloaded for powerful extension into the direction change. The relatively long ground contact time enables the stretch-shortening cycle to be optimally effective in producing high power outputs through the inside and front of the foot to push the athlete forward and laterally, aided by the trunk, which is already leaning in the direction of travel.

### Inside Foot Cut

An inside foot cut (figure 8.41) is a high-velocity movement that, when executed well, requires little decrease in the athlete's forward momentum. The movement requires the athlete to plant and pivot off the outside of a foot that is planted medially to a defender whilst swinging the inside foot across the defender to plant it on the outside of the defender's foot. This place is a great offensive position from which to accelerate. But the execution of this skill and the requirement to provide forceful directional change through the outside of the foot make it one of the hardest movement skills to execute in open play.

# Inside Foot Cut

For the inside foot cut, the planted foot is placed more medially to the athlete (i.e., more under the hips), optimizing the positioning of the hips to allow the trunk to lean in the direction of travel while maintaining vertical propulsive forces.

The trunk lean also facilitates an optimal position for recovering the swinging (inside) leg across in front

of the body, whilst adopting a position that enables maximal extension of the planting leg before toe-off.

As the leg swings across in front of the body, it is moved so that it can drive backwards into the ground to contact the ground below the centre of mass.

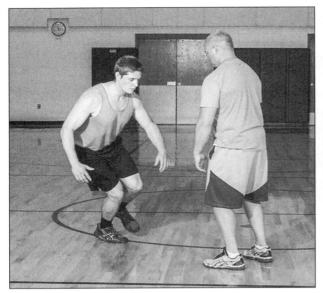
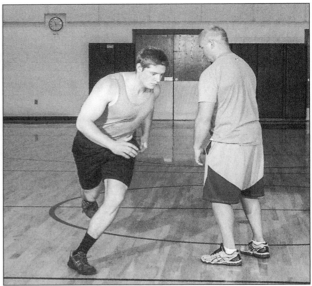
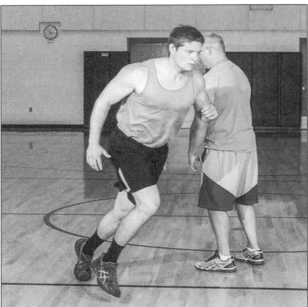

**Figure 8.41**   Inside foot cut.

Normally, these evasion skills would be learned in closed situations, developed in more open situations and refined as agility skills through practices in which decision making and application of the skill in reaction to the changing environment are the keys to success.

## Summary

Ground-based speed and the ability to accelerate in different directions are qualities that distinguish high-performing athletes from the rest. To develop high-velocity movements, athletes must have a range of underpinning technical skills as well as the appropriate physio-mechanical qualities to execute these techniques effectively.

Speed is a skill that can be developed by practitioners who understand what produces high-speed movements and know how to develop these qualities through progressive programming. Acceleration, maximal velocity and direction change mechanics typically depend on the athlete's ability to manage the centre of mass and get in position to optimize ground reaction forces. The practitioner must understand the relationship between stability and mobility and the management of forces to maximize an athlete's speed and directional change capabilities.

Similarly, agility is an athletic quality that combines cognitive and physio-mechanical skills like few others in sport. The practitioner must use a holistic and multifaceted approach to the athlete development programme to link functional strength, plyometric ability, technical execution and decision-making skills into an integrated package. Change-of-direction skills should initially be developed and then progressed in complexity to incorporate high-velocity execution. The perceptual and reaction aspects of the movement should be developed through sport-specific aspects of training.

Speed and agility practices need to be short and sharp to maintain the speed and quality of movement. Speed is a quality movement, and quality is a function of perfection (as opposed to intensity, which is a percentage of maximal). Therefore, intensities are high, volumes are low, and rest periods need to be relatively long.

Total session volume typically is limited by the extent to which high-quality adaptations to both technique and the neuromuscular system can be promoted and sustained. Recovery times within sets should be high, and a low total number of repetitions should be performed within a session.

# CHAPTER 9

# Developing Jumping and Plyometric Skills

Jumping is a fundamental locomotive skill that underpins many sport-specific skills and athletic movements. In executing a jumping action, the athlete is required to exert forces into the ground or take-off surface from either one or both feet, followed by a substantial flight phase, typically of longer duration than a running gait, and a landing action. Such actions in sport can take many forms, and the components of approach, take-off, flight and landing are associated with skilled athletic performance and specific training actions that maximize the physio-mechanical properties of the musculoskeletal system to optimize power development and reduce associated injury risks. These actions, known as plyometrics, form a core component of any athlete development curriculum.

This chapter looks at the specific requirements for jumping actions within sport and advances the practitioner's understanding of how and why to develop these actions within an athletic development programme. This understanding will enable a broader analysis of plyometric training methods and techniques, and give reasons for incorporating them into both generic and sport-specific training schemes to enable the athlete to exploit the mechanical potential of the stretch-shortening cycle mechanism.

## Jumping Actions

In many classification systems, jumps are classified according to the means of foot transfer that occurs before or subsequent from the flight phase of the action. Most of these actions occur in chaotic movement sports, in which the athlete is required to react to a dynamic stimulus (space, opponent or ball), although some sports (for example, track and field) define the requirements for jumping actions very stringently. Indeed, all versions of the common jumping action are seen in the triple jump, which requires the athlete to hop, step (leap) and jump.

A jumping action is usually regarded as any action in which the athlete takes off from or lands on two feet. In many sporting situations, such as a defensive header in soccer or a block in volleyball, the athlete uses a two-footed take-off, and in some sports a transfer to a single-leg landing occurs, such as in the tennis serve. Jumping may also originate from a split stance. Practitioners need to acknowledge that a two-footed take-off doesn't necessarily mean that the feet are parallel.

At a fundamental level, leaping or bounding is defined as the transfer of weight from one foot to the other. Surprisingly, an analysis of a wide variety of sports shows that few have this movement skill as a sport-specific requirement. Similarly, the ability to take off on one foot and land on the same foot (hopping) does not appear as a defined skill in many sporting contexts. But the qualities of motor control required to coordinate single-leg take-offs and landings are essential in chaotic and multidirectional sports, in which high-force and high-velocity single-leg movements and the ability either to stabilize in this position or to transition into another movement commonly occur as performance features. The ability to control such landings is especially associated with a reduction in common injuries in athletes, such as ACL injuries in which the knee is forced into flexion and valgus positions, usually without contact or collisions.

Equally important, the ability to generate sufficient impulse into the ground through ground reaction forces either to accelerate (take off) or to decelerate (land) the centre of mass through a single-foot contact is an important athletic quality. Force application in jumping mechanics is a vital component of the skill. The amount of force applied and the timing of force application are crucial in achieving a change in the direction of the athlete's centre of mass. The required vector is determined by whether the athlete needs to jump as high as possible, as far as possible or to an optimum height to intercept a travelling object, such as a basketball or a baseball hit towards the far wall. As discussed in chapter 4, the flight path of the athlete's centre of mass is determined by the amount of horizontal and vertical impulse applied into the take-off stride.

This critical moment of force application can be influenced by a number of variables. Predominantly, these variables are the velocity of the centre of mass at take-off, the angle of take-off and the height of the centre of mass at take-off. The relative importance of each of these variables changes depending on the athletic context. For example, in a standing maximal vertical jump, the height of the centre of mass at take-off can account for between 40 and 44 per cent of the variance in the resultant jump height,[1] which is influenced by both the athlete's physique (which cannot be changed) and the body position at take-off.

Dynamic contexts, in which the athlete transitions into the take-off from either a run or another jump, occur more frequently in sport than static take-offs. In these instances, the athlete's actions immediately before and during take-off significantly influence take-off velocity and angle, which relates to the concept of optimal velocity introduced in chapter 8. Indeed, the analysis of the long jump by Hay, Miller and Cantera[1] found that horizontal take-off velocities in the fourth- and third-to-the last strides before take-off were the most significant factors influencing flight distance. These factors in turn influence the height of the athlete's centre of mass and so are arguably the most important considerations for technical development.[2] Indeed, relative height of centre of mass at take-off was the second most significant factor in flight distance, indicating the importance of postural control and ground contact mechanics in the progression of jumping skills.

The athlete must practise and master approach transitions to jumping situations, the forceful application of single- and double-foot take-off mechanics, the management of posture during flight and, essential for most sporting contexts, control of landing mechanics. Mastery means that the athlete either maximizes the jump (for example, in a long jump context, in which the length of the jump is determined by the last point of body contact) or can transition efficiently into the subsequent movement.

# Plyometrics

As with most powerful actions in sport, jumping relies on the stretch reflex to optimize the elastic properties of the muscle. As discussed in chapter 2, the stretch reflex allows the protective mechanisms of the neuromuscular system to be overridden to produce powerful reflex actions and allows the elastic energy stored within the serial elastic components of the musculotendinous and myofascial structures to contribute to powerful performance. The need for the protective mechanisms of the stretch reflex (or stretch-shortening cycle) within the muscle arises from the consideration that, as a body falls towards the ground from a height, it constantly gathers momentum as gravity accelerates it. Landing from a jump requires the athlete to control ground reaction forces of 3 to 14 times body weight or more, depending on the flight trajectory, flight time and velocity of the centre of mass. This exceptionally high level of force may need to be controlled through a single-leg ground contact.

Therefore, the first consideration for jumping progressions relates to the athlete's postural strength and his or her ability to be robust enough in postural integrity to control the ground reaction forces from landing. But this robustness doesn't necessarily relate to the athlete's force-producing capabilities purely from a musculoskeletal sense, because the requirements for force expression are typically quicker than can be voluntarily expressed.

This need has led to the evolution of specialist training methods known as plyometrics that change the body's neural recruitment characteristics rather than the muscle's structural characteristics to reflect the functional demands for peak power outputs in landing and rebounding situations. The word *plyometrics*, popularized by the American Fred Wilt in his writings in the 1960s and 1970s, is derived from the Greek words *plethyein* (to increase) and *isometric* (in relation to the muscle action).[3]

Understanding the term helps the practitioner understand the methodology of the training. Most of the work in this area was pioneered by the Soviet scientist and track coach Dr Yuri Verkoshansky throughout the early 1960s. It was based on the idea of causing a shock (in its purest form, plyometrics is known as shock training) that results from the collision of an athlete's body with the floor. As the athlete accelerates towards the floor from a height, the body accumulates kinetic energy. As the body lands, a sharp and instantaneous increase in eccentric muscle tension occurs, caused by the external opposition (i.e., the ground) to the body's direction of travel. This increase in muscle tension stimulates the intrafusal muscle spindle fibres to initiate a reflex contraction that uses the elastic potential of the muscle to produce a powerful and involuntary response to the ground reaction forces.

The rapid transition between the eccentric and concentric phases of muscle action in this circumstance is marked by the amortization phase. As this chapter explains, the length of this phase is largely determined by the athlete's landing mechanics. The very rapid increase in

muscle tension arising from ground reaction (contact) forces stimulates the muscles to produce high-impulse forces during the subsequent take-off. For the kinetic energy to play a major role in stimulation, the amortization phase has to be as fast as possible, which has major implications for the athlete's landing technique to minimize ground contact time yet maximize ground reaction force. Balancing the inverse relationship between these two movement outcomes is a planning and coaching skill that needs to be mastered in the effective delivery of plyometrics within a programme.

Let's analyse two rebound jumping methods: the depth jump and the drop jump. Each of these training exercises has a different objective. The objective of the depth jump (figure 9.1) is to achieve the highest possible vertical height. Contrast this with the drop jump (figure 9.2), which has the objective to achieve the highest possible vertical jump but with minimal ground contact time (i.e., the emphasis is on short ground contact rather than the resultant jump height).

In an activity that is not time constrained and for which greater power output is desired (as in the depth jump), the athlete typically starts from a higher jumping height to achieve greater vertical displacement through the dropping phase. Descending from a higher starting point enables the body to accelerate through a greater distance and store more kinetic energy. A longer ground contact time, however, is needed to achieve maximal vertical impulse and enable ground reaction forces to achieve maximal vertical acceleration of the body against gravity. The longer the force is applied (whilst still be able to use the stored kinetic energy within the musculoskeletal network), the greater the rebound action is. Therefore, in coaching a depth jump, the concept of optimal ground contact time is discussed. With the drop jump, the concept of short ground contacts is promoted. In the drop jump, the athlete's ability to control the landing and increase the rate of reactive force development is the key consideration in determining how high the drop should be.

This principle is important, because it underpins the potential athletic development

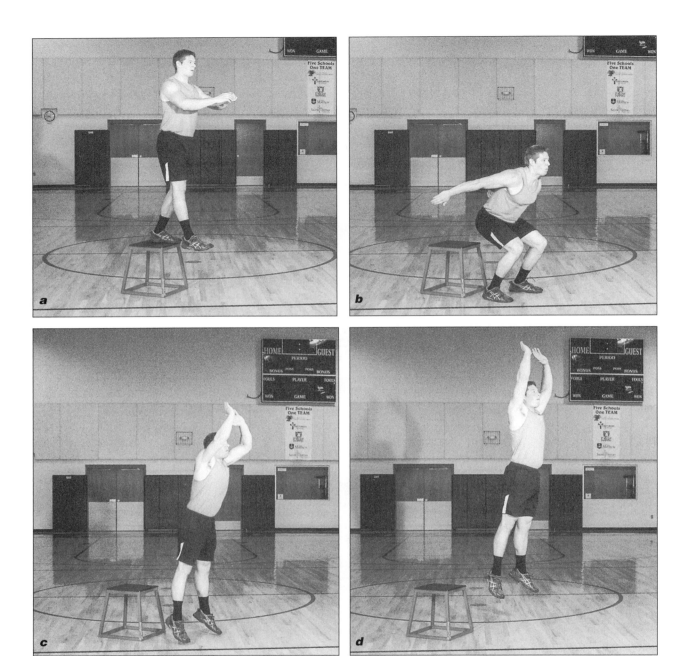

**Figure 9.1** Depth jump: *(a)* start position; *(b)* land on floor; *(c)* take-off after relatively long ground contact time; *(d)* maximal vertical height.

progressions that can be put in place. For example, if the objective is to increase maximal vertical power, the athlete should be encouraged to perform rebound jumps that have an overhead goal (for example, a maximal reach height). To enhance power with reduced ground contact times, however, consider the use of low hurdles to jump over. Note that each of these qualities should be developed

within the athlete's overall programme. If the aim is to increase the athlete's ability to generate impulse (as discussed in chapter 4), the rate of force development with optimal foot contact times will aid activities such as starting acceleration (in which inertia needs to be overcome when the athlete has less momentum and therefore is in in contact with the ground longer). Contrast this scenario with maximal

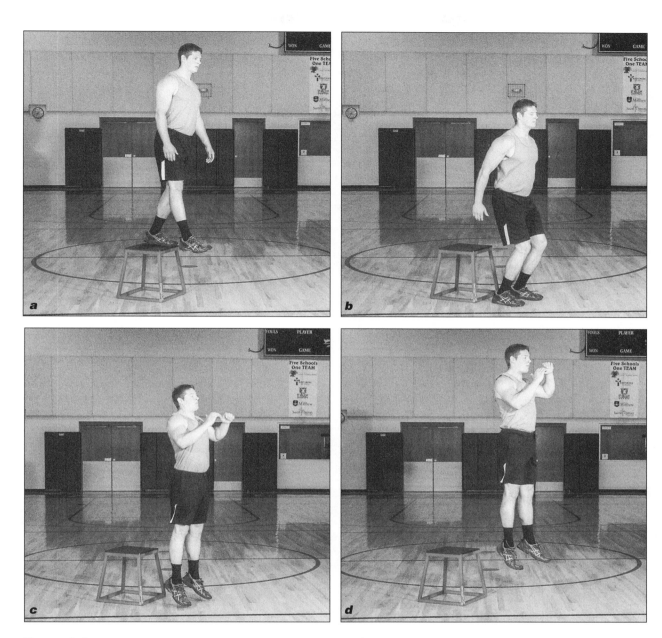

**Figure 9.2** Drop jump: *(a)* start position; *(b)* land on floor; *(c)* take-off with minimal ground contact time; *(d)* maximal vertical height.

speed running, in which the horizontal velocity of the athlete means that optimal forces have to be applied in minimal ground contact times, which requires the athletic qualities developed by activities such as the drop jump.

Initiating a stretch reflex requires proper landing and rebounding techniques. Effective ground contact techniques enable the athlete to optimize reactive force production. For this reason, landing mechanics are usually the

first skill component taught in a plyometric or jumping-skills progression. If the foot placement during approach and landing mechanics is optimized, potentiation (an enhancement in contractility and excitability of the contractile components in the athlete's neuromuscular system) caused by the stretch reflex can occur (table 9.1). As the athlete approaches the landing, the ankle is dorsiflexed so that the toes are pulled up towards the knee and the

**Table 9.1**  Landing Mechanics Enhance the Stretch-Reflex Actions of the Lower Limbs

|  | **Eccentric phase** | **Amortization phase** | **Concentric phase** |
|---|---|---|---|
| Action involved | The prime mover (agonist muscle) is stretched. | This transition phase between eccentric and concentric phases should be as short as possible for the action to be effective. | The muscle fibres in the prime movers are shortened. |
| Results of action | Potential energy is stored in the muscle and connective tissue. Stretch receptors within the muscle are stimulated. | Stretch inhibitors send signals to the central nervous system, which stimulates concentric contraction of the agonist muscles. | Basic energy is released from the muscles and connective tissue. Prime movers are stimulated to contract forcefully and concentrically. |

athlete lands with an active flat foot. The gastrocnemius and soleus muscles and the Achilles tendon are therefore prestretched during the landing approach. Immediately before ground contact, the athlete should forcefully plantarflex the ankle so that the foot attacks the floor. Although this action might seem to reduce the pretension in the posterior muscles of the shank, it will in fact enable a more forceful landing and rebound action.

As the foot contacts the ground, active plantarflexion means that the athlete contacts the ground aggressively with a large portion of the foot (although the heel does not contact the ground). As in speed work, the credit card rule is a good one to apply; the coach should be able to swipe a credit card, and nothing more, under the heel at the point of foot contact. Weight is distributed evenly through the middle of the foot, rather than towards the rear, as can happen if the heel is on the ground. Having most of the foot in contact with the ground means that the athlete has a relatively large surface area through which to apply reactive force into the ground.

Proper timing and attacking the floor with aggressive plantarflexion immediately before ground contact prevents the effect of pretension in the ankle from being lost. Indeed, in time-constrained activities, this must occur as a means of reducing the amount of time that the foot is in contact with the ground. The action of gravity and downward vertical momentum causes the gastrocsoleus complex (calf muscles) to be eccentrically lengthened on ground contact, which stores energy in the serial-elastic components of the muscle and stimulates the muscle spindle fibres within these muscles. Indeed, actively contracting to plantarflex increases the resultant stretch on the lower leg muscles on ground contact, which increases the rate of stretch in these muscles and the effect of the stretch reflex in the subsequent rebounding action.[4]

In untrained people, the golgi tendon organs within the myotendinous junction also are stimulated to inhibit a contractile response to the external load (i.e., multiples of body weight going through the muscles). This protective response can be inhibited through repeated exposure to the relevant stimulus, another reason for including high-force, high-velocity rebound jumps in a range of training programmes.

The amortization phase represents the transition from eccentric lengthening to reflex concentric actions. This phase needs to be as quick as possible to maximize the plyometric action. If the amortization phase is too long, the stored elastic energy within the serial-elastic components will dissipate through heat and the stretch-reflex action will not be as effective in increasing the muscle activity during the subsequent concentric phase of the action.[5] For this reason, this phase of the jumping technique is critical and needs a heavy focus in training athletes to jump.

The responsive concentric muscle action occurs throughout the push-off phase of the jump, during which the agonist muscles, those primarily responsible for the movement, contract with more activation than would normally occur during a voluntary muscle contraction. The reaction is assisted by the release of stored energy within the muscles, resulting in an efficient transfer of ground reaction forces into the jump. But this efficiency can be achieved only with an optimal technique that enables all the actions to be coordinated in a way that ensures the appropriate sequencing of force and energy transfer.

A plyometric response underpins most powerful actions within sport. Therefore, the response must be developed through the appropriate introduction of jumping and rebounding to the athletic development programme. The need to coordinate such actions is an important aspect of athletic performance. This learned process will benefit any sport performer.

# Biomechanics of Jumping

Jumping mechanics are influenced by the position of the body relative to the foot contact with the ground. For example, in the countermovement jump, in which the aim is to achieve maximum vertical height from a static two-footed take-off, the shoulders should be in line with the knees at the bottom of the

countermovement (figure 9.3). This alignment brings the trunk upright and the centre of mass over the middle of the foot, enabling the athlete to push as hard and as long as possible into the ground to create as much vertical force as possible, which is important because the athlete will travel in direct opposition to gravity.

Analysis of the maximal countermovement jump[6] indicates that three major factors influence the overall height of the jump or the height that the centre of mass will achieve: physique, skill and neuromuscular power (figure 9.3). The height of the centre of mass at take-off accounts for approximately 44 per cent of the total jump height and largely depends on the athlete's physique. The athletic development coach can do little to influence the athlete's physique or arm length as the athlete reaches tall towards the apex of the jump.

Essential skill components, however, can be practiced. Proper timing ensures that the trunk is tall as the foot leaves the floor and that the arms travel forwards to reach maximal height at the apex of the jump when the centre of mass is at its highest point. Indeed,

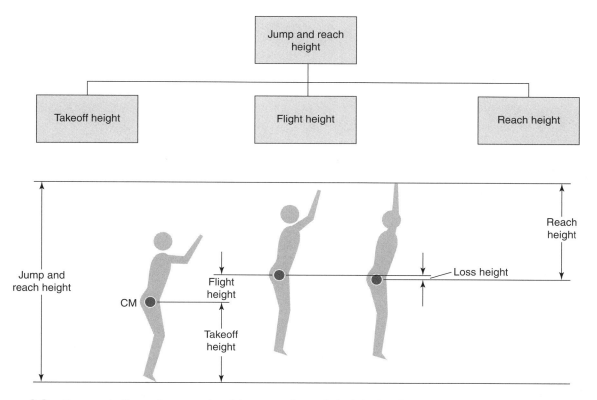

**Figure 9.3**    Factors influencing maximal jump and reach height in the countermovement jump.

arm reach height—the distance between the centre of mass and the top of the fingertips at maximum vertical displacement—accounts for up to 42 per cent of the total jump height. Therefore, arm action is important. As the athlete descends through the preparatory counter-movement to initiate a slow stretch-shortening cycle and store energy in the muscle's serial-elastic components, the arms are brought backwards behind the hips. As the athlete begins to extend the hips and the knees, he or she brings the arms forwards. In a skilled action, the arms reach the lowest point as the body weight is moving through the middle of the foot. Transferring weight to the front of the foot too soon reduces the time over which the ground reaction forces can occur or the surface area through which forces can be exerted, which will significantly influence the impulse of the take-off action. As the push transfers towards the front of the foot and the ankle plantarflexes, the arms continue their forward movement. The segmental momentum that the arms gain contributes to the upward momentum of the body as it leaves the ground and carries on through the flight.

The net force exerted by the combined extensor actions of the hip, knee, ankle and shoulder extensors are the largest determinants of the vertical velocity of the centre of mass at take-off. This force, minus the losses in flight height because of the action of gravity on the athlete's mass, determines the rate of change in velocity of the centre of mass during the flight phase of the jump. Training these muscles to develop and express large forces rapidly through coordinated actions is an important part of developing the biomechanics of the athlete when jumping.

The postural control muscles in the trunk are also vital during the vertical jump. Unless the torso is rigid and erect during take-off, the centre of mass height will not be maximized and the structure through which ground reaction forces can be transferred will not be rigid. This will significantly reduce the vertical impulse and therefore the momentum of the body in flight. Postural rigidity throughout the action is an important concept to transfer from other progressions within the athletic development programme (chapter 10).

Horizontal jumps within sport and related plyometric training methods usually involve single-foot take-offs because of the horizontal momentum that the athlete usually has coming into such actions. In a single-foot take-off, the arms and the unsupported (non-take-off) leg serve to counter the rotational forces that occur when a force is offset (i.e., through one side of the body).

Single-leg horizontal jumps across a variety of sports can generally be broken down into four key components related to the approach, take-off, flight and landing phases of the movement. As with all jumps, landing mechanics are important, and these will be discussed in detail as the first stage in progressing a jumping teaching sequence, although the sport-specific techniques for landing in sandpits (e.g., the long jump) or on the back on a crash mat (e.g., high jump or pole vault) are best explored through sport-specific coaching resources.

The approach phase brings the athlete to take-off with a large horizontal velocity and with the dominant foot appropriately placed for take-off, usually requiring the athlete to adjust the length of his or her final strides. The location of the optimal take-off point differs with the context of the jump. For example, in the long jump, the optimal take-off point is a fixed point, and athletes will have a preferred take-off leg, which influences the length and stride patterning of the run-up. In the basketball lay-up, however, the take-off point is determined by the athlete's velocity and distance from the backboard, a situation replicated across many sports; the situation may require the athlete to take off from either foot with a short approach (for example, a soccer player may have two to six strides to approach an attacking header towards goal).

During take-off, the flight parabola of the centre of mass is determined. If the objective is to attain maximum horizontal displacement as in the long jump, the athlete needs to achieve lift (vertical velocity) with little loss in horizontal velocity by using an active foot plant with a down-and-back motion in the planted foot (see figure 9.4), following which the ankle, knee and hip joints are fully extended. As the take-off leg is planted, the nonplanted foot rotates under the hips so that it rises to a horizontal

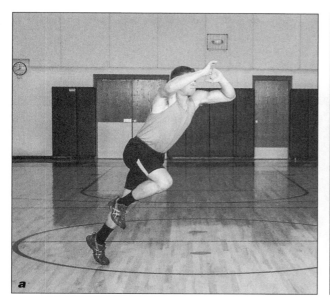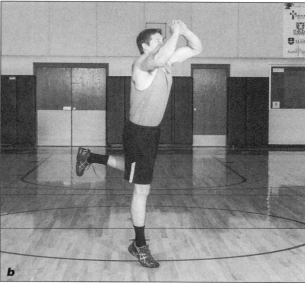

**Figure 9.4**   The take-off for single-leg *(a)* horizontal and *(b)* vertical jumping actions.

position immediately before the take-off foot loses contact with the ground. The direction in which the knee of this leg points influences the direction of travel in the jump. Simultaneously, the opposite arm moves forward, similar to the sprint running action described in chapter 8, to counter rotations that could otherwise exist between the upper and lower bodies because of the leg actions.

If vertical height is the objective, the approach movement needs to be slower. The horizontal velocity at take-off is less, and the planted foot has a longer ground contact time and is able to apply more vertical impulse. The hips are directly above the planted foot as the major drive into the ground occurs, and the active flat foot pushes downwards into the ground rather than down and back as in the horizontal jump. The arm action is also slightly different; the arm movements are upwards in a vertical jump rather than forwards as in the horizontal jump.

The action of the non-take-off leg is also important in single-limb take-offs. Basketball coaches encourage players performing lay-ups to jump for the hoop with the outside knee bent and driving upwards as the inside arm drives upwards. Other single-leg sporting actions are the same; the ankle, knee and hip joints of the take-off leg fully extend during the process at the same time that the thigh of the contralateral leg drives to a horizontal

position with the knee and ankle flexed. The opposite arm also moves forward to counter any rotations in the trunk because of the actions of the legs.

The take-off (figure 9.4) is essential to achieve a flight that permits the athlete's centre of mass to travel through the optimal flight time and pattern for the skill whilst enabling the optimum position for landing. For example, in the high jump, the athlete attempts to maximize vertical velocity and initiate rotations to clear the bar with a flop technique. In soccer, the defender may need maximal vertical velocity to outjump an attacking player and head the ball clear, but all rotations must be avoided. Conversely, in the long jump, in which horizontal flight displacement is essential, the aim is to take off tall to maximize the height of the centre of mass, yet the athlete needs to minimize any losses in horizontal velocity generated in the approach phases to the jump.

Learning to land from a jump is probably more important than learning to take off in terms of the safe progression of jumping exercises. Landing requires the athlete to decelerate a body travelling towards the ground at a speed being accelerated by gravity at 9.81 metres per second. Safe landing means positioning the centre of mass relative to the base of support and aligning the joints appropriately to absorb the load.

In most sporting contexts, landing from a jump is not only a discreet skill but also a transitional skill that links to another movement such as rebound jumps, landing and running or landing and cutting. Chapter 5 identified the potential for knee injuries in situations of high force loading through rapid decelerations achieved through the incorrect alignment of the ankle, knee and hip. Acute (i.e., traumatic) injuries to these joints are a major concern in landing mechanics, but the repetitive nature of landing in sport also means a risk for long-term consequences. Athletes need the motor skills and strength to prevent chronic injuries.

As figure 9.5 illustrates, the landing techniques required for different movement situations show many similarities but also subtle differences, and these differences needs to be reflected in the athlete's learning progressions. In all situations, the shoulders should be in line with the knees to bring the centre of mass over the base of support, stabilizing the athlete and reducing the chance of overbalancing forwards. The ankles, knees and hips flex to absorb the impact forces generated through ground reaction. No internal rotation at the knee should be evident. A high-impact knee valgus (inward collapse) is a major precursor to knee injury in many sporting situations. Therefore, the knee must track the line of the toes as the athlete lands.

The major differences between an athlete stopping and an athlete reaccelerating relate to the weight distribution through the foot and the amount of flexion in the joints in response to ground reaction forces. As illustrated in figure 9.5, when the athlete is landing, the hips and knees flex to absorb and dissipate ground reaction forces that otherwise transfer up through the musculoskeletal chain. Conversely, to rebound, the key focus is on maintaining the stiffness at the ankle and knee joints that allow the stretch reflex to occur, thus optimizing the ground contact time.

Athletes should be coached to land towards a flat foot (i.e., prepare for impact with the ground with the ankle stiff and dorsiflexed) and attack the ground. Immediately before ground contact, the athlete forcefully and aggressively plantarflexes the foot to increase the tension through the gastrocnemius, soleus, and Achilles tendon. The athlete is actively plantarflexing at ground contact, leading to several positive consequences for performance.

The active muscular contraction is resisted by ground reaction forces and the tension level in the local neuromuscular system rises rapidly, engaging the stretch reflex more rapidly and therefore more effectively. If timing and coordination are appropriately developed, the other positive consequence is that the athlete makes contact with the ground with the heel raised

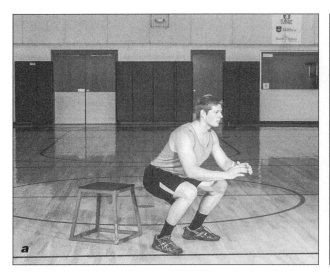 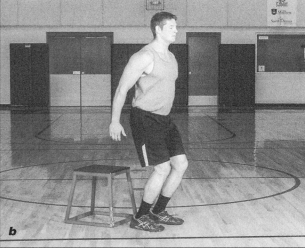

**Figure 9.5**   Proper landing technique: *(a)* to decelerate and stop; *(b)* to land and take off again.

but a large proportion of the foot in contact, providing a large surface area through which to express forces into the ground.

Although the technique for establishing ground contact remains the same, the contact time varies depending on the objective of the rebound jump (table 9.2). These ground contact times are influenced by the relative height of the required rebound jump and the ankle and knee stiffness achieved in landing preparation. If the objective is to develop fast stretch-shortening reflexes with short ground contact times, drop jumps, repeated stiff-leg rebound jumps and repeat tuck jumps are ideal. Conversely, if high forces at rapid rates of force development are the objective, repeated squat jumps and depth jumps are recommended. The specific coaching points and developmental progressions for these exercises are considered in this chapter. What is important to understand now is that within the breadth of an athletic development progression, the spectrum of exercise to develop both fast and short ground contact times typically should be considered.

Experienced coaches will be able to evaluate the quality of ground contact by observing the action, a skill that takes time and practice to develop. Observation also includes listening for a crisp, clear ground contact rather than a heavy or thudding landing. Ground contact time can be quantified in a laboratory setting using an expensive and sensitive force platform or a jump mat. These devices are reasonably accessible and measure the amount of time between the foot making contact with the floor and the foot leaving the floor. These data can be immediately fed back to the athlete, and a corrective intervention can be applied to enable

the athlete to achieve (for example) a faster ground contact (if this is indeed the desired outcome).

Plyometric actions are quick, and some athletes, especially in the early stages of learning, are not able to distinguish between a good ground contact and one that is too slow. Feedback about ground contact times is extremely useful in such situations and can guide learning as well as provide an effective monitoring tool. Feedback might be particularly effective within a session if the practitioner wants to monitor the quality of the movement, something that will be retarded by fatigue. If the quality of ground contact (or indeed other aspects of skill execution) begins to deteriorate during a session, or indeed even during a set, the practitioner may wish to consider stopping the work or revising the rest period to preserve the intent of the movement.

# Mature Model for the Horizontal Jump

As a developmental skill, a mature model for horizontal jumping can be developed early in childhood and be fully evident around 9 years of age. The skill of horizontal jumping is linked to gaining distance from a single- or double-foot take-off and is often associated with running or clearing an obstacle.

The basic technical model for the horizontal jump relies heavily on the stretch-reflex mechanism to generate the power necessary for lift when the athlete is starting from a static position and has no horizontal momentum.

The mature skill has several important features that need to be incorporated into skill development programmes. The first is a balanced starting position, which enables maximal force transfer (impulse generation) through ground reaction forces to facilitate the movement.

Following the countermovement, the jump is initiated by a forcible extension of the hips, knees and ankles whilst at the same time bringing the arms forward from behind the body. A common mistake in young athletes is that

**Table 9.2** Typical Ground Contact Time Varies With Jumping Objective

| Type of jump | Ground contact (ms) |
| --- | --- |
| Tuck jump | 150 to 200 |
| Drop jump | 200 |
| Depth jump | 500 |
| Repeated squat jump | 300 to 400 |
| Stiff-legged rebound jump | 150 to 200 |

# Basic Technical Model for the Mature Skill of Two-Foot Horizontal Jumping

- Stand up straight and look forward. Start with good posture and feet hip-width apart.
- Bend from the knees and hips and keep the arms straight. Perform a countermovement into take-off by swinging the arms backwards from the shoulder. The trunk moves into a forward lean so that the centre of mass begins to move forwards.
- Push through both feet evenly. Force is generated by straightening the knees and hips, and pushing down into the ground through the feet as the ankles plantarflex.
- Arms swing through with force and stretch forwards and upwards. Hips and knees fully extend as the feet leave the ground. The trunk leans forward.

- At the top of the flight, bend the hips and knees and bring the thighs forward to a position parallel with the ground.
- Simultaneously, the trunk comes forward, putting the body in a jack-knife position.
- Land on the balls of the feet, followed by the rest of the feet. Flex the ankles, knees and hips to absorb the landing. Arms reach forwards. Centre of mass moves forwards over the feet (squashy landing).

---

the dipping action of the countermovement is too shallow or too slow; the athlete cannot benefit maximally from the stretch reflex and stored elastic energy of the ballistic action. During the countermovement, the movement of the arms behind the trunk should be high. Their subsequent forward movement is an important part of the skill often neglected in coaching the action. Learning to coordinate this action is part of the practice development, and in immature actions it is not always evident. Indeed, the arms may be seen to move sideways and downwards or rearwards and upwards, often to maintain balance, not to aid forward momentum.

The body should be fully extended, allowing the force to be pushed through the floor for as long as possible to provide maximal impulse for forward momentum. Extension should be completed with the trunk moving into a significant forward lean (maybe as much as 45 degrees) as the athlete leaves the floor. The head lifts and focuses forwards. The arms move forward as the legs extend and reach their highest, or furthermost forward, point at take-off. The arms are held high throughout the jump. In flight, the hips and knees bend to

bring the legs through under the body before the descent. The thighs are held parallel to the floor during flight. Bending the legs too early will retard forward momentum, a common error in many athletes.

The legs should be extended through and in front of the body in preparation for landing. The lower legs land vertically. The degree to which this forward movement occurs depends on the context in which the jump might be used (maximal distance versus landing in a specific spot). The landing should be light; the athlete absorbs the landing forces through flexed hips and knees. Two-foot landings are obviously more stable than single-foot landings, and flat-foot landings are more stable than toe landings, a common error.

## Mature Model for Skipping

At first glance, skipping may seem to be a strange skill to consider in the context of jumping. Skipping, however, is a transitional, rhythmical movement skill that involves alternating steps that in sport are often followed by a hop, jump or run. At a mature skill level, skipping is a complex bilateral activity that involves coordination between both sides of the body working in alternation. Skipping is also a prerequisite skill for a specific class of plyometric activities known as bounding (figure 9.6) that develop powerful horizontal movements in athletes through single-leg take-off and landing actions.

Throughout the skipping action, the trunk should be upright and the feet hip-width apart. From a standing balanced start, the athlete steps forward and transfers weight forward through an active driving action in the rear leg. The front leg is flexed as it moves forward,

and the arms work in opposition to the legs. The opposite arm and leg action is important; as the high knee comes forward, the opposite arm drives backwards from the shoulder. The use of the arms should be rhythmical, but the observer will see reduced arm movement through the phase of weight transfer between the feet.

After the initiation step, the nonsupporting leg is brought forward with a high forward knee lift and the ankle is dorsiflexed ('Pull the toes up to the knee'). As this leg comes to land, ground contact should be active. The person lands and pushes through the balls of the feet. In more advanced athletes, ground

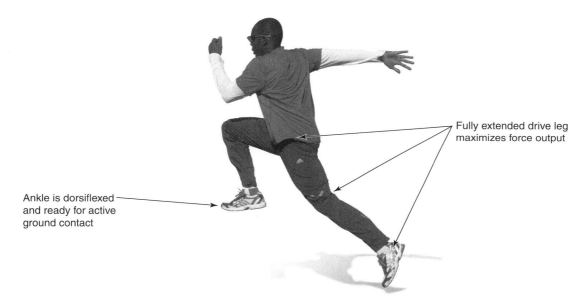

Fully extended drive leg maximizes force output

Ankle is dorsiflexed and ready for active ground contact

**Figure 9.6**   Bounding is a highly effective plyometric skill for power development.

# Basic Technical Model for the Mature Skill of Skipping

- The body is upright. The feet are shoulder-width apart.
- Step forward onto one foot, moving the weight forward. Keep the leg flexed. The arms work in opposition to the legs.
- On the supporting leg, perform a small, springing hop, pushing through the ball of the foot and landing on the ball of the foot.

- As the hop occurs, bring the nonsupporting leg through with a forward knee lift. The toes are pulled up towards the knees.
- Step forward onto the other foot, moving the weight forward. Keep the leg flexed.
- Ensure smooth transitions. Keep the head up and trunk erect, and do not rotate the shoulders or hips.

contact can be developed into an active flat-foot action with the heel staying off the floor. After making ground contact, the athlete performs a springing hop, pushing through the floor with the balls of the feet to propel the body farther forward. The weight transfer alternates between left and right feet. A low vertical lift occurs at the top of the hop. The aim is to develop a fluid and smooth repetitive and consistent transition into the weight transfer through each foot, keeping the trunk erect and with no rotation through either the shoulders or the hips as the athlete moves forward.

# Mature Model for Vertical Jumping

A vertical jump is a coordinated action that can be used in many sporting contexts or as a test to measure explosive power in an athletic context.

The start should be balanced, and the weight should be evenly distributed between the feet. An athlete who is off balance often ends up pushing through only one foot, leading to rotational imbalances and reducing the force transferred through the feet into the ground. Again, the countermovement should be rapid

and full. Typically, a preparatory bend of 60 to 80 degrees of flexion in the knees brings about optimum stretch-reflex actions,[7] although in some people this bend may be as much as 110 degrees.

It is thought that preferred angle for knee flexion is individualized in such actions. The body intuitively optimizes the angle of knee flexion to eccentrically load the individual's neuro-physio-mechanical structures in the lower limb so as to maximize the resultant power production.

In a mature action, the child's trunk remains vertical as the arms reach backwards. The vertical trunk as the athlete begins to take off will bring the centre of mass above the middle of the foot, the optimum position for creating vertical lift through ground reaction force. In slight contrast, as demonstrated in figure 9.7, an advanced athlete passes through this position into take-off but reaches it through a different movement pathway. The advanced athlete begins with flexion from the hips as the knees extend, stretching the hamstrings and initiating a stretch reflex in these muscles as the hips start to extend. This unloading of the hamstrings causes the knees to rebend under the trunk. At the point immediately before

# Basic Technical Model for the Mature Skill of Vertical Jumping

- Stand in good posture, with arms by the sides.
- The feet are hip-width apart. Perform a counter-movement—hips come up and back, shoulders move forwards with the back straight, and arms come back behind the body. As the hips extend, the knees bend under the body as the trunk is brought into a vertical orientation in preparation of the jump. The arms stay back behind the body.
- Forcibly extend the knees, hips and ankles by pushing into the ground with both feet. Both feet leave the ground at the same time. The arms swing up and reach upwards during flight.
- Reach high with the body and arms for as long as possible.

- Bring the toes up towards the knees (flex the ankles) before landing.
- Cushion the landing by flexing the hips and knees as the balls of the feet land on the ground. Visualize using a flat-foot landing, even though the heels aren't really contacting the ground at the same time as the balls of the feet.
- The feet are shoulder-width apart. The trunk is upright, and the head is up for good balance.
- Land lightly in a flexed body position, absorbing the force. Two-foot landings are more stable than one-foot landings.
- Finish by standing up.

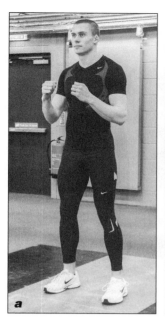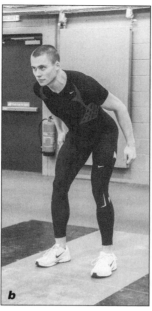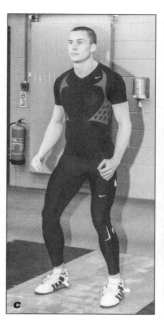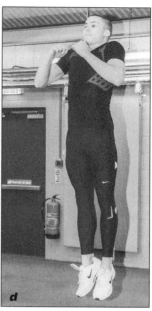

**Figure 9.7** Advanced athletic vertical jump from a static two-footed start encompasses a more effective stretch-reflex action in the leg extensors.

take-off, the trunk comes to vertical and the athlete is able to push into the ground with maximum force through the hips, knees and lastly ankle joint extensors.

The jump needs to be full and forceful. The trunk extends as the arms swing forwards and upwards in a simultaneous, coordinated and forceful action that continues through the vertical lift. The arms reach as high as possible, achieving maximum height at the top of the flight. The body should be fully extended at the apex of the flight trajectory. This position indicates that the centre of mass is optimized in its vertical movement. An exaggerated forward lean of the body on take-off or in flight will cause horizontal displacement during flight, which will detract from vertical climb.

Arm actions are the source of many errors in the skill execution of young children. Arms may be uncoordinated with legs, may wing to the sides or may even move backwards rather than forwards and upwards as the centre of mass rises. The head position is also important in aiding flight. The head should be tilted upwards to lead the movement, and the eyes should be focused on hitting the target (e.g., ball, basket) at the highest point of the flight trajectory.

A balanced, stable landing also is an important feature of the mature jumping action in a child. If maximum vertical height is the aim of a jump, it should occur close to the point of take-off. To establish a cushioned and stable landing in which the ground reaction forces are absorbed through the body, the child needs to prepare for landing. The development of proper landing technique is explored more fully later in the chapter.

# Developing a Mature Jumping Action in Younger Children

Most fundamental movement skills reach the mature stage by 7 years of age. The child can integrate all the component parts of the movement pattern into a coordinated, mechanically correct and efficient act.[8] The child has a platform from which to jump higher and farther, progressing towards more specialized and sport-specific actions at later stages of development.

Practitioners working with young children must understand that without a mature action for a skill, children will be limited in their ability to acquire and apply fundamental skills later in life.[9] This circumstance is detrimental to sport performance and, arguably more important, can limit the choice to participate in sport and physical activities later in life. Before looking at more specialized and demanding jumping tasks, the discussion here needs to consider how mature skills might be developed in young athletes.

Significant development can be achieved through games and activities that challenge the child to explore jumping and hopping skills in relation to the environment. For example, in the early stages of learning, a child may discover various ways to jump or hop by participating in small team relay races during which the child is given specific instructions—such as jump like a frog or have only one foot on the ground at a time—by which to cover the distance to a teammate. These basic games can be progressed to activities that focus on practicing specific aspects of jumping skills (for example, a horizontal or a vertical jump) and finding out what arm and leg actions produce the most height or distance. Questions and challenges are an important part of this coaching strategy, as illustrated by the jumping long practice.

As the jumping action becomes more coordinated and mature, progressions can be used to develop specific aspects of the jump. For

# JUMPING LONG

### Coaching Points
- Stand up straight and look forward. Start with good posture and with feet hip-width apart.
- Use a fast knee and hip bend to start the jump.
- Push hard into the ground with both feet evenly.
- Swing the arms backwards and then stretch forwards and upwards.
- Aim to jump far as well as high.

### Equipment
Four to six dish cones per child to mark distances jumped

### Organization
Arrange children into pairs. Try to match children of similar size or skill level. Each child should have a start (take-off) position marked on the ground and a cone to mark the distance he or she jumps at each attempt.

When instructed, one child at a time should stand at the take-off line and jump. Variations include the following, among others:

- Straight legs at take-off, arms by side
- Bent legs at take-off, arms by side
- Bent legs at take-off, arms swinging forwards and upwards
- Bent legs at take-off using arms, back straight, jumping long and low
- Bent legs at take-off using arms, back straight, jumping long and high

As the child lands, place a marker cone by the heel to identify the distance jumped. If possible, use a different colour for each jump so that the child has a record of which jump covered the distance. Make sure that everyone in the group has a chance to jump

After a series of jumping techniques, encourage the children to think about and show which combination of take-off and landing positions allowed them to jump the farthest. Encourage them to think about the distance jumped relative to the technique used for that jump.

Competition can be added by awarding points. For example, give a point for beating a previous jump distance. (Encourage the child to think about what he or she did to jump farther.)

# HOPPING MAD

## Coaching Points

- Land on a flat foot with the knee and hip bent to absorb the force.
- Keep the head up and still and the eyes level to aid balance.
- Have an upright trunk.

## Equipment

Markers to define a boundary area

## Organization

Spread the children out within the playing area, which can be adapted to accommodate the size of the group. If spatial awareness is important for the level of athlete being coached, then constrain the space available as appropriate. Divide the group into pairs or groups of three. Choose one child per pair or group to take the lead. The lead invents a short sequence of hops (up to a maximum of eight) that his or her partner or partners copy, which can include the following:

- Hopping on one leg for a certain number of hops before changing to the other leg
- Varying the height of the hops
- Varying the speed of the movement or the timing between hops
- Changing direction within the sequence
- Altering the distance of the hops

The role of leader should be alternated between the pair or around the group for an appropriate number of rotations. The children can be encouraged to invent a scoring system for the game, such as 1 point for every hop in sequence that is executed correctly.

example, a lot of practice jumping with bent legs and no arm action encourages leg propulsion.

As children reach a mature stage of skill level, they need to be exposed to activities that continue the practice of jumping, leaping or hopping, and they should be encouraged to apply these skills to various contexts, whether temporal, spatial or even sport-specific in some instances. The hopping mad practice encourages children to remain stable whilst hopping with different intensities and when transferring weight from one foot to another.

# Advancing a Specialized Action: Developing Plyometric Technique

The stretch-shortening cycle is a physio-mechanical phenomenon that underpins performance of any competitive sport that involves aspects of running, jumping or direction change. Therefore, any athletic development programme that seeks to improve sport-specific performance should enhance the stretch-shortening cycle. A major purpose for plyometric activities is to heighten the excitability of the neuromuscular system for improved reactive ability. In short, plyometric exercises provide the link between speed and strength in the athletic progression.

The progressive approach to developing plyometric capabilities needs to be linked to the athlete's ability to manage force development and expression progressively and competently and cope with a range of increasingly complex movements. The foundation consists of repeated jumping and landing skills. There has been much debate about other power development movements such as upper-body actions and medicine ball throws and whether they should be considered plyometric. Although these activities are not wholly plyometric in the truest sense, they are given consideration later in the chapter and can be seen to have a rightful place in the athletic development curriculum.

# Understanding Plyometric Intensity

Jumps from increasing heights or landings with high horizontal velocities can induce significant reactive forces and high levels of stress within the athlete's neuromuscular system. Force output is regulated by the number of motor units being fired and the frequency of action potentials arriving at these motor units within a muscle or group of muscles. Specific recruitment of muscle groups within a coordinated movement sequence is a function of both the central nervous system and musculoskeletal system positioning of the joints. Joint position determines whether the muscles are aligned in an optimum position for length–tension–velocity relationships to produce efficient movement. The practitioner must emphasize appropriate technique (postural control) in the execution of a movement and a progressive approach to overloading this technique.

Plyometric training is extremely demanding on the neuromuscular and musculoskeletal systems. Therefore, the practitioner must absorb and understand the principles and considerations behind the competence-based progressive delivery of these highly effective exercises if they are to be prescribed safely and correctly.

The intensity of a plyometric action is determined by the amount of stress placed on the musculoskeletal system based on the assumption that the action is undertaken with maximal intent (maximum effort). The stress applied to the athlete's system is a function of the athlete's mass, the velocity of the centre of mass and the height of the centre of mass at landing, all of which influence the ground reaction forces experienced through the landing. But not everyone has the same response to a defined load (in this case, ground reaction force). The person's ability to tolerate or indeed overcome the resistive load has a significant effect on the relative intensity of an exercise.

Therefore, when considering progressions, the practitioner should consider the athlete's characteristics (biological and training age, strength, technical ability, body mass and gender) in conjunction with (not separate from) the intended movement programme (volume, drop height, movement complexity, number of points of support and consequential muscle actions). Case by case, the relative importance of each of these aspects should be evaluated to determine whether an athlete is ready to undertake a particular exercise within a programme or whether caution might advise against its use. The answer will become evident as the exercises and their progressions are explored in more depth.

# JUMP ONTO A 60-CENTIMETRE BOX

## Coaching Points
- The athlete uses a two-footed take-off and landing.
- Movement is initiated with a countermovement.
- The athlete needs to achieve maximum extension before flexing the hips and knees to land on the box. This action ensures maximal vertical propulsion.

## Equipment
A 60-centimetre box that is very stable and has an even, nonslip surface

## Caution
The athlete must be able to generate sufficient vertical force to enable him or her to land on the box. The height of the box can be adapted to the individual strength demand.

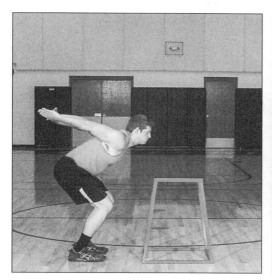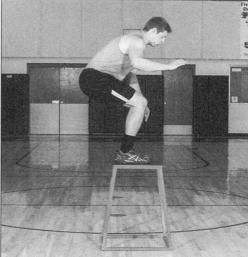

**Figure 9.8**    Jump onto a 60-centimetre box.

## Organization

Stand in front of the box at a comfortable distance, usually 50 to 70 centimetres. Use a two-footed take-off to jump onto the box (figure 9.8). Land evenly on both feet.

## Activity Consideration

The athlete is accelerating against gravity to land, therefore the landing demand (reactionary force) will be less than body weight and the landing will be low velocity. For this reason, this exercise typically has a low plyometric intensity rating.

# JUMP ONTO A 1-METRE BOX FROM A 60-CENTIMETRE BOX

## Coaching Points

- Step off the box with the ankles dorsiflexed.
- Use a double-foot landing with an active flat-foot contact.
- Use rapid yet forceful ground contact.
- Maintain an upright trunk.

## Equipment

Two boxes (1-metre and 60-centimetres) that are stable and have nonslip surfaces

## Organization

Place the two boxes 1 to 2 metres apart, depending on ability. Step off the first box with the ankles dorsiflexed. Land on both feet simultaneously, using a forceful and active flat-foot contact, and then jump onto the second box, landing with a double-foot contact (figure 9.9). As you land, drive into the standing position. Perform sets of four to six repetitions.

## Activity Consideration

This low-complexity double-foot movement has no external loading beyond body weight. But the athlete is stepping off a relatively high height and will accelerate towards the floor

*(continued)*

## Jump Onto a 1-Metre Box From a 60-Centimetre Box *(continued)*

(at 9.81 meters per second) with gravity for a long time. This activity places very high demand on the eccentric muscle actions to brake the action and high demand on the concentric muscle actions to produce rapid reaction forces that will propel the athlete back through the 60-centimetre height onto the landing box.

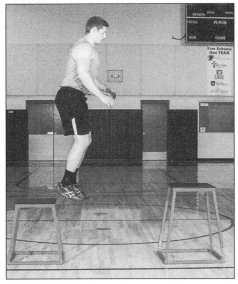
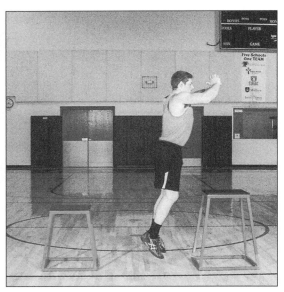
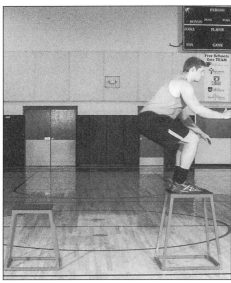
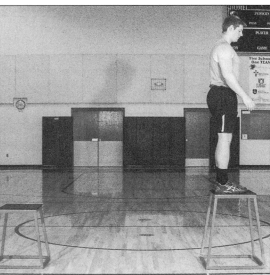

**Figure 9.9** Jump onto a 1-metre box from a 60-centimetre box.

### Programming Consideration

Four sets of 3 to 5 repetitions = 12 to 20 foot contacts

A high-intensity exercise such as this requires the athlete to be unfatigued to execute high-quality movements. Fatigue will detract from coordination and force production. High numbers of repetitions (e.g., more than six) within a set may cause fatigue that is counterproductive to the objective of the exercise. Similarly, if the athlete is fatigued from cumulative work within a training week or if the exercise is being used late within a high-volume session, proceed with caution.

### Athlete Consideration

The athlete needs to be technically competent in performing a squat landing from a 1-metre height before being considered for this exercise. Athletes who are not able to control their landings consistently should not be considered for this exercise.

This exercise requires high levels of both eccentric and concentric strength, particularly in the lower limbs. Therefore, the major consideration is the athlete's ability to overcome the ground reaction forces of many times body weight going through the hip, knee and ankle joints and to apply concentric force reactively to reaccelerate the body against gravity in the subsequent concentric action. Body mass is an important consideration in whether an athlete undertakes this exercise; heavy individuals with a body mass over 120 kilograms would be advised to undertake this exercise with caution. Body weight also influences the number of repetitions performed: Five repetitions for a 70-kilogram athlete has a significantly different volume load from three repetitions in a 100-kilogram athlete.

This exercise lends itself to strong people who can apply reactive forces in short periods. Therefore, any person who cannot perform a squat with one and a half times body weight might not be strong enough for this exercise.[10] Likewise, those who can't complete five repetitions of a squat with 60 per cent of body weight as an additional load[11] might not have the reactive strength capabilities to perform this exercise competently.

---

# MULTIDIRECTIONAL HURDLE HOP

### Coaching Points

- Use single-foot landings with an active flat-foot contact.
- The ankle remains dorsiflexed throughout the activity.
- Maintain alignment of the hips, knees and ankles throughout the activity.
- Maintain hip, knee and ankle stiffness in extension and dorsiflexion throughout the sequence.

### Equipment

Four minihurdles

### Organization

Four minihurdles are placed equidistant apart (the distance depends on athletic quality) in a square (figure 9.10). Start in the middle of the square. Hop over a hurdle and back to the middle. Continue hopping in sequence around the four hurdles. This sequence can be adapted to forward, back, left and right movements or the sequence can go forward, left, back, right in sequence, as required by the programme objectives.

### Activity Consideration

The multidirectional hurdle hop is a complex single-foot movement. Directional change is required through a single-foot take-off and landing, which requires advanced single-foot landing and take-off skills. The landing height for each jump isn't great, so the vertical ground reaction forces aren't large relative to other movements. But the mediolateral and anteroposterior forces that need to be controlled in landing are relatively high. The direction change from transverse plane to sagittal plane needs to be achieved without a long ground contact time through which to reapply force, so this drill is challenging to execute. The height and distance of the hurdles can be altered to increase or decrease the concentric force challenges of the movement.

*(continued)*

## Multidirectional Hurdle Hop *(continued)*

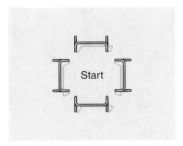

**Figure 9.10**   Multidirectional hurdle hop.

### Programming Consideration
Four sets of 3 to 5 repetitions = 12 to 20 foot contacts

A highly complex single-limb exercise such as this one requires the athlete to be unfatigued to execute high-quality movements. Fatigue will detract from coordination and force production, manifesting as increased ground contact time between each hop. High numbers of repetitions (e.g., more than 6) within a set may cause fatigue that is counterproductive to the objective of the exercise. Similarly, if the athlete is fatigued from cumulative work within a training week or the exercise is being used late within a high-volume session, proceed with caution.

### Athlete Consideration
This exercise has low eccentric demand, so body weight may not be as significant a factor to consider as training age. This complex exercise is for an intermediate-level athlete who has plyometric experience and conditioning.

The athlete needs to be able to control a single-leg landing and take-off from different directions, including jumping away from the line of vision. Sagittal plane and frontal plane forces require the athlete to have high levels of ankle, knee and hip stability. The athlete should be able to execute a well-controlled single-leg landing from a small drop height as well as be stable in a single-leg hop landing from both the sagittal and frontal planes. Stable posture is key, because inappropriate rotations through the upper body might induce transverse movement forces through the hip, resulting in a valgus movement at the knee that may cause injuries at the knee joint. Competence in performing multiple single-foot linear hops and in performing double-foot multidirectional movements is essential. The success of the exercise depends on the athlete's ability to execute the skill without prolonged ground contact, which is a potential in such complex movements.

In terms of plyometric progressions, the movement demand is a function of loading, support and complexity. Mechanical loading, or the physical stressor to the body, is a function of the influence of gravity on the athlete's system mass during the movement. System mass is used, because plyometrics exercises are often performed with an external load, such as a weighted vest or a barbell. When a vertical jump is performed, the athlete is resisting gravity, and therefore the body decelerates as the athlete rises.

In contrast, a body moving towards the floor will be accelerated by gravity, at a rate of 9.81 metres per second. Any athlete dropping from a height will be landing with forces many times body weight. These forces must be resisted and reacted to quickly if the plyometric exercise is to be successful in achieving the required training benefit. The longer the athlete's flight time is, the greater the influence of gravity will be. Therefore, the acceleration pattern (determined by the drop height, the velocity of the body and the hang time of the jump) plays a major role in determining how much stress the athlete's musculoskeletal system will be subject to per repetition. As an example, a triple jumper landing from the hop and taking off for the jump may have in excess of 15 times body weight being transferred through a single leg during the ground contact phase.

The acceleration pattern and the system mass determine the eccentric demand during the landing. The objective of the take-off determines the concentric muscular demand of the exercise. For example, jumping rope in place, which is a basic plyometric exercise, requires little vertical displacement of the body. The drop height is low, and the subsequent rebound jump is not very high. Both the eccentric and concentric strength demands are relatively low for the athlete. In-line repetitive hops for distance have high concentric demands, because the athlete must propel the body forwards using a single limb. But the eccentric demands on the supporting leg during landing are reasonably low because the acceleration drop is, relatively speaking, not significant, and the athlete is seeking to decelerate and reaccelerate in the same direction. The demands are very different in a depth jump, in which the athlete decelerates and then reaccelerates in the opposite direction.

In comparison, a drop from a 1-metre box that is followed by jumps over 70-centimetre hurdles will have a high eccentric demand but a reasonably low concentric muscle action focus. Adding a 15 per cent external load to the body (for example, by adding a weighted vest) increases the concentric muscle action requirement and the eccentric demand. Most researchers[12] agree that drops from heights in excess of 1.2 metres may retard plyometric response because the eccentric demand can exceed the capabilities of the neuromuscular system to maintain a quick enough amortization phase. For athletes of more than 100 kilograms of body mass, this height may be significantly less; a maximum height of 50 centimetres might be considered for a drop. Although these guidelines represent the majority of athletic populations, some elite power athletes exceed these parameters. Later in this chapter, guidelines for the appropriate calculation of drop height for shock plyometrics are introduced.

A common criticism of practitioners who are seeking to increase the intensity of plyometric drills is that they use equipment such as hurdles to progress a drill without thinking critically about how this will achieve or influence the objectives of the exercise. For example, consider the double-foot jump over a minihurdle. The objective of the drill is to maintain an extended hip and knee and use the stiffness in the ankle joint to achieve vertical clearance of the hurdle.

The hurdle increases the vertical force needed to achieve a jump by providing a target height to clear. A young or inexperienced athlete, however, is focused less on the technical points (toes pulled up, ankles stiff, hips and knees stiff and straight) and more on clearing the height of the hurdle, causing him to bend his knees so that he can clear the hurdle, toes pointing downwards, which compromises his preparation for effective ground contact. Therefore, increases in intensity of an exercise should be matched to the challenge it provides and the athlete's movement competency. Note as well that the level of challenge does not change the specific objective of the movement.

Practitioners make a similar mistake when they identify that an athlete needs to work on reducing ground contact time. They correctly recognize that a drop jump might be a sound means of achieving this objective, but after a while they think they need to progress the exercise and therefore introduce a high box for the athlete to land on following the rebound jump. This change requires the athlete to produce greater concentric force, which necessitates a longer ground contact time. Thus, the exercise selection is counterproductive to the athlete's needs!

Many people have traditionally underestimated the additional demand created by an activity when changing from a double- to a single-leg action. Often they think that most basic sporting movements are plyometric, and many single-leg plyometric actions, such as running, do not impose significant demands on the athlete. Likewise, a simplistic action such as repetitive jumping on the spot can easily be turned into a single-leg cyclical action without undue demand on most athletes, despite the fact that the exercise places twice the demand on the athlete, because the load through the support leg has instantaneously doubled. In few training activities would coaches likely be happy to prescribe a training load exactly twice as much as the previous one.

Yet this type of progression is common in training arenas around the world. For example, a young child has been performing double-foot jumps over a series of six minihurdles. When the coach thinks that the athlete is able to do this with sufficient competence, often the next step is to repeat the activity as a single-leg drill even though this exercise is wholly different. The surface area through which to transfer ground reaction forces is vastly reduced, and much less musculature can be used to generate ground reaction forces. Likewise, the reduction in the base of support means that the athlete has to work much harder through the hip and lumbar–pelvic region to remain in balance during the movement.

When planning the plyometric development progression, practitioners may consider double-leg and single-leg progressions occurring in tandem. Single-leg activities are not merely progressive variations of double-leg exercises but rather a family of exercises in their own right that can and should be developed as athletic competence rises.

Plyometric movement complexity is also often underestimated in terms of imposed neuromuscular and musculoskeletal demand. The introduction of equipment or direction changes to a drill can exponentially increase the relative intensity of the exercise. Simplistic movement patterns and in-place or in-line drills are ideal for inexperienced athletes or those who have a relatively low training age

or current training status. These exercises can be progressed through increased repetitions, greater vertical heights, longer linear dimensions and so on so that the athlete is challenged in a single movement plane whilst controlling rotations and maintaining balance.

The introduction of directional changes to the movement significantly alters the nature of a drill, as does the use of some types of equipment, such as boxes, hurdles or bungees. These changes need to be thought through so that the additions to the drill do not significantly alter the nature of the ground contact. The more complex the drill is, the higher the quality of coaching the athlete will need to maintain the quality of skill execution. The practitioner needs to have advanced observational skills to determine whether the nature of ground contact remains the same with the drill progression. Highly complex drills that require many directional changes or responses to different stimuli should be used with caution and only with advanced athletes with well-developed reactive plyometric skills.

## Measuring Plyometric Volume

In sport training, the amount of work undertaken needs to be quantified to make an accurate estimate of the load being placed on the athlete at a given time. By quantifying the volume and the intensity, the volume of load of an exercise or series of exercises can be determined. In plyometrics (or sport-specific jumping activity) this volume is measured by the number of foot contacts in the drill. For example, four sets of 10 bounds is 40 foot contacts. Another less common means of quantifying loads is to look at the distance a drill covers; for example, an athlete may be required to hop 10 metres or 40 metres depending on experience.

Normally, the relationship between volume and intensity in most training activities is inverse (i.e., the more work that is done, the less intense this work is, or the lower the quality of the movement is). For example, although a mile (1,609 metres) may be run maximally (a world-class male athlete may do this in around 3 minutes, 55 seconds, a female in 4 minutes, 25 seconds), the quality of the work done is not comparable with that required to run 100 metres maximally (world-class time less than 9.9 seconds for a male, 11.2 seconds for a female). The male mile runner is averaging 6.85 metres per second, compared with 10.1 metres per second for the male 100-metre runner. Although the intensity of both activities may be maximal, the quality of the work output in a sprint cannot be maintained for long distances or high volumes.

As with speed work, the quality of plyometric actions is paramount. Although intensity may be a function (or percentage) of maximal, quality is a percentage of perfect! Therefore, high volumes need to be approached with caution. Practitioners do not always understand caution; some misinterpret some of the popular volume guidelines published for athletes (table 9.3).

These guidelines illustrate that as the athlete's level of experience increases, so does his or her ability to tolerate a loading regime and that to facilitate overload, the programme volume can be increased. More work can be achieved before a fatigue threshold is reached that may retard the quality of the work.

What often isn't recognized is that the range of plyometric options available to the beginner is far different from the options for the advanced athlete. Low-intensity plyometric exercises—simple exercises like skipping or jumping rope that have low concentric and low eccentric demand and no acceleration drops—may be performed by a beginner for many more than 100 repetitions in a session with no injurious effect. A drop jump from a 30-centimetre box may fall into the limits prescribed in table 9.3.

Contrast this with a depth jump from 1.2 metres. The eccentric demand of this exercise means that beginner and intermediate athletes should not be exposed to it, and advanced athletes should approach it with caution depending on their strength levels, current training status and technical ability. With such a demanding exercise, volume is likely to be limited to three to five sets of three to eight repetitions (9 to 40 foot contacts) both to maintain the quality of the movement and to prevent an overreaching injury because of fatiguing the body beyond the tolerance of the motor system. Generally, the more demanding the exercise is, the lower the volume (number of sets or repetitions) performed should be, even by experienced athletes.

In conjunction with those cautions is the importance of recovery between sets. High-quality movements require complete rest for the athlete to be maximally effective. Active recovery periods of 1 to 5 minutes between sets, depending on the volume and relative intensity of the exercise, are suggested. Maximal intensity requires maximal recovery. If the athlete feels residual fatigue between sets, the rest break should be appropriately extended. Movement quality should not be compromised for quantity as the athlete's power production develops. Even in sports in which athletes are required to perform powerful movements under fatigue (for example, basketball or soccer), the opportunities to develop power endurance will be found elsewhere within their training schedules. When it comes to speed, strength and power, practitioners should remember that submaximal efforts become relatively easier (more efficient) as maximal capabilities are raised. Therefore,

**Table 9.3** Appropriate Plyometric Volumes for a Session

| Plyometric experience | Beginning volume (foot contacts) |
|---|---|
| Beginner (no experience) | 80 to 100 |
| Intermediate (some experience) | 100 to 120 |
| Advanced (considerable experience) | 120 to 140 |

Reprinted, by permission, from D.H. Potach and D.A. Chu, 2008, Plyometric training. In *Essentials of strength training and conditioning*, 3rd ed., edited by T.R. Baechle and R.W. Earle for the National Strength and Conditioning Association (Champaign, IL: Human Kinetics), 421.

the quality of the movement should be the main objective at all times.

## Athlete Considerations

Within the athletic development curriculum, a number of factors should be considered for the athlete before prescribing plyometrics. Biological and training age, gender, strength, body mass, technical ability and coachability of the athlete need to be considered.

As with resistance training, the appropriate biological age for the athlete to begin plyometrics training has been contentiously debated. Much of the debate stems from the philosophical approach that equates plyometrics with formalized and organized training activities. Although disciplined coaching of form, structure and volume load are important within an athlete's power training development, practitioners should also recognize that many basic forms of human movement are plyometric in nature. Plyometric activities are fun, and children will naturally want to participate in them. Kids will run as well as hop, skip and jump as often as they can without any formalized coaching intervention. If these activities are considered safe for play, the same can be applied to practice.

In the early years, the concepts of play and practice should be inextricably linked to reinforce the emphasis on developing mature skills through games and play-based challenges in childhood. Jumping and landing technique and the development of the stretch-reflex mechanism have so many potential benefits for performance and injury reduction in sport that they should be the pillars of a well-rounded physical education process for any child. The key question moves from 'Should children do plyometrics?' to 'How quickly should I formalize and progress plyometric training with children?' The answer is found by considering the interaction of a number of key variables at an individual level.

The two key variables that should lead this debate relate to the child's strength and technical ability. These aspects are particularly important because the major concern related to the safety of jumping and rebound exercises is the ability to manage ground reaction forces in the landing phase of the movements.

The point to consider here is the ability of the neuromuscular system to tolerate the force demands whilst maintaining the integrity of joint alignment during imposed landing tasks. For example, a high-velocity landing either from a height or through a horizontal leap in which the knees deviate laterally or medially from the desirable alignment of tracking over the toes can potentially result in a catastrophic injury to one or more of the four ligaments that maintain the integrity of the knee joint. Practitioners leading such programmes need to ensure that the athlete has high technical proficiency before undertaking movement patterns that involve landings from high accelerations.

The ability to generate concentric and eccentric forces through the hip, knee and ankle musculature should be developed in conjunction with technical competence in landing and take-off mechanics. For that reason, wholly integrated programmes provide speed training, jump training and strength-training stimuli. As the athlete's neuromuscular system develops, technical competency increases. The athlete can then be exposed to a greater range of stimuli, which will further develop technical and physical abilities, and so forth. Risk of serious injury increases significantly when the athlete is subjected to tasks that exceed his or her technical and physical tolerance limits. In an activity such as plyometrics, these two factors are inherently interlinked, explaining why the strength levels have been emphasized in relation to perceived exercise intensity.

A well-designed plyometric progression enables athletes to develop the correct landing and ground contact mechanics and the coordinated expression of concentric forces following an appropriate amortization phase. The progression must require the athlete to demonstrate learning or competence at each successive stage of complexity and intensity. This approach also enables the athlete's training age to be developed so that his or her neuromuscular system can develop the resilience to increased volumes and intensities that progressions will invariably bring. Practice should be about preparing the athlete to transition to the next level of development. The following sections cover a number of progressive plyometrics activities for practitioners to build on.

If the objective of the plyometric training is to maximize learning, it should be delivered by experienced and qualified coaches who are willing to invest time in achieving technical mastery in the athletes they work with. A consistent and effective technique must be developed from the athlete's first formalized introductions to plyometric practices.

As with adults, children need to be protected from fatigue if they are to develop the appropriate reactive strength qualities through their training experiences. As with speed activities, plyometric activities should be undertaken following an appropriately structured warm-up but early enough within a session that fatigue, both physical and mental, does not interfere with the quality of the movements.

Practitioners should carefully consider the relative training and biological ages of people who are undertaking plyometric exercise at later stages in life. For example, many people return to recreational or competitive sport following a period of inactivity. These weekend warriors often return to ballistic and explosive activities such as basketball, five-a-side soccer or road running without undertaking any preparatory work. The tendency is for these people to engage in regular training with a group of people who have been undertaking this activity for a number of months or years.

As athletic careers progress, athletes typically pick up injuries and develop chronic conditions. Injury is an inevitable consequence of sport participation, regardless of how well planned and structured the person's athletic preparation is. Athletes who are joint compromised (i.e., have had injuries requiring surgical repair) are advised to consider higher intensity plyometrics as contraindicated and perform activities in accordance with their clinical history.

Note that plyometrics themselves are not contraindicated, and most medical professionals consider the use of some plyometric activities as essential at different points of rehabilitation and protective against future injury. For example, reactive drop jumps or repetitive hops into hold may be considered beneficial as advanced rehabilitation or strengthening for a chronic injury in an athlete who has a history of ACL rupture.

Master athletes need more careful consideration for conditions relating to joint degradation or depletion in bone mineral density. These conditions require a much more cautious approach to plyometric prescription. Although most osteological conditions respond well to mechanical loading, the rapid rates of ground reaction forces, coupled with the need for a highly reactive neuromuscular system, potentially preclude all but the lowest intensity plyometric activities.

Regardless of age or stage of development, the athlete's training status is an important consideration for the coach when determining the level of plyometric activity that the athlete should perform. The importance of strength has been highlighted, but other generic athletic qualities such as balance, coordination and reactive speed can be developed by plyometrics. These qualities are also important for an athlete to have to take part in and derive benefits from plyometrics that involve reactive accelerations.

In particular, single-leg and multidirectional explosive movements challenge the athlete to remain in dynamic balance with the centre of mass above a small base of support. With this in mind, many of the movement competency analyses (such as the hurdle hop and hop and single-leg squat) described in chapter 6 might be considered important indicators of an athlete's preparedness to undertake certain plyometric actions.

Similarly, reactive athletic qualities are essential if the rebound actions are to be optimized and training benefits maximized from repetitive jumping activities. Many strong athletes have well-developed ballistic movement qualities that enable them to produce dynamic forces. These qualities are different from the reactive qualities required from fast plyometrics, in which the forces need to be exerted in minimal time. If an athlete does not demonstrate high levels of reactive strength, the practitioner should consider spending time developing this quality through activities that challenge technical competence in the execution of ground contact rather than focusing on plyometric activities that might have other emphasis (e.g., depth jump, multidirectional jumps).

To develop efficient plyometric technique, the athlete needs to be coachable and responsive to correction. The movements are very quick; therefore, the athlete's sensory skills need to be reasonably well developed to be responsive to feedback on technique. Small changes in technique, particularly in relation to the action of the foot and ankle joint on ground contact, can make significant differences to the outcome of a plyometric exercise. Athletes who do not respond quickly to directional feedback will not progress as well as those who are better able to accept and act on feedback.

The final characteristic of the athlete to be considered in progressing plyometrics is the athlete's gender. Practitioners should maintain the approach to gender that has been advocated throughout this text; that is, every individual should be evaluated on athletic qualities rather than on stereotypes of certain populations. That said, specific considerations apply to planning plyometric programmes for male and female athletes.

The primary mechanical consideration to be considered when coaching postpubertal female athletes is the high Q-angle that results from the widening of the hips during puberty. The implications of the Q-angle for the potential malalignment of the femur relative to the support foot in landing were discussed in chapters 3 and 5. Not surprisingly, in the recent past, female basketball players in the NCAA were six times more likely than their male counterparts to incur a rupture in the anterior cruciate ligament,[13] and most knee injuries in females occur in noncontact situations (landing, deceleration, turning).

The plyometric programme for a female athlete needs to have a bias, especially in the early stages, towards developing the ability to execute stable landings. This emphasis will not only develop a sound technical model but also help train the neuromuscular system to activate high levels of motor units within the gluteus medius, hamstrings and quadriceps to fire instantly, increasing the stability of the knee joints and maintaining femoral alignment with the feet. Appropriately progressed training with respect to this objective has been demonstrated to show a 70 per cent decrease in noncontact ACL injuries in female soccer players.[14]

Evidence from historical studies[15] illustrates that the leg extensor muscles in males can sustain higher eccentric loads than those of females. This finding correlates with the understanding that, because of different morphologies, females typically have lower absolute strength levels than their male counterparts do.

This differential in strength also carries over into the expression of power. Women's power output in explosive lifting exercises is approximately 63 per cent of the output of their male counterparts,[16] and similar trends have been observed in maximal vertical and horizontal jumps. The rate of developed force also typically is slower in females than in males, although anecdotal evidence suggests that training may reduce this differential. Indeed, with training, female athletes who undertake jumping activities may be able to use a greater portion of the stored elastic energy in their muscle fibres than male athletes can.

Female athletes are also increasingly susceptible to injury because they have higher joint laxity, primarily because of increased amounts of oestrogen and other hormones following the onset of puberty. The practitioner must be cautious about prescribing activities that require joint stiffness for successful performance and that can magnify the consequences of any instability in joints. Similarly, the changes in hormone levels that occur naturally in a female who is not on hormonally regulated birth control influence the ability to execute high-force, high-velocity movements.

## Safety in Delivering Plyometric Activity

The practitioner needs to know and understand a number of general safety considerations before commencing plyometric exercises. The most important of these is the surface onto which the athlete jumps. The surface must not be wet, slippery or unstable in any manner. Athletes travelling at high velocities need to be confident that the surface they are transitioning across is consistent and will not cause them to deviate from their optimal landing technique in any way.

Besides being consistent, the hardness of the landing surface needs to be carefully considered. Plyometric activities use the stretch-shortening cycle to develop power, and a rapid amortization phase is crucial to skilful execution of the repetitive actions. Therefore, the coach should consider carefully how the landing surface will both transmit ground reaction forces and enable a rapid and natural amortization phase in the movement. For example, very hard surfaces such as concrete or tiled floor should be avoided. These surfaces have no shock absorption properties, so the resultant impacts are potentially injurious to joints, particularly in the leg and lumbar–pelvic regions. Conversely, a surface that is too springy may interfere with the natural transmission of ground reaction forces, influencing the athlete's stretch-shortening cycle action and preventing efficient use of the stretch reflex. Surfaces that are more appropriate include synthetic tracks or even natural grass if it is not wet and the underlying soil is dry and compacted. These surfaces provide marginal shock absorption without dampening the myotatic reflex.

The athlete's footwear is an extension of the landing surface and is therefore an important consideration. The sole of the shoe must be nonslip. Shoes without sufficient cushioning provide no dissipation for the ground reaction forces, potentially causing injury higher up the kinetic chain in the lower limb. Conversely, training shoes with excessive cushioning extend the amortization phase whilst the athlete is in contact with the floor, reducing the effective transfer of training benefits. Ideal shoes provide mid- and rear-foot support to aid ankle stability and stiffness in the landing.

If the session plan requires equipment for the athlete to jump onto, off or over, the equipment must be robust enough to satisfy the demands imposed by the task. The equipment must also be appropriately set up. A box that the athlete is to jump onto needs to be set at a realistically challenging height. Providing an appropriately challenging height will focus the athlete's mind on the task, but practitioners might expect the occasional bruised or cut shin from athletes who do not make a particular box jump! Another recommendation is to set up boxes with space behind them, preferably with a crash mat, in case the athlete does trip on the edge of the box and fall over the top.

As expected, any box being used needs to have a wide enough base to be stable in all circumstances and robust enough to cope with the mass of the athlete landing on it. The surface of the box or platform should be nonslip as well. Small details such as ensuring that a hurdle is facing the correct way also make a big difference to the safety of a drill. In nearly all exercises involving hurdles, the legs of the hurdle point away from the direction in which the athlete travels. That way, if the athlete makes contact with the barrier, it will easily fall and not cause any injury.

The spacing between equipment also needs to be carefully planned. The equipment provides a target for the athlete to jump onto or over; therefore, the spacing of the hurdles or boxes, as well as the respective height, determines the horizontal and vertical components of the flight trajectory of each jump. Taller targets spaced more closely together encourage more vertical displacements; lower ones more widely spaced encourage more horizontal acceleration. The objective of the exercise and the athlete's capabilities determine how the equipment should be arranged. If in doubt, coaches should use caution in the initial setup and then expand on it as necessary and appropriate. Keeping accurate records of progress from every session enables a practitioner to identify the measurements for object height and spacing achieved within a drill.

Space is a key consideration for plyometric activity. For example, athletes transitioning into and from a series of high-speed alternate-leg bounds require acceleration and deceleration runways on either side of the bounding sequence, so 30 to 100 metres of runway may be necessary. Similarly, vertical space should not be ignored. Although jumps onto boxes may not require a lot of floor surface area, the athlete needs at least 1.5 metres of clearance above head height whilst standing on the tallest box. Other ballistic activities, such as throwing medicine balls, require adequate ceiling height clearance as determined by the weight of the ball and the athlete's force-producing capabilities. The size of the clear space must be adequate for the medicine ball to land in without fear that it will land on another athlete in training.

## Developing Landing and Ground Contact Technique

The appropriate technical model for landing was presented earlier in this chapter. A number of potential drills can be used progressively to promote mastery of correct landing mechanics. Each drill or variation subjects the athlete to increasingly higher horizontal velocities or vertical impact forces. The athlete needs to demonstrate a sound technical base for two-footed landings before these practices are adapted to a single-foot landing. The progression from landing into preparation for landing into low-intensity plyometric jumps involves a number of simple stages that can be developed as competence increases. As figure 9.11 suggests, although each related skill has its own progression, these can be simultaneously introduced after some level of prerequisite competence has been achieved.

The key consideration to progressing the landing is that the athlete is able to maintain lumbar–pelvic alignment, weight distribution and hip–knee–toe alignment at each successive stage of exercise difficulty. Each progression of landing drills sees a rise in either exercise intensity (such as an increase in horizontal velocity or vertical height) or movement complexity. For example, the landing following a backwards double-foot jump requires the athlete to move in a plane away from the field of vision, requiring the proprioceptive mechanisms to control the landing. In such an exercise, control of the landing is far more important than the distance jumped. Similarly, the 180-degree turn in mid-air is designed to be relatively low impact, but the turn significantly reduces the

time available for the athlete to prepare for landing. Therefore, the athlete needs to find the landing position quickly and effectively.

The transitional drills highlight appropriately the key progression of emphasis from landing only to a repetitive landing–take-off–landing sequence. The core theme of these exercises is executing a solid and competent landing before moving to another activity. Exercises in this progression do not focus on rebounding from the floor or making a fast transition to other movements, but on executing a correct landing before reaccelerating to another movement. Emphasizing the subsequent movement rather than the landing may be potentially detrimental to learning. The theme should reflect the premise that without a sound landing, the athlete will not be in an appropriate position to transition into another movement. The athlete should be encouraged to hold the landing position and then transition into the subsequent movement rather than stand up and then perform another countermovement to a following jump (for example). The length of time between the landing and the subsequent movement can be gradually reduced if the integrity of the landing technique is maintained.

Exercises that enhance plyometric ground contact technique need to emphasize a number of component technical factors and movement quality. As shown in figure 9.11, every exercise with this objective should be performed with stiff ankles, knees and hips, as seen in the sequences from jumping rope through multiple flat-foot bounces to drop jumps. The idea is for the ankle to remain stiff, attacking the floor only immediately before landing. In flight, the ankle should be dorsiflexed (or cocked) with the toes pointing up towards the knees.

At every stage of the progression, correct postural alignment on ground contact should be maintained and emphasized. If posture begins to break down, the drill should be regressed so that the athlete can maintain postural control. The other quality to be addressed is the need for a quick and crisp foot contact. If the drill complexity progresses beyond the athlete's ability to maintain rapid ground contact (less than 0.2 seconds), the drill should be regressed

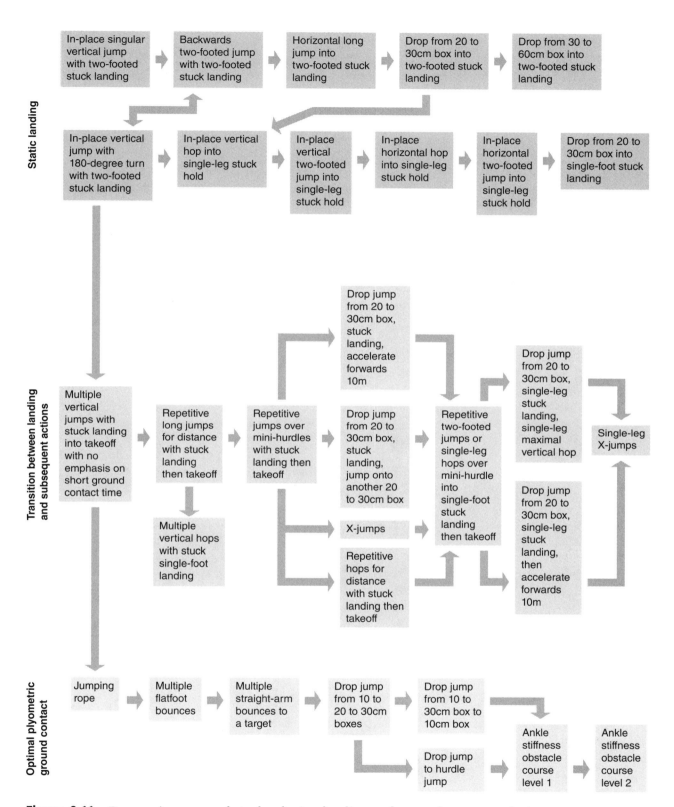

**Static landing**

In-place singular vertical jump with two-footed stuck landing → Backwards two-footed jump with two-footed stuck landing → Horizontal long jump into two-footed stuck landing → Drop from 20 to 30cm box into two-footed stuck landing → Drop from 30 to 60cm box into two-footed stuck landing

In-place vertical jump with 180-degree turn with two-footed stuck landing → In-place vertical hop into single-leg stuck hold → In-place vertical two-footed jump into single-leg stuck hold → In-place horizontal hop into single-leg stuck hold → In-place horizontal two-footed jump into single-leg stuck hold → Drop from 20 to 30cm box into single-foot stuck landing

**Transition between landing and subsequent actions**

Multiple vertical jumps with stuck landing into takeoff with no emphasis on short ground contact time → Repetitive long jumps for distance with stuck landing then takeoff → Repetitive jumps over mini-hurdles with stuck landing then takeoff

Multiple vertical hops with stuck single-foot landing

Drop jump from 20 to 30cm box, stuck landing, accelerate forwards 10m

Drop jump from 20 to 30cm box, stuck landing, jump onto another 20 to 30cm box

X-jumps

Repetitive hops for distance with stuck landing then takeoff

Repetitive two-footed jumps or single-leg hops over mini-hurdle into single-foot stuck landing then takeoff

Drop jump from 20 to 30cm box, single-leg stuck landing, single-leg maximal vertical hop

Drop jump from 20 to 30cm box, single-leg stuck landing, then accelerate forwards 10m

Single-leg X-jumps

**Optimal plyometric ground contact**

Jumping rope → Multiple flatfoot bounces → Multiple straight-arm bounces to a target → Drop jump from 10 to 20 to 30cm boxes → Drop jump from 10 to 30cm box to 10cm box

Drop jump to hurdle jump → Ankle stiffness obstacle course level 1 → Ankle stiffness obstacle course level 2

**Figure 9.11** Progressive approach to developing landing and ground contact technique.

259

to enable this quality to be maintained. Practitioners need to ensure that the quality of the movement doesn't deteriorate because of fatigue; the emphasis needs to remain on the quality of the movement. Complete recoveries and a low number of repetitions are important at all stages of learning these movements.

Especially in the early progressions, the athlete must not be challenged to jump too high in rebound jumps. The temptation is to introduce a wide range of hurdles or boxes at the early stages, but this changes the activity from one that emphasizes the landing technique to one that emphasizes vertical force production, which typically requires a longer ground contact time. Vertical height in the reactive jump can still be a challenge, but successful execution of the exercise should not be determined by it.

The focus should be on a crisp and reactive foot contact. In plyometrics, the rate of stretch rather than the magnitude of the stretch is important in creating powerful movements. Knowing this may help focus the athlete on performing quality foot contacts rather than jumping high.

The importance of the active flat foot through ground contact (to produce forces through the majority of the foot to enable a rapid take-off) is emphasized in exercises such as the multiple straight-arm bounces. Maintaining a posture in which the arms remain straight throughout a movement prevents their contribution to upward momentum as the athlete rises. Similarly, if the hips and knees remain stiff, the only possible joint that contributes to upward movement is the ankle joint as the ball of the foot attacks the floor. Using a target such as a block against a wall encourages the athlete to push hard into the floor to generate rapid vertical forces that can be quantified by the reach of the arms.

The practitioner should reinforce the importance of keeping the ankles dorsiflexed during the flight phase of such movements. The progression to stepping off from boxes begins with the first stepping movement. As described in figure 9.11, the athlete must pull the toes up towards the knees as he or she steps off the block to place the foot in an optimal landing position from which to attack the floor as the foot contacts the ground. Beginning the movement by stepping off from a low box reduces not only the initial impact forces but also the drop time, forcing the athlete to focus on correct foot placement before ground contact. A jump mat provides the athlete immediate feedback about ground contact times and a target to focus on in seeking to enhance this.

Even though progressions develop towards multiple obstacles, these activities can still be regarded as low-impact plyometrics. The emphasis on the ground contact means that the drop heights will be reasonably small; likewise, the minihurdles and rebound boxes will be relatively low to the ground. Alternating a box with a hurdle on an obstacle course (figure 9.12, obstacle course level 1) allows the athlete to reset the foot between jumps, ensuring that he or she has the best opportunity for optimal ground contact. The early overuse of successive hurdles sometimes means that this opportunity is lost as the athlete progresses down the course; ground contacts becomes progressively longer with each hurdle. As the athlete's competence and plyometric conditioning improve, boxes can be replaced with an increased numbers of hurdles (as illustrated by the level 2 obstacle course shown in figure 9.13).

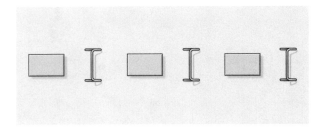

**Figure 9.12**    Ankle stiffness obstacle course level 1.

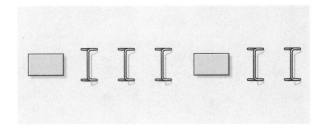

**Figure 9.13**    Ankle stiffness obstacle course level 2.

## Plyometric Progressions

Plyometrics are typically classified within one of four movements: jumps, hops, bounds and shock movements (table 9.4). This classification is useful for describing the nature of a movement, and it provides a framework for determining progressions. Some jumps, however, may have higher plyometric demand than some hops, for example. Also, not all movements are easily classified; for example, a standing triple jump isn't really a bound (according to the definition in table 9.4) but a combination movement that involves a hop followed by a bound leading into a single-leg take-off, double-foot landing, which is only a jump because the landing is on two feet. But this movement is complex enough to be regarded as a bound, and it does involve weight transfer from one foot to the other.

Practitioners are encouraged to think about progression not simply within a classification of plyometrics and then between plyometrics; they should also think about the factors that influence plyometric intensity. Progression should be from simple movements to complex ones, single-plane movements before directional changes, double-leg movements to single-leg movements and low-impact demands (low eccentric force) to high-impact demands (high eccentric force). Technical emphasis exercises should precede those involving obstacles and shock or depth jumps. In any coaching context, when the quality of plyometric movement begins to deteriorate through either fatigue or progression beyond the athlete's competence, the session should end.

# Jumps

Many types of jumping movements can be readily arranged into a progressive curriculum by the imaginative coach who is able to link the principles of sound technique to the jumping context. As long as the athlete is able to generate the required level of concentric force through a countermovement, jumping upwards onto an object is often less demanding than jumping onto the same level, perhaps because many jumps onto an object are singular efforts interspersed with recovery as the athlete steps down from the box. This jump is in contrast to many other jumps that involve multiple and successive repetitions with no recovery between reps because ground contact needs to be minimized.

Some of the exercises introduced in the ground contact context are obviously jumps. The key differential between these and some of the exercises described in this section (figure 9.14) is the objective of the exercise. Figure 9.11 introduced exercises in which the key deliverable was an efficient and effective ground contact technique that is transferrable to all jumping situations. Contrastingly, other jumps require this technique as a foundation to build on, because the objective of the jump moves to developing horizontal or vertical forces to maximize the height or distance of the jump.

**Table 9.4** Plyometric Classification

| Classification | Description | Example drill |
|---|---|---|
| Jump | Movement that starts and finishes on two feet | Split squat × 8<br>Box jump × 5<br>Split-stance countermovement × 8 |
| Hop | Single-foot take-off with landing on the same foot | Lateral minihurdle hop × 6<br>Speed hop × 40m |
| Bound | Single-foot take-off with landing on the other foot | Standing triple jump for distance × 2 to 4 sets<br>Speed bounds × 60 m |
| Shock | Highest intensity plyometrics; acceleration drop from a height into a rebound jumping movement | Depth jump to box jump × 3<br>Depth jump to multiple-hurdle jump × 5 |

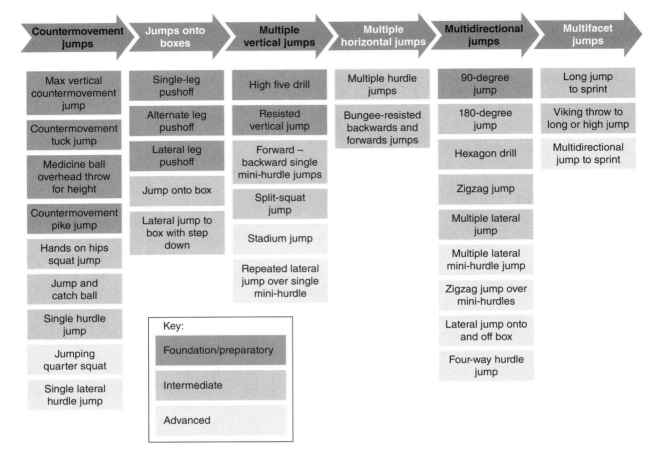

## Countermovement Jumps in Place

| FOUNDATION/PREPARATORY | | | |
|---|---|---|---|
| **Max vertical countermovement jump**: Perform rapid quarter squat countermovement before jumping as high as possible | **Countermovement tuck jump**: Perform rapid quarter squat countermovement before jumping as high as possible, bringing knees to chest in the air and landing on both feet | **Medicine ball overhead throw for height**: Hold medicine ball in both hands in underhanded grip and perform countermovement followed by launching ball over head as high as possible | **Countermovement pike jump**: Perform rapid quarter squat countermovement before jumping as high as possible, hinging from hips in midair and lifting straight legs to hands before landing on both feet |

| INTERMEDIATE | | |
|---|---|---|
| **Hands on hips squat jump**: Hands on hips, squat until thighs are parallel to floor, trunk upright, pause a second, then jump as high as possible | **Jump and catch ball**: Perform vertical jump to catch ball thrown overhead at highest point possible | **Single hurdle jump**: Stand in front of hurdle, perform countermovement jump and jump over hurdle, landing on both feet |

| ADVANCED | |
|---|---|
| **Jumping quarter squat**: Start in back squat position, feet hip-width apart and perform rapid quarter squat countermovement before jumping as high as possible, keeping bar in contact with shoulders | **Single lateral hurdle jump**: Stand beside hurdle, perform countermovement jump and jump sideways over hurdle, landing on both feet |

**Figure 9.14**   Progressive approach to developing jumping skills that are transferable to a multisport context.

## Jumps Onto Boxes

| FOUNDATION/PREPARATORY | | |
|---|---|---|
| **Single-leg pushoff**: Stand in front of box with one foot on floor, heel slightly up, one foot hovering just above box, ankle dorsiflexed and drive foot down onto box, jumping as high as possible, landing with same foot on box and floor | **Alternate-leg pushoff**: Stand in front of box with one foot on floor, heel slightly up, one foot hovering just above box, ankle dorsiflexed and drive foot down onto box, jumping as high as possible, switching feet in midair, and landing with opposite foot on box and floor | **Lateral-leg pushoff**: Stand sideways to box, outside foot on floor, heel slightly up, inside foot hovering above box, ankle dorsiflexed and drive foot down onto box, jumping as high as possible and travelling sideways across box, landing with opposite foot on floor |

| INTERMEDIATE | |
|---|---|
| **Jump onto box**: Perform rapid quarter squat countermovement then jump as high as possible to land with both feet on box | **Lateral jump to box with step down**: Stand sideways to box and perform rapid quarter squat countermovement before jumping sideways to land with both feet on box then step down and repeat in other direction |

## Multiple Vertical Jumps

| FOUNDATION/PREPARATORY | |
|---|---|
| **High-five drill:** Face partner, arms stretched above heads, perform repetitive vertical jumps and high five with straight arms at peak of each jump | **Resisted vertical jump:** Perform maximal vertical jumps against the resistance of a bungee or resistance band |

| INTERMEDIATE | |
|---|---|
| **Forward-backward single mini-hurdle jumps:** Perform multiple jumps forward and backward over a mini-hurdle | **Split-squat jump:** Start in a split stance and perform a countermovement to jump as high as possible, switching legs in midair and landing in opposite split stance |

| ADVANCED | |
|---|---|
| **Stadium jump**: Perform two-footed jumps up stadium stairs | **Repeated lateral jump over single mini-hurdle**: Stand sideways to a mini-hurdle and perform lateral jumps over the hurdle |

## Multiple Horizontal Jumps

| INTERMEDIATE | |
|---|---|
| **Multiple hurdle jumps**: Jump over a series of hurdles lined up 1 to 2 metres apart, maximizing height of centre of mass and minimizing ground contact time between hurdles | **Bungee-resisted backwards and forwards jumps**: Perform maximal distance forwards and backwards jumps against resistance and assistance from a bungee cord held from behind |

*(continued)*

**Figure 9.14**  *(continued)*

As figure 9.14 illustrates, a number of jumping exercises can be included in a curriculum. Note the complexity that can be applied to developing a plyometric curriculum that will develop competence in jumping skills. As figure 9.14 proposes, a progression occurs between the different classifications of jumps. In-place jumps with little horizontal displacement typically precede gravity-resisted (jumping-upward) movements to movements in which

## Multidirectional Jumps

| FOUNDATION/PREPARATORY | | | |
|---|---|---|---|
| **90-degree jump**: Perform repetitive maximal countermovement jumps, turning in midair to land at right angles to the direction of takeoff | | | |

| INTERMEDIATE | | | |
|---|---|---|---|
| **180-degree jump**: Perform repetitive maximal countermovement jumps, turning in midair to land facing the direction opposite takeoff | **Hexagon drill**: Stand in middle of hexagon marked on floor (about 1 metre diameter) and perform two-footed jumps, outside then inside, around diameter of hexagon, facing same direction | **Zigzag jump**: Perform diagonal two-footed jumps (forward and diagonal), alternating to the left and right side of a 10 to 20-metre line | **Multiple lateral jump**: Perform repetitive lateral jumps over a line, minimizing ground contact time |

| ADVANCED | | | |
|---|---|---|---|
| **Multiple lateral mini-hurdle jump**: Perform repetitive lateral jumps over a mini-hurdle, minimizing ground contact time | **Zigzag jump over mini-hurdles**: Perform diagonal two-footed jumps (forward and diagonal) over a series of mini-hurdles over a 10 to 20-metre course | **Lateral jump onto and off box**: Stand sideways to a box then jump laterally onto the box, land, then jump laterally off the box | **Four-way hurdle jump**: Stand inside square of four mini-hurdles and jump forward over first hurdle, land, and immediately spring back to middle of square, continuing around the square, facing the same direction |

## Multifacet Jumps

| INTERMEDIATE | |
|---|---|
| **Long jump to sprint**: Perform maximal long jump, landing on feet and immediately sprinting forwards | **Viking throw to long or high jump**: Hold medicine ball in both hands in underhanded grip and perform a countermovement jump then launch the ball as high as possible followed by a long jump (if throw is in front) or maximum vertical jump (if throw is behind) |

| ADVANCED | |
|---|---|
| **Multidirectional jump to sprint**: Perform series of jumps over a line or hurdle until coach signals to transition from landing to maximum sprint | |

**Figure 9.14**  *(continued)*

the take-off and landing happen on the same level. The next obvious level of progression is towards gravity-assisted drops from a height, which are explored later in this chapter when shock jumps are presented. Multifaceted jumps add complexity because they mix movements and integrate skills and are therefore typically higher level exercises.

To view jump progression in this manner, however, would be oversimplistic. With the inclusion of external objects, movement requirements in frontal or multiple movement places, or the requirement for higher levels of concentric force application, the practitioner can begin to differentiate or individualize prescription of each classification of jump. A programme can be planned that encompasses a range of jump types, adding variation to the practice at an appropriate level of challenge for the individual.

To explain this concept in more detail, let's analyse in-place countermovement jumps as an example. The take-off mechanics for each jump are similar; a countermovement should initiate the stretch reflex to aid the explosive vertical movement that precedes a powerful push into the floor from the hips, the knees and then the ankles extending in sequence. The arms also rise to assist in the upward momentum. This vertical force and upward arm action can be emphasized through activities such as a medicine ball throw for maximum vertical height. As figure 9.15 illustrates, to emphasize maximal vertical ground reaction forces, the instructions to the athlete need to be related to throwing the ball to maximum heights ('Can you hit the ceiling with the 5-kilogram ball?'). Inevitably, some minimal horizontal displacement will occur (typically in a backwards direction), but this movement is much less than what occurs in a throw that has the joint aim of reaching maximum height and horizontal distance. Such actions might typically be used as a precursor to horizontal jumping or linking actions such as jumping or throwing forwards into running.

A squat jump is different from the more advanced jump squat (figure 9.16). Squat jumps are often used for testing maximal vertical impulse of the leg extensors. The start of the squat jump typically takes the athlete to a point where the muscles exceed the optimal length–tension relationships for the stretch reflex to occur. Similarly, the position is reached slowly and held in pause (compared with the very rapid countermovement dip and drive, which is also typical of the jump squat; usually it is a quarter-squat action), which means that the myotatic reflex is typically negated in the squat jump action; it is simply too slow. But some elastic energy is stored in the muscle fibres, and this will aid vertical propulsion.

In both the squat jump and the jump squat, the arm action is negated by the hand position on either the hips or a bar. But the jump squat is characterized by the fact that the athlete has an external load located a long way above the centre of mass, which requires greater concentric force and postural control in the jumping action. Similarly, in landing from the jump squat, the athlete needs to be able to control large eccentric forces, rapidly brake these forces and use the stretch reflex to perform a repeated action.

The depth of the squat in the jump squat action and the load on the bar typically vary with the athlete and the objective. In repeated high-velocity movements, rebounding relies

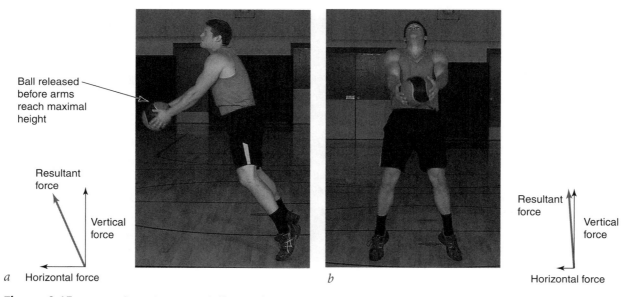

**Figure 9.15** Launch actions are different for maximum medicine ball throws with different objectives: *(a)* ball thrown for maximum height and forward distance; *(b)* ball thrown for maximum height.

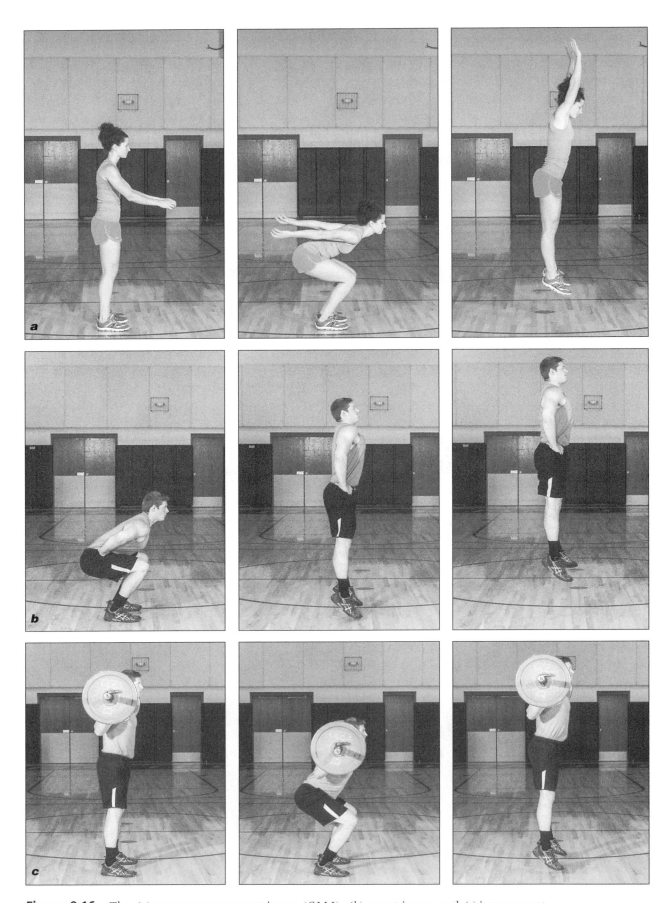

**Figure 9.16** The *(a)* countermovement jump (CMJ), *(b)* squat jump and *(c)* jump squat.

on the stretch-reflex mechanism. Therefore, the squat depth is reasonably shallow and the external loads are typically light. The exact formula to use to calculate system mass loading (weight of the athlete plus weight of the bar) is the subject of an ongoing debate among researchers; estimates are between 0 and 70 per cent of maximum load on the bar.[17] If the objective is a high-force movement, the squat depth will be greater, the load will be higher, but the plyometric effect will be less; an elongated amortization phase will occur as the athlete lands and descends into the squat position. For this reason, such movements are often done as singular rather than repeated efforts.

Coordination with an external object is also a feature of advancement. For example, the jump and reach to gather a ball repeatedly thrown is an extension of the maximum vertical jump. The feed to the athlete needs to be of sufficient frequency to prevent slowing of the repetitive jumping action. The athlete should be encouraged to catch the ball at the maximum obtainable height of flight trajectory, which provides opportunity for positive transfer of skills to specific sporting situations such as the volleyball smash, a backboard rebound in basketball or interception of a crossed ball in soccer by a goalkeeper.

The height of the hurdle in an isolated hurdle jump depends on the athlete's ability to generate vertical force. The height simply needs to be significant enough to challenge the athlete to jump high enough to clear the hurdle. The drill should be set up so that the athlete is able to execute the jump with full-body extension, rather than clearing the height by performing a tuck jump. If the exercise is performed with a lateral movement rather than a forwards movement, it is significantly more challenging (hence the classification as an advanced movement) and the height of the hurdle may be lower.

The use of single-leg movements in the box jump provides not simply a basic tool for developing jumping force but also a way to prepare for hops and bounds. The height of the box should be sufficient so that the knee of the leg on the box is approximately level with the hip when the foot is flat on the box and the heel is close to the edge of the box. This position

enables the athlete to optimize all of the leg extensor musculature in this ballistic action.

Whether the athlete lands with the legs in the same position, switches legs in midflight or stands laterally to the box, the aim is the same: to achieve maximum height and reach by pushing down into the box. Lateral movements can be made more challenging by requiring the athlete to travel laterally across the box so that the legs can be switched between jumps. Because the aim is to achieve maximum vertical force, the ground contact time in these actions is usually relatively long, so the actions can be regarded as ballistic rather than necessarily plyometric.

The height of the box to be jumped onto depends on the athlete's ability to perform a countermovement jump. Another factor that cannot be ignored is the athlete's confidence in being able to achieve the jump without hitting the shins on the side of the box. A progressive approach to increasing height is essential in these actions.

Typically, repeated vertical jumps are introduced before horizontal jumps, because the movements are easier to control. Stadium jumps illustrate this principle well. The athlete continually accelerates against gravity, which requires large concentric forces, but successive landings are on a higher level; therefore, eccentric demand is low. The athlete can therefore focus on landing mechanics and quickly applying the vertical force through a quick amortization that doesn't require the eccentric strength that a repeated shock movement (e.g., repeated box jumps) would involve.

The height of hurdles and the number of planes that the athlete is required to jump through typically determine the relative difficulty of the movements within any progression. The principle of adding resistance is useful to explore in this context, because the nature of the resistance can affect the execution of the jump. For example, the addition of a load such as a weighted vest increases the mass of the athlete, which requires higher concentric forces to accelerate against gravity. Because the mass is constant, a higher load is accelerated towards the floor in landing, so the athlete needs to have higher eccentric strength capacities in landing. Ground contact times may be increased between repeated jumps. Practitioners using this strategy need to understand whether they are seeking to increase force production capacities or to develop explosive forces through short ground contact times to maximize the plyometric response.

Variable resistances provide a differential level of resistance throughout each stage of the jump. For example, a simple resistance bungee cord anchored around the athlete's waist provides increasing resistance as it stretches. This method may not necessarily be useful for developing acceleration, because the point of the jump at which the rate of acceleration is greatest is the point that is least resisted (as the athlete accelerates from the floor, the bungee is least stretched). At the point where vertical momentum is lowest (the apex of the jump), the resistive load is greatest. But this variation does assist acceleration towards the floor, and it may be a useful strategy if the objective is to focus on landing and ground contact mechanics. Devices with accommodating resistance, such as the Vertimax, control this phenomenon by decreasing resistance as the athlete leaves the floor.

A tightly held bungee cord also provides resistance to horizontal jumps, resulting in the firing of more motor units (multiple horizontal jumps, figure 9.11). Jumping horizontally from a starting point to a number of cones at different angles means that the drill becomes both multidirectional and resisted in one direction, assisted in another. This method may be useful for an athlete jumping backwards to a starting point, because typically less force is produced in backwards jumping actions of this nature. Alternating between a number of resisted efforts (e.g., four) should enable the neuromuscular system to be potentiated (i.e., increase the motor unit recruitment over that achievable voluntarily) in an unresisted effort.

In such drills, athletes should initially be instructed to jump around the cones in number order, but to progress the exercise, the sequence can be altered by the coach calling out a colour or number sequence. This progression forces the athlete to think and make decisions while moving. But if the coach seeks to make the drill reactive (i.e., by presenting the jumping sequence as the athlete performs the drill), ground contact time must not be prolonged by the time delay between the verbal cue and the reactive decision, because this interruption would change the nature of the activity.

Repeated or cycled split jumps may seem to be reasonably simple. But the coordination of the take-off from and landing in a split stance, with the switching of legs in midair, makes this a challenging movement to do effectively. As a single movement, the split jump can be a simple way to practise jumping from a contralateral stance and achieving a stable landing with this stance. In a repeated action, however, achieving a short ground contact time and generating vertical height requires a good level of plyometric skill.

Practitioners often ask why repeated double-foot horizontal jumps typically are not included in a plyometric progression. These actions generate a lot of forward momentum in landing, which causes forward rotations in the trunk as the legs contact the floor. In running or bounding actions, these rotations are countered by the contralateral arm and leg actions of the movement. In the absence of these actions, controlling repeated two-footed long jumps is extremely difficult, so they typically are not a natural progression in a jumping programme. Including a series of hurdles, however, forces the athlete to increase the vertical component of the movement, which changes the nature of the jump significantly.

Most athletes need a reasonable jumping background before they can competently execute repeated multidirectional jumps. As with directional changes in running, these actions require forces to be exerted through different parts of the foot, typically increasing ground contact time, especially when the athlete has to jump over obstacles. When planning the integration of these drills into a programme, the practitioner needs to establish the balance between the height of the hurdles, the scale of the directional change required and the need to maintain the integrity of the ground contact.

The greater the change in direction is, the more challenging the drill typically is. But this rule is not observed when the athlete turns and jumps over a hurdle a number of times; in that circumstance, the athlete is continually jumping forwards. Although drills such as the 90- and 180-degree jumps enable athletes to develop and control transverse rotational forces as part of a jump, typically the athlete needs to remain facing in one direction whilst the frontal (side to side) and sagittal (forward and backwards) movement components are altered.

The inclusion of these movements in a curriculum is important if the programme is to facilitate a transfer of training benefit to a multidirectional sport. Performing training movements that occur only in the sagittal plane will inevitably contribute to the injury risk posed when the athlete is subjected to transverse and frontal plane movements within the sport. In particular, the musculature around the hip and ankle joints needs to be prepared for rapid and forceful directional change in most chaotic and contact sports.

## Single-Leg Actions: Hops and Bounds

Most jumping actions can be performed as a single-leg hop, although the practitioner should remember that this action doubles the load going through leg and hip musculature, and the intensity level is therefore typically much higher. The offset and smaller base of support can also mean that high-intensity hopping movements become a balance and coordination challenge for many athletes, so ground contact times often significantly increase.

The key to effective progression is to avoid presenting the athlete with a challenge (e.g., a hurdle) that exceeds his or her capacity for effective single-foot ground contacts that are protracted in length. Often, the principle that less is more is appropriate for these exercises in terms of heights to jump over or distances to travel over. Because many sporting actions require power through single-leg movements, hopping actions represent a significant contribution to the suite of functional power exercises for the sport performer.

A simple and fun introduction to single-leg work can be achieved through the choo-choo trains drill (figure 9.17). This exercise is excellent for working with groups of athletes. The challenge is for the athletes to form a chain by having the right (or left) foot held by the right hand of the following athlete. The train must then move 20 metres without the chain being broken. Holding the leg behind forces the athlete to push the hips forward while hopping.

Typically, the chain will not move far with each foot contact, so the flight time in which to reposition the foot in preparation for landing is short. The athlete is forced to push off and reposition the ankle very quickly in preparation for landing. The next set should be done with the other foot working. Interactive and fun drills such as this encourage athletes to communicate and work together, and the drill can provide competition if two trains compete against each other. Besides being perfectly functional, drills such as this are a refreshing break in training from the disciplined and individualized drills that often characterize plyometric training.

The key to generating vertical power often lies in the assistance provided by the nonsupporting leg in a hopping action. As the athlete performs a countermovement to initiate the exercise, the unsupported leg is drawn backwards to provide a counterbalance and increase the stretch to the musculature around the hip. From here, as the supporting leg joints extend, the nonsupporting leg is brought forward with

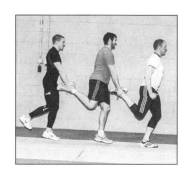 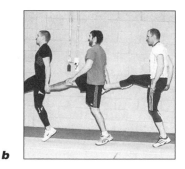

*a*    *b*

**Figure 9.17**    Choo-choo trains: *(a)* leg held behind; *(b)* leg held in front.

both of the arms. This movement adds mass to the upwards-moving body segments, increasing vertical momentum. As the athlete accelerates towards the floor, the unsupported leg is lowered in preparation for the next repetition. Exercises such as the maximum single-leg tuck jump develop this action in athletes and are ideal to introduce early in a hopping programme (figure 9.18). At this point, the athlete should be able to execute single-leg landing technique drills consistently and should have progressed towards intermediate-level jumping activities.

As activities become more demanding through the progression illustrated in figure 9.18, and the athlete is required to execute efficient ground contacts at high velocities and with more impact, the level of physical and skill competence required increases significantly. For example, the multiple hop for height and distance is often regarded as a single-leg bounding exercise and has the aim of improving stride length. This activity places enormous strains on the supporting limb and requires very high levels of single-leg reactive strength to be performed effectively.

With imagination and application of basic principles, multidirectional hopping movements can be added to a programme at a number of levels. For example, agility ladder hops or hexagon drills teach pushing off through different parts of the sole of the foot in a single-leg stance. With no predetermined heights to clear, the concentric and eccentric demands are low and ground contact can be focused on.

Contrast this with an arrangement of hurdles that need to be hopped over with a direction change at each foot contact (for example, four-way minihurdle hops). If the distance between the hurdles is too great or the hurdles are too high for the athlete's skill or strength,

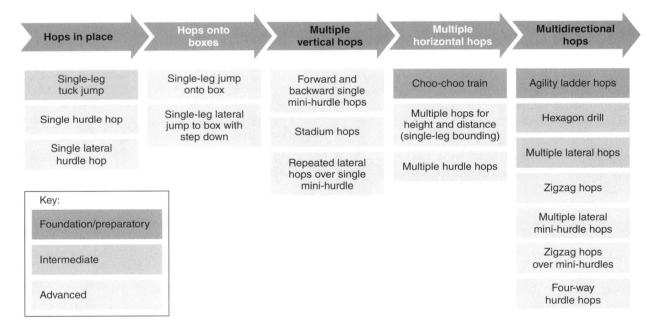

## Hops In Place

| INTERMEDIATE | |
|---|---|
| **Single-leg tuck jump:** Off one leg, perform a rapid quarter squat countermovement then hop as high as possible, bringing knees to chest in the air, landing on both feet. | |
| ADVANCED | |
| **Single hurdle hop:** Stand on one leg in front of hurdle, perform countermovement then hop over hurdle | **Single lateral hurdle hop:** Stand on one leg beside a mini-hurdle, perform countermovement then hop over hurdle, landing on same foot |

**Figure 9.18**  Hopping progressions.

## Hops Onto Boxes

| ADVANCED | |
|---|---|
| **Single-leg jump onto box**: Off one leg, perform rapid quarter squat countermovement and jump as high as possible, landing one- or two-footed on box | **Single-leg lateral jump to box with step down**: Stand laterally to box and perform rapid quarter squat countermovement then a single-leg takeoff, jumping as high as possible, landing one-or two-footed on box |

## Multiple Vertical Hops

| ADVANCED | | |
|---|---|---|
| **Forwards and backwards single mini-hurdle hops**: Hop over hurdle, landing on takeoff then hop back over hurdle to start position | **Stadium hops**: Hop up stadium steps | **Repeated lateral hops over single mini-hurdle**: Stand sideways to hurdle, one leg raised and perform explosive lateral hops over hurdle, minimizing ground contact time |

## Multiple Horizontal Hops

| FOUNDATION /PREPARATORY | |
|---|---|
| **Choo-choo train**: Form a train with other athletes by holding the right foot of the athlete behind you in your right hand and together the train moves 20 metres without being broken | |

| ADVANCED | |
|---|---|
| **Multiple hops for height and distance, single-leg bounding**: Perform repetitive hops with minimal ground contact, using the arms and opposite leg to counterbalance rotations | **Multiple hurdle hops**: Hop over 3 to 8 hurdles lined up about 1 metre apart, minimizing the height of the centre of mass and minimizing ground contact time |

## Multidirectional Hops

| FOUNDATION/PREPARATORY | | | |
|---|---|---|---|
| **Agility ladder hops**: Hop through the rungs of an agility ladder in sequence | | | |

| INTERMEDIATE | | | |
|---|---|---|---|
| **Hexagon drill**: Stand in middle of hexagon marked on floor (about 1 metre diameter) and perform repetitive hops, outside then inside, around diameter of hexagon, facing same direction | | **Multiple lateral hops**: Perform repetitive lateral hops over a course 10 to 20 metres long | |

| ADVANCED | | | |
|---|---|---|---|
| **Zigzag hops**: Hop diagonally forwards, alternating direction of successive hops to the left and right | **Multiple lateral mini-hurdle hops**: Stand on one leg laterally to a mini-hurdle, perform a countermovement, then hop over the hurdle, immediately returning to the start | **Zigzag hops over mini-hurdles**: Diagonally hop (forwards and diagonally) over a series of mini-hurdles laid out over 10 to 20 metres | **Four-way hurdle hops**: Stand inside a square of four mini-hurdles, face forward, and hop over the front hurdle, immediately springing back to the middle of the square on landing and continuing around the square |

**Figure 9.18**   *(continued)*

the ground contact time between each jump increases significantly and the nature of the skill in practice is altered.

With experience and careful planning, however, an individual multidirectional exercise such as zigzag hops can be manipulated to provide variable intensities. In figure 9.19, the athlete is challenged to change direction by hopping over minihurdles. Less advanced athletes might need discs on the floor instead of hurdles to remove the need for a high vertical force component so that they can focus on achieving direction change in the hop. Similarly, the height of the minihurdle can be changed, as can the distance between the hurdles.

The ability to differentiate a singular drill when working with a group of athletes is a useful quality for the coach. For example, by aligning the minihurdles perpendicularly to the direction of travel (figure 9.19*a*), the predominant movement remains in the sagittal plane. By turning the hurdles through 90 degrees from this point (figure 9.19*b*), the movement is subtly increased in complexity to one that is predominantly frontal plane, which requires significantly more lateral hip and ankle stabilization in landing, as well as increased lateral propulsive actions in take-off. An intermediary stage between these exercises may be a bounding action (figure 9.19*c*), in which the athlete takes off from one foot and lands with the other.

The transfer of weight through a take-off from one foot into a landing on the other is a more common action in everyday life than hopping. Indeed, such actions in a plyometric sense are often an extension of the running movement. Therefore, a reasonable approach is to programme some basic bounding exercises such as skipping variations earlier in an athlete development programme than the majority of hopping exercises. Preparatory jump work has also typically been done in exercises such as alternate-leg push-offs and split squat jumps. Advanced-level bounds, however, are performed with the athlete moving at high velocity. The athlete needs high levels of eccentric and concentric single-leg strength to execute this exercise safely and effectively.

Bounding exercises are used predominantly for horizontal locomotion and should be performed with forces high enough to stimulate the myotatic reflex. The ground contacts are then short enough to minimize the amortization phase between eccentric lengthening and concentric shortening on landing. The athlete should accelerate through a course with each successive stride. For this reason, bounding drills are typically performed at much higher horizontal velocities than other plyometric exercises. To emphasize the horizontal component of an action, and therefore the speed over the ground, the time to cover a 25-metre course is often used for athletes who are significantly competent in the bounding action. Table 9.5 presents an indicative structure for evaluating athlete performance in such a test.

As figure 9.20 illustrates, bounding exercise progressions typically start with simple skipping skills. In achieving a mature skill action in the skip, the child learns to push off from one foot and land on another while using an opposite arm, opposite leg action. The flight phase is longer and higher than in running, although

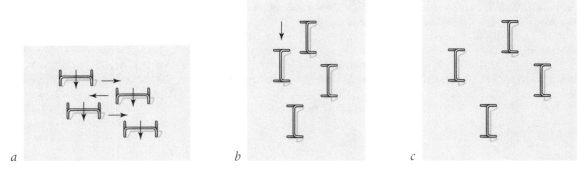

*a*        *b*        *c*

**Figure 9.19** Single-leg zigzag exercises: *(a)* hurdles aligned perpendicularly to the direction of travel; *(b)* hurdles turned 90 degrees; *(c)* hurdles farther apart for a bounding exercise.

the action is similar, albeit exaggerated. This basic action can be developed to one in which the knee is driven forward with a much more powerful action over time, so that it rises past vertical (power skipping). The coordination of the skill can be challenged simply by altering the direction of travel and asking the athlete to skip backwards.

Although a triple jump is normally associated with a hopping action, starting from

**Table 9.5** Time Standards for 25-Metre Bounding

| Rating | Time (sec.) |
|---|---|
| Excellent | 3.03 or less |
| Good | 3.04 to 4.00 |
| Average | 4.01 to 5.07 |
| Fair | 5.07 to 7.03 |
| Poor | 7.04 or longer |

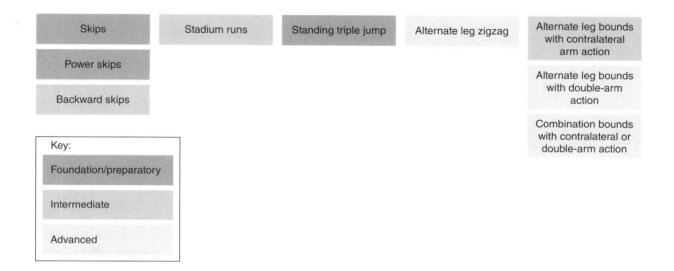

## Bounding Exercises

| FOUNDATION/PREPARATORY | | |
|---|---|---|
| **Skips**: Skip rhythmically along 20- to 60-metre course, alternating leading foot | **Power skips**: Skip rhythmically along 20- to 60-metre course, getting as much height and distance in each skip as possible | **Standing triple jump**: From standing start, hop, immediately step, then jump, landing on both feet trying for maximal height and distance with each movement |
| **INTERMEDIATE** | | |
| **Backward skips**: Skip backwards rhythmically along 20- to 60-metre course, alternating leading foot | **Stadium runs**: Run up stadium steps, pushing off each step as quickly and powerfully as possible | **Alternate leg bounds with contralateral arm action**: Perform exaggerated running action, with lead leg attacking and contacting floor with shin vertical, driving for height and distance with each step |
| **ADVANCED** | | |
| **Alternate leg zigzag**: Leap from foot to foot in exaggerated forwards and diagonal movement for 20 to 40 metres or defined number of contacts | **Alternate leg bounds with double-arm action**: Perform bounding action, both arms driving forward with each foot contact | **Combination bounds with contralateral or double-arm action**: Bound but do not alternate the lead leg, combining a number of movements with one leg forward at a time |

**Figure 9.20** Bounding exercises.

a double-foot stance naturally makes it a bounding progression. A two-footed take-off leads to landing on one leg (end of hop) and then transferring weight to the other (step) before a final take-off for maximal distance to a double-foot landing from the jump. As the athlete's competence increases with the action and ground contact becomes more forceful and quicker, targets for each phase of the action can be set to aid the athlete's progress. Also, changing the nature of the start to introduce increased horizontal velocity (for example, by walking or jogging into the first take-off step and making it a proper hop) significantly increases the demands of the drill.

The fact that the gait pattern in these exercises goes (for example) left, left, right, left should not worry the practitioner. Although strictly speaking, this is not the textbook definition of bounding, the ability to push forcefully off either foot and land on the same one or transfer weight effectively to another is an important skill for any athlete. Progressive actions should not be defined by conformity to a textbook definition. This argument is well illustrated by looking at advanced combination bounding sequences in which the athlete may be challenged to make foot contact according to a predetermined sequence, such as left, left, right, right, left, right.

In bounding, the lead leg needs to attack the floor as the athlete works into the bounding action. The resulting force pushes the driving leg forward. From there it accelerates forward. The heel tucks tight towards the buttocks, and the thigh drives forward to become the lead leg in flight.

The arm pattern that the athlete uses in alternate-leg bounding also can be altered. The contralateral arm action of running is usually adopted as the athlete becomes familiar with this action. As the rear leg pushes off to begin another stride, the opposite arm moves forward following a powerful rear-driving action from the shoulder (see chapter 8). Double-arm actions enable the athlete to achieve much greater horizontal velocities and longer stride lengths, because the combined mass of both arms swinging contributes to both ground reaction and forward momentum. The arms could be thought of as delivering a blow to the runway during the action. By increasing the downward force into the surface, the energy return is magnified, which in turn increases the stride length of the movement.

The athlete obviously needs time to adjust to double-arm actions. In flight, as the lead leg is accelerating towards the track, the arms should be moving forward forcibly, maintaining a long or straight position so that they act as force multipliers in the movement. In contrast, in running, the bent arms are speed multipliers that can travel through distances in less time. The distinction is more readily acceptable by recognizing that the flight phase in bounding is longer than that in sprinting or other forms of movement.

## Shock Plyometrics

Because gravity accelerates the body mass to the floor from a vertical height, shock plyometrics are the highest intensity plyometrics that an athlete can perform. Within this category, progressions and regressions enable practitioners to differentiate between athletes. Key differentiating variables relate to the height from which the athlete drops and the required movement that follows the dropping action.

The higher the drop height is, the greater the acceleration to the floor is, and the more eccentric strength the athlete will need to maintain the quality of the plyometric rebound through a minimized amortization phase. The athlete can develop eccentric strength by practicing landing and absorbing force eccentrically (figure 9.21). The integrity of the plyometric movement must not be lost by having the athlete drop from too great a height. The longer the ground contact is, the longer the amortization phase is, and the less reactive the training response is. The objective of the shock action needs to be clearly understood; if minimal ground contact is the aim, then drop jumps from smaller heights should be used.

If vertical force is the required outcome, ground reaction times may be longer to enable the athlete to apply greater forces for longer. This concept may help distinguish between a depth jump to squat jump movement (longer absorption of eccentric forces, longer ground contact, reduced plyometric effect) and a normal depth jump for height, in which force absorption through the hip, knee and ankle joints is minimal and ground reaction times are reduced (although they will still be higher than in a drop jump from an appropriate height). An advanced technique and strength base is important, as discussed earlier in this chapter.

Shock exercises should be used only with advanced athletes who are competent in landing techniques. When complexity significantly exceeds the athlete's capacity to execute a mechanically sound landing, the injury risk increases exponentially. The athlete also needs to have a well-developed sense of the

countermovement to develop reactive forces into the floor. This action is important, because the maximum height that an athlete can achieve in a countermovement jump plays a role in determining the appropriate height from which a shock plyometric should be undertaken.

Two variables are important for the practitioner to monitor in assessing both the quality of the depth jump and the appropriate height from which to perform a shock plyometric. The first is jump height; the second is ground contact time. If suitable equipment, such as a jump mat or force platform, is available, quantitative data relating to both variables should

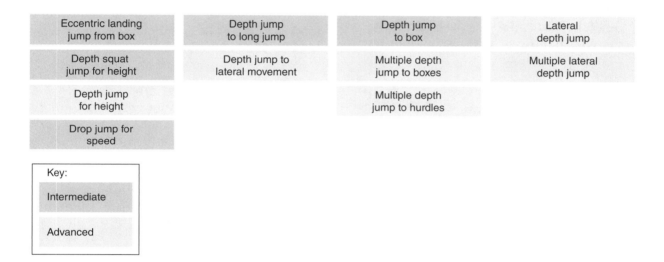

## Shock Progressions

| INTERMEDIATE | | | | |
|---|---|---|---|---|
| **Eccentric landing jump from box**: Drop from high box to stable two-footed landing, decelerating into a static hold | **Depth squat jump for height**: Drop from box to two-footed landing, descend into squat then jump as high as possible | **Drop jump for reactive speed**: Step off box then jump off floor as quickly as possible, minimizing ground contact time | **Depth jump to long jump**: Drop from box to two-footed landing then jump as far as possible, minimizing ground contact time | **Depth jump to box**: Drop from box to two-footed landing then immediately jump onto second box 1 to 2 metres away, minimizing ground contact time |

| ADVANCED | | | | |
|---|---|---|---|---|
| **Depth jump for height**: Drop from box to stable two-footed landing then immediately jump as high as possible | **Depth jump to lateral movement**: Drop from box to two-footed landing, immediately decelerate then jump as high as possible, minimizing ground contact time | **Multiple depth jumps to boxes or over hurdles**: Place a series of boxes or hurdles in a line then perform depth jumps from box to box or over each hurdle | **Lateral depth jump**: Step laterally from side of box to two-footed landing then immediately jump sideways as high and far as possible | **Multiple lateral depth jumps**: Perform multiple lateral depth jumps over a series of boxes or hurdles |

**Figure 9.21** Shock progressions.

be instantly available. Without such technology, jump height can be measured either by a simple reaching test with the arms or by a jump onto or over a box or hurdle of known height. Although not an exact science, ground contact time can be observed with an experienced coaching eye, and it can be heard as well.

The use of video aids this process enormously, particularly when the practitioner is developing a coaching eye and can benefit from the opportunity to review high-speed actions repeatedly. The athlete also can benefit from the visual feedback to support the proprioceptive feedback he or she experiences. The quality of the ground contact (length of time, stiffness in the joints, weight distribution through the foot and so on) plays an important part in whether the action looks and sounds to be of the desired quality. Sound is important, because a crisp, aggressive and active flat-foot contact sounds very different from one that occurs with technical errors.

Because of the influence that gravity-assisted movement has on the eccentric lengthening of the muscles, a rebound jump following a depth jump from a low height (for example, 10 centimetres) should always be higher than the athlete can achieve with a simple countermovement jump. Starting with low box heights, the practitioner can simply increase the drop height by small and known increments until the athlete either cannot maintain or match the jump height achieved in a maximal countermovement jump or until the ground contact time is observably increased or the quality is decreased.

This concept is illustrated in figure 9.22, which shows how reactive jump height can change with the height of the box from which the movement is initiated. The variation in box height used within the spectrum of training progressions depends on the quality of the ground contact exhibited, whether the desired training outcome is based on maximum reactive strength or maximal reactive speed, and the nature of the following movement.

As with previous progressions, single landings are less demanding than multiple landings and movements in a sagittal plane are less demanding than movements in a frontal plane, because of the complexity of the movements.

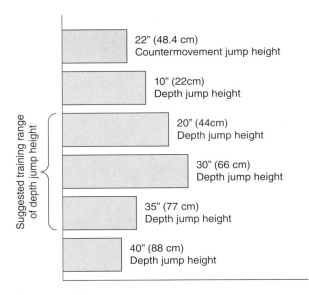

**Figure 9.22** Determining effective drop heights for depth-jumping movements.

When multiple repetitions are performed, using boxes in a jumping sequence enables the athlete to re-establish a solid foot position between efforts even with minimal foot contact on the top of the box, something not possible in jumps involving multiple hurdle clearances. Single-leg shock jumps are possible, but the practitioner needs to be confident in the athlete's qualities before having him or her attempt such movements. Even then, the height of the box from which the movement occurs will be much lower (relatively speaking) than that used in double-leg movements.

# Related Ballistic Movements

Practitioners have widely debated the relative merits of classifying upper-body ballistic actions as truly plyometric. The same debate often occurs about the use of medicine balls to perform ballistic or reactive throwing, jumping or kicking actions. This debate centres on whether the amortization phase in such actions is truly minimized to maximize concentric (reactive) force production.

For example, the explosive press-up (figure 9.23) is often given as an example of an upper-body plyometric action based on the realization that the athlete's acceleration towards the floor

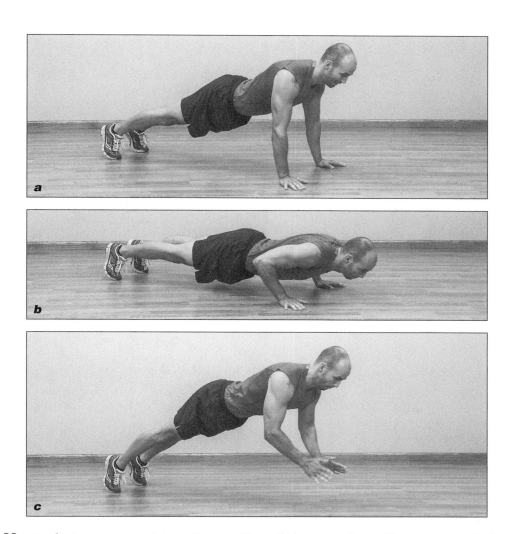

**Figure 9.23** Explosive press-up: *(a)* starting position; *(b)* lower to floor; *(c)* press-up explosively.

is retarded because there is an eccentric loading of the elbow and wrist extensor musculature as well as the horizontal adductors of the sternoclavicular joint, followed by a forceful concentric action in these muscles. The key determinant of whether these are truly plyometric lies in the analysis of the amortization phase. If the amortization phase is to be truly minimized, elbow flexion under gravity would cease as soon as the athlete's palms touch the ground.

As shown in figure 9.23, however, analysis of the point of ground contact in the clap press-up indicates that the elbow and sternoclavicular joint flexion and adduction continue long after the hands contact the ground. During this time, the neuromuscular system is undoubtedly storing elastic energy that will benefit the following concentric action, but ground contact time is long, as is the amortization phase in the movement. This argument may be somewhat academic, because although these movements are probably not truly plyometric, they are definitely ballistic and play an important function in training the upper-body force–velocity capabilities of an athlete.

As with the differentiation between jumps and shocks, the athlete is required to achieve competence in a basic movement (the clap press-up) before progressing to multidirectional movements such as the alternating-arm medicine ball press-up (figure 9.24*a*), in which the athlete moves explosively and laterally across the ball between repetitions, and the shock drop-in plyometric press-up (figure 9.24*b*), which requires tremendous upper-body strength as the athlete drops into and out from an explosive press-up from either

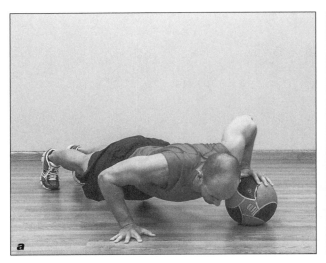 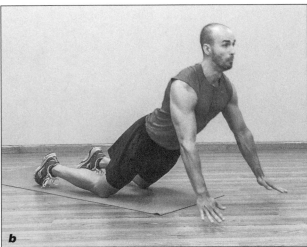

**Figure 9.24**   Variations of the explosive press-up: *(a)* alternating arm medicine ball press-up; *(b)* drop-in plyometric press-up.

a kneeling (advanced athletes) or standing (highly advanced) starting position.

Dynamic medicine ball actions (figure 9.25) should be considered similarly ballistic rather than strictly plyometric. These exercises are extremely adaptable to a wide range of ages and experiential progressions. One key to bear in mind is that the intensity of medicine ball throws is quite different from that of plyometrics. In a medicine ball exercise, the athlete accelerates a ball that weighs a percentage of his or her body mass. In a plyometric exercise, the athlete typically decelerates and reaccelerates multiples of his or her body weight. Thus, the strength requirements of the activities are very different.

Assuming that postural integrity is maintained throughout a movement, the potential range of dynamic medicine ball exercises is limited only by the practitioner's imagination. Typically, these exercises transfer forces from the floor up through the kinetic chain; thus, they mimic the sport-specific nature of the transference of ground reaction forces into an external object.

Games such as medicine ball tennis can be inserted into the athlete development curriculum as a means of variation in a challenge. This activity is not suggested as a sport-specific drill for tennis players, because although the movements may be biomechanically similar, the force–velocity components of the medicine ball throw are very different from, say,

a tennis forehand. But the athlete is required to move to intercept an object, twist to stretch the prime movers rapidly and exert large concentric forces in a reflex contraction. Power is transferred from the ground up through the kinetic chain, and the more impulse that the athlete imparts into the external object (the ball), the farther and faster it will fly. The game is a fun and worthwhile activity (the nature of a game increases the challenge to the athlete) to incorporate into an athlete's power development work as an alternative means of developing multidirectional power.

# Programming Considerations

Earlier in the chapter, the key considerations for programming were outlined, which identified the need for minimizing fatigue before and within these plyometric sessions. Plyometric sessions typically are scheduled at the start of a training week or after a recovery day when the athlete is relatively fresh. Plyometric activities normally take place towards the start of a session after an extensive warm-up when the athlete is similarly unfatigued.

Some training strategies have been shown to enhance the neuromuscular recruitment that underpins explosive movements. These techniques use postactivation potentiation

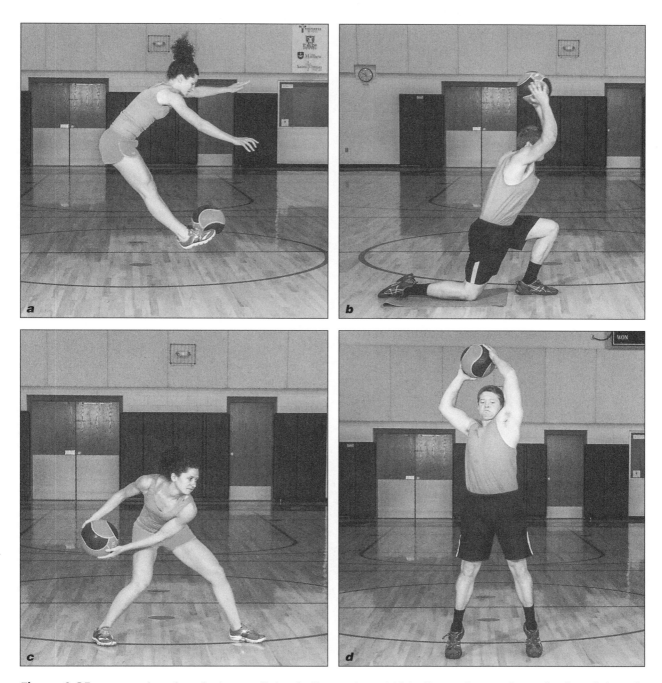

**Figure 9.25**    Examples of explosive medicine ball exercises: *(a)* hip flexor throws (lower body); *(b)* kneeling overhead throw (upper body); *(c)* medicine ball tennis (total body); *(d)* trunk rotation into ball slam (total body).

stimuli to enhance the acute power output, rate of force development or both in a following activity.[18] The basic premise is that a high force stimulus (for example, a three-repetition maximum squat) requires the neuromuscular system to recruit the maximum number of motor units to perform the action. When the athlete then performs a biomechanically similar movement (for example, a depth jump to box jump), the neuromuscular system is already potentiated (primed) to recruit a greater percentage of motor units than the athlete would be able to recruit voluntarily to perform the action.

This principle has been applied in many techniques, such as using resistance sleds in a sprinting action (see chapter 8). It has also been used in reverse situations such as when a speed–strength (high-velocity) action has been used to potentiate a higher force action. An example is maximal countermovement jumps onto a box to precede snatch lifts (see chapter 10).

Two common strategies can be used with advanced athletes to make the best use of this phenomenon to maximize the benefits of plyometric training. The key consideration that underpins both strategies is the need to maximize neural recruitment whilst not inducing fatigue that will interfere with the movement quality.

Complex training involves alternating maximal strength exercises with high-velocity exercises on a set-by-set basis (for example, heavy clean pulls from the floor with alternate-leg bounds). Research has demonstrated that to be maximally effective, the resistive load on the maximal strength exercise has to be in excess of 90 per cent of the athlete's one-repetition maximum (1RM) to activate a response.[19] A rest period must occur between the heavy and explosive exercises, typically 2 to 5 minutes, although the optimum duration for this rest appears to be highly individualistic.

A similar strategy grounded in the same theory is contrast training, in which an athlete performs multiple sets of a maximal strength exercise before performing multiple sets of an explosive exercise or performs an explosive jump before performing a high-force lift. For example, the athlete performs four sets of three reps of a clean before performing four sets of a depth jump into four hurdle jumps, or performs three sets of four reps of maximal box jumps before performing four sets of three reps of behind-the-neck push jerks.

# Summary

This chapter illustrated that jumping and related actions are fundamental movement skills that underpin the development of power within a multitude of sporting actions. The physio-mechanical mechanism that underpins the development of power within such actions is the stretch-reflex or stretch-shortening cycle, essentially a protective action that creates powerful concentric contractions in fibres that have been forcibly and rapidly stretched in preceding actions. Plyometric techniques are specialized training methods developed to train rebounding actions that use the stretch reflex to establish powerful movement capabilities in athletes.

Many basic running, jumping, hopping, leaping and bounding activities rely on the stretch-reflex action. Therefore, plyometrics shouldn't be regarded as the preserve of the advanced athlete. A wide variety of single- and double-leg activities can be modified to be included in an athlete development programme to achieve various objectives according to the person's skill level and training programme requirements. Variation can be achieved through the contact pattern between the feet and the ground (double-foot contacts, single-foot contacts, alternate-foot contacts), the relative demand of the exercise and the vertical displacement of the activity (jumping up, staying on the same level, dropping down from a height).

In determining the appropriate level of intensity of a plyometric progression, the practitioner must consider a number of factors related to the athletic capacities and physical characteristics of the individual athlete, the relative complexity and physical demand of the exercise, and the environmental considerations that underpin the delivery of safe coaching practice.

Plyometric activities may be effective in any training programme. Care needs to be taken, however, to ensure that exercise demand does not exceed athletic potential, especially in terms of the athlete's technical competence or strength. As with many training methodologies, the introduction of such situations may significantly increase the potential for traumatic injuries to the lower limb or lumbar–pelvic region. With the appropriate emphasis on technical development in conjunction with strengthening of the neuromuscular system, the athletic development professional can achieve significant and lasting improvements to an athlete's movement skills that will enhance sport-specific performances over time.

# CHAPTER 10

# Developing Functional Strength Progressions

Strength is a concept derived from the management of forces. In a sporting context, strength is about developing or resisting both internal and external forces to create either accelerations or decelerations. Movement quality (skill) in athletics is about the person's ability to manage the transfer of forces through the posture whilst executing a given technique under pressure.

This chapter analyses the concept of strength training in relation to athletic skill and brings together much of the information from previous chapters to provide a framework for the development of this fundamental quality in such a way that it can underpin other movement and sporting skills. A number of exercise progressions are introduced, providing a toolbox of techniques for the practitioner that can be developed within the practical context of an athlete development programme.

## Absolute Strength and Relative Strength

Strength (force) can be evaluated in an athlete in a number of ways. The most common means of evaluating strength is the one that many coaches refer to in conversation with athletes: How much can you bench press, squat, clean and so on? These questions refer to the concept of absolute strength or the athlete's ability to lift an external load. Often, absolute strength is normalized to enable comparisons between athletes or athletic groups to look at the concept of relative strength, in which force generation capabilities are related to body mass. For example, a 98-kilogram athlete who squats 200 kilograms (system mass is 98 kilograms plus 200 kilograms on the bar equals 298 kilograms, equating to 3.04 times body weight) is considered relatively stronger than a 120-kilogram athlete who squats 215 kilograms (system mass of 335 kilograms, or 2.7 times body weight). Absolute strength can be important in collision sports in which a key performance requirement is the ability to manage the impact of external forces colliding with the athlete.

The concept of relative strength isn't necessarily related to how much external load can be managed. In many sports, the concept of force application is about moving only the athlete's mass over the floor or through the air, such as in running, jumping and gymnastic activities. Therefore, the strength-to-body-weight ratio (or power-to-body-weight ratio) is an important consideration for most sports.

Strength relative to body mass has a number of related considerations. Body mass comprises the entire mass of a person, inclusive of mass that has no positive correlation with athletic performance (i.e., fat mass). By reducing fat mass, a person can enhance his or her relative strength without getting any stronger! Similarly, an increase in lean body mass can be brought about by an increase in muscle mass; the change might not improve the strength-to-body-mass ratio significantly, but it will almost certainly improve the athlete's absolute strength. In few cases has a gain in lean muscle only had a negative effect on strength levels, or indeed sporting performances, as long as the overall balance of training was maintained.

The real key to understanding the importance of strength to athletic movements lies in the concept of transfer of strength to performance. The key question to ask an athlete isn't necessarily, 'How strong are you?' but 'How much of your strength can you access in performance?' As chapter 4 explains, power is a function of force production and velocity of movement, and it is related to acceleration. The greater the rate of force that the athlete is able to produce, the better he or she will be at generating accelerations. The ability to develop acceleration is probably the biggest determinant of an athlete's performance in a sporting context. Therefore, the power-to-body-weight ratio is an important concept in evaluating athletic movement.

After the practitioner understands this concept, the question 'How strong is strong enough?' becomes rhetorical. The question 'How strong does this athlete need to be to realize peak power in performance?' should drive programme design, leading to the concept of functional strength, a term used in many marketing and income generation schemes recently. As with many aspects of training, the successful practitioner is able to differentiate between best practice and good marketing by referring back to underlying scientific principles.

# Introducing Function to Strength Training

In biology, function is related to the successful advancement through which an organism has evolved to survive a natural selection process.

Understanding function requires looking forward along a chain of causation (related events that cause the next thing in the sequence to happen) to achieve the goal or outcome (i.e. if this happens, it will cause this, which will enable that).

In sport, the interaction of forces acting on and within the body must be positively adapted and strengthened. The most prominent forces are gravity and ground reaction force, although collisions with and the propulsion of external objects are also common in many sports. Within the body, ensuring that forces can be transferred effectively in the direction of intention (rather than dissipating forces through uncontrolled rotations or compensations) is also an important strength development outcome. The process is aided by giving the athlete the appropriate training stimuli to facilitate the greatest positive adaptation.

Engineering literature provides some understanding of the concept of function. The requirements for an engineering project outline the most important attributes for the product. The specifications document details which processes or functions will best deliver the requirements. Coaches should operate in a similar way in sport. After determining the athlete's role (i.e., the performance requirements), the coach develops training specifications to guide the adaption process to deliver the specifications. For example, in the NFL the cornerback is probably the best all-around defensive athlete. Analysing physical performance profiles for this position based on the NFL allows performance norms to be established to provide targets for development. Based on these records, a cornerback being considered for the NFL needs to be able to run 10 yards (9.1 m) in 1.45 seconds and 40 yards (36.6 m) in 4.4 seconds, jump over 36 inches (91 cm) and complete the 5-10-5 shuttle in less than 4 seconds.

Unlike in engineering, in sport we do not work with mechanistic processes but with individuals, and all are different. Many sports have a natural selection for body type at the highest levels. For example, high jumpers and swimmers are tall because height provides a performance advantage in terms of centre of mass and leverage. But many sports, despite having an ideal shape for performers, have successful performers who have a wide range of shapes and sizes. Consider the differences between Serena Williams and Justine Henin in tennis, Wayne Rooney and Cristiano Ronaldo as world-class strikers in soccer, or baseball pitchers Steve Cishek (standing 6 feet, 6 inches [198 cm] and weighing 220 pounds [100 kg] and Tim Collins (5 feet, 7 inches and 170 pounds [77kg]).

To achieve natural selection in sport, the concept of function must be connected to the athlete's structure. Indeed, the correlation between structure or form and function is one of the central themes in biological and physical sciences. Programmes must incorporate four major stages of thought to achieve strength-training benefits that can be transferred into athletic performance:

1. What is the functional requirement for the sport (anthropometry, force and velocity characteristics and joint and musculature actions)?

2. What is the form, shape or physical characteristics of the athlete?

3. What physio-mechanical properties need to be influenced in this person?

4. What training mechanisms will best deliver the sporting function for this athlete's form?

Chapters 1 to 5 introduced the broad progression of objectives for an athletic development programme. First, the athlete needs to learn to generate large forces and develop this ability. He or she progresses to being able to generate these large forces quickly (i.e., generate impulse) and ultimately to express this impulse at the right time and in the right direction through sport-specific technique. The training progression that influences the impulse and timing through movement skill execution is based on a broad spectrum of methods differentially applied to meet objectives.

Remember that training objectives identify training priorities, which will influence the balance of programme design. Not all methods employed at any time need to be exclusively focused on achieving an objective. This concept is explored in detail later in this chapter, and applied examples are provided in chapter 11.

# Strength Performance Requirements in Sport

The first requirement for any sport performance is for the athlete to be strong enough for his or her posture to exert ground reaction forces effectively and overcome gravitational pull. Without this athletic quality, movements will not be efficient or effective and injuries will occur. Postural strength is a fundamental quality that underpins everything else presented in this chapter. Beyond postural strength, every sport has fundamental strength, power or speed requirements that determine success at a given level of performance. Chapter 4 explained the relationship between force and velocity and identified training methods to develop specific outcome qualities. In contact sports such as rugby and American football, power (force times velocity) depends more on the magnitude of the strength component. Success in sports such as running, tennis and soccer depends more on the speed (velocity) component.

Beyond postural strength to transfer forces efficiently, the strength performance requirements of a given activity need to be developed to prevent injuries and provide the appropriate basis for long-term power production in an athlete's activity. As figure 10.1 illustrates, the basic aim is to influence the athlete's joint positioning (i.e., correct technique), functional hypertrophy (i.e., growth and arrangement of fibres within the contractile proteins of the muscle[1] rather than fluid cell volume increases within the sarcoplasmic reticulum of the cell) and the neural recruitment processes of the motor units within the muscle.

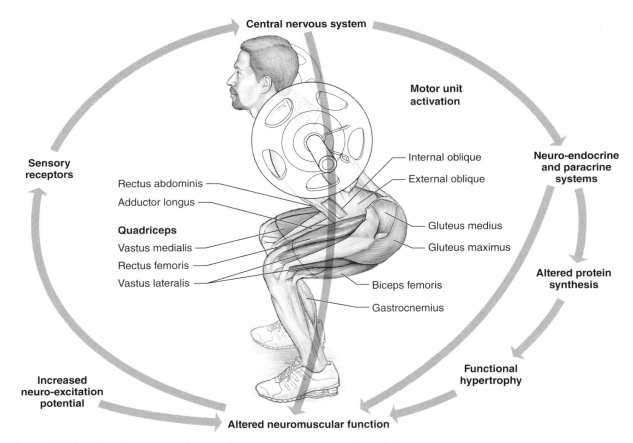

**Figure 10.1**    The physio-mechanical responses to strength training.

# Functionality of a Training Movement

To be considered functional, training should have a number of conditions that can be influenced to target specific objectives in terms of training adaptation. Practitioners should not regard exercise, or more appropriately a training programme, as being functional or not. Considering this as an area with absolutes or definitive outcomes is unwise. A better approach is to consider a sliding scale of functionality in which some exercises may be more functional than others, depending on how the exercise is prescribed, set up and executed.

## Principle 1: Train Movement in Multiple Planes

Strength training should involve all three movement planes and multiple joints in simultaneous action. This method develops and enhances the key aspects of multiple-muscle synchronization and postural control. The principle that joint positioning determines muscle recruitment and function is a guiding philosophy of functional strength work.

Therefore, triplanar movement, not the muscles themselves, should be the focus of strength training. Training the correct movements with acceptable technique enables the targeted muscles to develop. The neural firing sequences enable appropriately coordinated actions to occur so that the muscle is activated in sequences that mirror the nature of the muscular actions in sporting or everyday movement. To illustrate the importance of training movements over training muscles, let's consider the role and training needs of the quadriceps muscle.

In sport, the quadriceps is the principal knee extensor. Rarely, however, does the quadriceps perform this function in isolation of other joint or muscle actions. When generating acceleration through the triple extension of the hip, knee and ankle—previously identified as the basis for most powerful accelerations in sport—the quadriceps actions are simultaneous with the prime movers for hip extension (gluteus maximus, hamstrings) and ankle plantarflexion (gastrocsoleus complex). This movement provides the basis for pushing actions in cycling and rowing as well as locomotor actions in sports based on running and jumping. In landing mechanics, the quadriceps cocontract with the hamstrings to stabilize the knee joint.

Similarly, when kicking, the quadriceps contract to extend the knee before contact with the ball and extend the knee and shank through contact with the ball. Note that this action follows from a position in which the hip and knee have been forcefully extended (hamstring and gluteal contraction), initiating a stretch-reflex action in the quadriceps. As the knee begins to extend, the hip joint decelerates and the knee is both stabilized throughout the extension action and decelerated towards the end of the action. All these actions, mostly a function of the hamstrings, are controlled by proprioception. These coactivation sequences need to be mirrored and reflected in the appropriate strength-training mechanisms.

If, as in bodybuilding, the focus of training is muscle growth, a leg extension would provide an appropriate training stimuli. But this isolated joint exercise involves only concentric sagittal plane quadriceps contractions in knee extension and eccentric resistance in knee flexion. Postural control is not required because the athlete sits in a machine that supplements muscle action to position the trunk and hip, making the movement uniplanar. Indeed, because the seated position is not replicated in many sports, the functionality of the position could be debated.

Another important consideration in the setup of the leg extension is the lack of support for the knee. Because the hip and thigh are supported, hamstring activation is not required. The unsupported knee is a pivot midpoint between the load at the feet and the effort in the quadriceps, which means that the leverage about the patella tendon is pronounced. This leverage and the lack of muscular stabilization in the knee make the leg extension a questionable exercise in terms of applicability.

Similar discussion can be made about the leg press, a double-joint movement with sagittal plane flexion and extension about the hip and knee. Working through a full range of movement means that some gluteal and hamstring coactivation occurs in the early stages of hip extension. Indeed, muscle action can be altered by altering the foot position. Placing the feet lower on the plate increases the emphasis on knee movement, thereby increasing quadriceps action. Raising the feet on the plate increases hip action, involving the gluteals and hamstrings more. Placing the feet wider than hip-width increases the training stress on the adductor muscles (adductor longus, adductor magnus). Although joint position can be manipulated to influence muscle function in this biarticular exercise, it remains a seated, trunk-supported exercise that does not require postural control and involves movement in a single plane of action. The foot position is constant throughout the exercise, and although hip flexion is deep at the bottom position of the movement, the extent of hip extension is typically limited to 90 degrees, which is not representative of many actions in field or court sports.

Contrast these exercises with the rear foot elevated split squat (figure 10.2). In this exercise, the powerful knee extension action is simultaneous with hip extension. The exercise is performed while standing, so forces are driven from the hip into the ground and postural control is required throughout the kinetic chain. The movement occurs predominantly in the sagittal plane, but significant muscular action is used to control rotations through the trunk (transverse plane movement) and forward and backward flexions at the hip (frontal plane movement). As a basic principle, raising the front foot in such an exercise emphasizes the posterior kinetic chain muscles (principally the gluteals in this instance). Raising the rear leg emphasizes the anterior kinetic chain, thereby increasing the demand on the quadriceps.

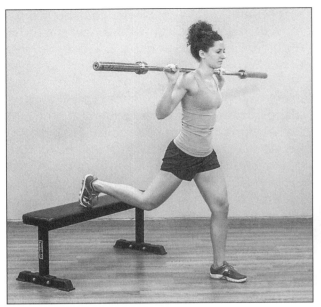 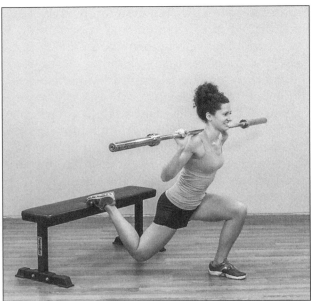

**Figure 10.2**   Rear foot elevated split squat.

Later in this chapter, consideration is given to whether these exercises can be made more functional by adding movement in other planes. Although the bar is moving predominantly in one plane, it is free to move in all planes, and trunk stabilization through isometric contractions in the postural muscles prevents mediolateral and anteroposterior movements. Similarly, these multijoint and therefore multimuscle, multiplanar actions require a full range of joint actions that use full flexions and extensions throughout the lower limb. Significant intermuscular coordination and proprioceptive control is needed throughout the entire kinetic chain.

Ground-based exercises such as pulls, squats and step-ups, in which the foot is fixed against the ground (an immovable object), as well as exercises in which the hand is fixed, such as pull-ups or press-ups, are known as closed kinetic chain exercises. The leg press, split squat, sled push and sled drag use compressive forces to develop strength (i.e., the posture is compressed between gravity and ground reaction forces from the floor). The leg extension exercise is an open kinetic chain exercise; the foot is not fixed. Open kinetic chain exercises tend to promote shearing forces such as through the patella in the leg extension, so

coaches should be cautious about overusing them in a programme.

Strength through contralateral stepping actions (which are important in most sports) can be developed through high force loads that are stable because they are on the ground and are uniplanar. Pushing loaded sleds from a low position enables a stepping action led by the extension of the knee, thus strengthening the quadriceps in the anterior kinetic chain. Reminding the athlete that forces are best transmitted through straight lines encourages him or her to maintain a rigid spine and straight-arm position during such a movement to maximize the transfer of forces from the push into the ground into the sled. Similarly, dragging a loaded sled backwards by using a harness is another exercise for developing quadriceps strength, primarily through extension of the knee. But the level of functionality that these high-force movements have relative to other exercises is something that the practitioner may wish to consider carefully.

As highlighted in figure 10.1, the focus should be on the motor cortex in the brain, a high-level regulator of the movements of the body. The motor cortex organizes the neuromuscular system to meet the environmental challenges imposed on the athlete. This system governs movement responses based on multiple inputs, not on isolated muscle qualities. Therefore, strength-training activities should involve multiple muscle actions to ensure that the motor cortex develops the coordination required for the athlete to produce appropriately forceful movement solutions to the problems presented in the sporting environment.

Closed kinetic chain exercises are typically body-weight exercises, although they may incorporate additional load. These exercises have higher levels of functionality because they replicate the sporting interaction that occurs between gravity, the athlete's body and the ground. The compound movements require interaction among all body segments to produce an efficient and coordinated movement.

Less direct load is imposed on target muscle groups in closed kinetic chain exercises, which many have argued will result in less direct stress on the muscle and therefore less hypertrophy within the fibres. Although this may the case, the relative importance of fibre hypertrophy in specific muscle groups needs to be carefully considered in light of the benefits that these exercises bring in terms of postural control and neuromuscular activation and coordination.

Emerging research is leading scientists to think that hypertrophy may not necessarily be a function of local muscle stress but more often a centrally regulated process related to the notion of cellular signalling mechanisms,[2] a concept first noted in cancer research. This concept is seeking to identify the specific conditions and genetic circumstances that cause cells such as muscle fibres to develop in a certain way.

One such signal comes from anabolic hormones, naturally occurring hormones that stimulate growth in muscles and connective tissue such as testosterone, IGF-1 and human growth hormone that are released in response to strength training. Significant evidence[1] demonstrates that these hormones are released in greater concentrations following compound exercises such as squats and deadlifts or heavy load stimulation (e.g., bench press) as opposed to following isolated joint exercises that involve fewer muscles and lower loads.

Strength training, however, is not just about overloading the neuromuscular system. Connective tissue needs to be developed so that it can adapt to the forces generated by muscles. Stress acts on the weakest part of a system, and therefore injuries to tendons are common when forces generated within muscles exceed the loading capacity of the tendon. Injuries are often a consequence when athletes use anabolic steroids that target muscle growth; the muscle's capacity to generate force rapidly exceeds the tendon's capacity to transfer those forces.

Similarly, ligaments need to be overloaded to maintain joint integrity during movements, especially when designing strength training for vulnerable joints such as the knee or the shoulder. This training is especially important when the joint will be subject to large impact forces, either from collisions with an opponent or from ground reaction forces in landing. Bones also respond to mechanical loading and develop because of appropriate strength training. The more multifunctional a strength-training programme is, the more all aspects of the neuromuscular and musculoskeletal system will benefit in terms of positive adaption towards performance demand.

Do not mistake this discussion about understanding functionality as a debate of free-weight (or free-standing) strength training versus training on machines. The key is to consider the level of functionality that an exercise provides to the overall training process. Indeed, many machines can be considered wholly functional, including many cable machines and jammer actions. The use of these machines and specific examples of functional exercises on such equipment are introduced later in the chapter.

## Principle 2: Transfer Force Through the Whole Kinetic Chain

Another consideration for determining the level of functionality of an exercise is how forces are transferred through the body during the execution of the movement. As identified in chapter 5, most forces in sport are generated from ground reaction forces with the floor that are then transferred through the legs, pelvic girdle and trunk to the extremities where they are expressed. Force transmission through the kinetic chain is characterized by deceleration at one joint and acceleration at the next joint in the chain, a process moderated by the central nervous system and proprioceptive mechanisms.

During high-force, high-speed movements in sport, the athlete needs to coordinate a number of muscular actions in various planes of motion to produce an effective action. The ability to recruit and produce multiplanar forces (i.e., strength) through multiple muscle groups around multiple joints involved in an action should be factored into the progression of skilled movements.

The other important characteristic in the successful transference of these forces is the requirement for stability in the major girdles of the body—the pelvis and shoulder—to provide an anchor for the limbs that are generating or expressing forces. Therefore, the more an exercise challenges pelvic control or shoulder stabilization, the more functional it might be.

Let's look at some traditional overhead pressing activities (table 10.1). Both the machine shoulder press and the seated dumbbell shoulder press are seated isolated joint exercises that require little from the kinetic chain in terms of neuromuscular activation to support the trunk or pelvis. Indeed, such isolation exercises may be seen to break the kinetic chain artificially, because the other musculature that would be used to impart force into the hands in a sporting action in the absence of the seat is not involved. Using dumbbells means that the arms operate independently, and the bar path in the pressing action is controlled by the athlete rather than the machine, which has a fixed bar path that the athlete cannot alter. These factors make the seated dumbbell shoulder press slightly more functional.

**Table 10.1**    Traditional Overhead Pressing Activities

|  | **Machine shoulder press** | **Seated dumbbell shoulder press** | **Behind-the-neck standing press** |
|---|---|---|---|
| Shoulder girdle control | Little control is required. The machine dictates the path of the movement with no deviation, and the upper back is supported by the seat. | Limited. Although the dumbbells add complexity to the movement because the arms operate independently, the upper back is supported by the seat. | Essential. The trunk and upper back are unsupported, and shoulder position must be maintained if forces are to transfer efficiently into the arms to keep the bar path vertical throughout the movement. |
| Pelvic girdle control | Not required because the trunk is supported by the seat. | Not required because the trunk is supported by the seat. | Essential. The pelvis needs to stay in neutral, and the trunk needs to remain upright. |
| Force transfer | Isolated joint exercise from the shoulders through the leverage of the machine. | Isolated joint exercise. The trunk is supported, and the seat provides a foundation for power transfer from the shoulder joint through to the dumbbell. | Compound exercise from the floor through the full kinetic chain, which is fully extended with the bar overhead at its farthest possible point from the base of support. |
| Planes of motion | Sagittal plane only. | Mainly sagittal plane flexion and extension, although the athlete needs to control transverse plane adduction in each shoulder and frontal plane flexion and extension at the shoulder. | Mainly sagittal plane, but the athlete has to prevent rotations about the hips, trunk and shoulders in the transverse plane and flexions and extensions in the frontal plane. |

If the seated dumbbell shoulder press is performed in a standing position, as in the behind-the-neck press, it might be considered a highly functional exercise; the athlete would experience significant postural challenge in maintaining the bar paths of each dumbbell while pressing the loads overhead. Indeed, with standing overhead pressing actions, athletes can often be seen to hyperextend their lumbar and thoracic spines (obvious by the increased lordotic curve in the lower spine) to increase pectoral involvement in the pressing activity that compensates for weakness in both the postural muscles of the trunk and the glenohumeral joint extensor muscles (deltoid group).

Arguably, the functionality of an overhead pressing action could be increased by adding a pushing action from the legs as in a push press or jerk. A push press or jerk starts from the same position as the behind-the-neck press (although the bar could be resting on the front of the shoulders instead) and uses a countermovement (rapid dip and drive) in the legs to initiate the upward movement of the bar and impart momentum into the bar as force is transferred through the legs and trunk from the floor, requiring less of a pushing action from the shoulders and arms. Because of the additional input from the legs, loads are usually increased to add to the neuromuscular challenge throughout the whole kinetic chain.

Another consideration for standing exercises is the challenge of maintaining a balanced position, a factor not required in seated or supported exercises. For an activity to be considered functional, it must have an element of dynamic balance, of maintaining equilibrium of the centre of mass relative to the base of support. In sport, movement involves a dynamic equilibrium with a constant interplay of mobility and stability. The athlete is constantly trying to retain balance to allow efficient movement. Strength training should reflect and recognize this purpose.

## Principle 3: Build Strength From the Ground Up but Challenge the Trunk Before the Extremity

The discussion so far has been about the importance of transferring forces through the entire kinetic or postural chain. In regard to overhead movements, this discussion has progressed to extending the kinetic chain to raise the athlete's centre of mass and maximize the distance of the centre of mass from both the base of support and the load that provides the challenge. That load challenges a movement response predominantly in a single plane and typically in a direction opposite to gravity. The strength challenge provoked by the movement must be met by the weakest link in the kinetic chain at the interaction of the axial skeleton with the appendicular skeleton at the major girdles in the body (i.e., the pelvis or shoulder girdle).

Because forces in sport are transferred from the ground up through the kinetic chain, a key requirement for a functional exercise is that it be a closed kinetic chain movement that requires a similar pattern of strength transfer. For example, the deadlift (figure 10.3) is a maximal strength activity that challenges the athlete to push into the floor as hard as possible to raise a relatively heavy load. The push from the floor comes from the simultaneous actions of the hip and knee extensors. The extension mechanics in the hip, and the ability to transfer the ground reaction forces from the ground into the bar so that the amount of lift in the bar is proportional to the extension range of the hip and knee, require the lumbar–sacral region to maintain its strongest position. Similarly, the scapula need to be retracted and stable for the shoulder girdle to remain stable and maintain integrity to prevent injury and transfer forces through to the arms holding the bar.

If these joints do not maintain their relationship, forces cannot be effectively transferred and movement compensations may occur. Ultimately, the load may be lifted, but at what cost? Complications such as disc herniation may arise from loaded movements when the integrity of the lumbar–pelvic alignment is not maintained. The athlete should focus on a challenge (in this case the load on the bar) that can be met at the girdles in the body rather than develop a compensatory movement. This advice applies to challenges from heavy loads as well as other strength challenges, such as movements in different planes within different body segments.

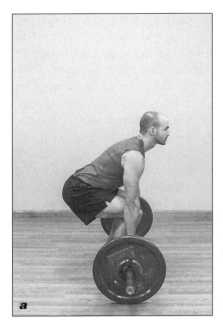
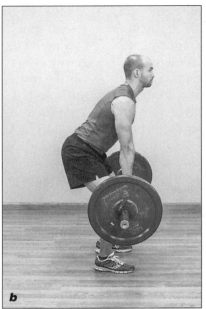
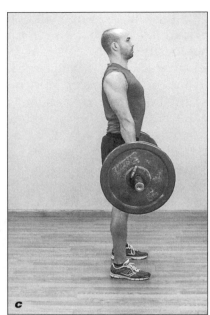

**Figure 10.3**   Deadlift: *(a)* starting position; *(b)* midlift; *(c)* standing.

## Principle 4: Sequence Muscle Actions to Produce High-Force, High-Velocity Movements

The concept of a functional exercise requires limited discussion, because training of all forms has to be incorporated and integrated into a programme. Functional strength training should complement the full spectrum of exercises incorporated into an athlete's routine, which means also focusing on the sequence of muscle actions that occur within a movement.

Most powerful actions within the body are based on the stretch-shortening cycle within the muscle. In the case of plyometric actions, predominantly fast stretch-reflex actions are used, but often strength movements cannot be executed within the 0.02-second period that characterizes such actions. But athletes can access the stored elastic energy that comes from eccentric muscle actions in slower strength actions, and therefore slow stretch-shortening cycles can be developed to assist in ballistic actions.

In executing multidirectional movement skills, eccentric muscle actions create decelerations, whether these are segmental (e.g., the hamstrings decelerating the knee in kicking

actions) or in the total body (e.g., gluteal, quadriceps and gastrocsoleus decelerating the lead leg for the body to pivot around the javelin throw). Eccentric muscle actions are an important part of strength programmes for all sports with the possible exception of cycling, one sport that has no eccentric muscle actions as part of the skilled movement requirements.

For the athlete to access his or her strength during performance, eccentric muscle actions need to be a consistent part of the training. A range of training modes and exercises that require maximal force production within 0.08 to 0.4 seconds should be used, depending on the skill being performed. Chapter 9 introduced plyometrics, which should be incorporated into a holistic strength-training programme for many athletes. Strength exercises with high levels of function should likewise enable the athlete to use stretch-shortening cycles to exert force rapidly and produce high-force, high-velocity actions.

Strength movements that use eccentric muscle actions to develop controlling and decelerating movements before explosive, concentric accelerations might be justifiably considered as having greater levels of transferability to sport performance than exercises in which the movement focus is on concentric actions before eccentric ones. Such contraction patterns are often associated with movements that have already been considered less functional, such as leg extensions and biceps curls. Conversely, squat or lunge movements (variations of which are explored later) use eccentric actions to lower the body under control before returning to the starting position with an explosive pushing action from the legs.

Other cornerstone strength exercises traditionally used within strength-training programmes can arguably be made more functional (i.e., greater transference of training benefits) by applying this principle. For example, the stiff-legged deadlift (or Romanian deadlift) is commonly used to develop eccentric strength in the hamstrings, but it can be executed in a number of ways, some of which are more functional than others.

The aim of the stiff-legged or Romanian deadlift is for the trunk to move forward with a hinge at the hip joint under load. With the shoulders retracted and the trunk braced, the hamstrings are eccentrically loaded as the weight is lowered. The trunk movement and bar lowering continue until the hamstrings 'sing' (i.e., reach lengthening capacity with a load), at which point the load is returned to the starting position. As figure 10.4 illustrates, the athlete often starts with reasonably straight legs, and the emphasis is on not moving the knees and hips throughout the movement. With no change in joint position, no real lengthening of the hamstrings occurs, so the muscle isn't actively stretched, but the eccentric muscle action resists the bar mass as it is lowered.

At the point where the bar cannot be lowered any farther, the trunk returns to the starting position. Many think that this action is led by the hamstrings, but the main functions of the hamstrings are to flex the knee joint and extend the hip through tilting the pelvis upwards.[3] No hip joint movement in the leg (hence the stiff-legged title) compromises the use of the hamstrings, meaning that the spinal erectors play a significant part in the lifting process.

Contrast this exercise with the execution shown in figure 10.5, in which the athlete begins in a position with the knees and hips more flexed. The first movement is the hip moving upwards and backwards, which immediately begins to lengthen the hamstrings. The upwards and backwards hip movement

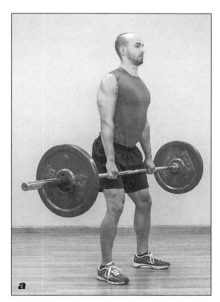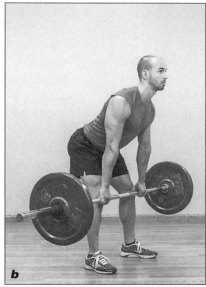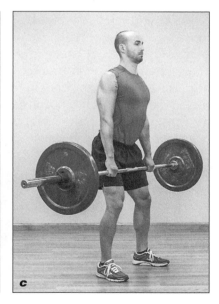

**Figure 10.4** Romanian deadlift method 1 with no stretch reflex: *(a)* starting position with legs straight; *(b)* midposition with the same knee and hip angle; *(c)* return to starting position with no change in knee and hip angle.

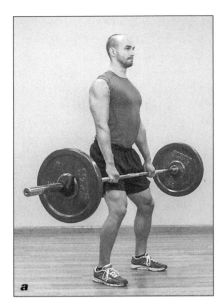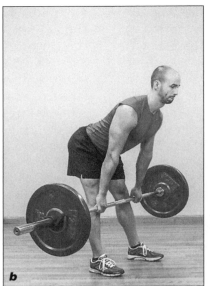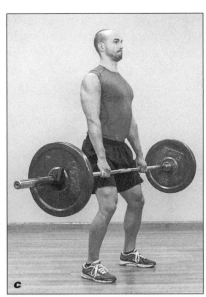

**Figure 10.5** Romanian deadlift method 2, incorporating the stretch reflex: *(a)* starting position with knees and hips flexed; *(b)* midposition as hips move upwards and backwards, knees extended; *(c)* return to starting position; hip extension unloads hamstrings, and stretch reflex drives knees forwards.

continues as the bar is lowered down the front of the thighs, lengthening the gluteus maximus in the process. A good coaching cue for athletes is to imagine they are trying to move their butts back to close a door that will never be closed. Another good cue for athletes is to feel the weight distribution towards the heels as the bar is lowered and the hips move backwards.

Because the feet are fixed to the floor, as the hips flex, the knees will be extended passively, an inevitability because the femur cannot change length. The combination of lengthening and load means that the athlete will feel the hamstrings 'sing', potentially early in the movement. Indeed, the trunk should not reach parallel to the floor, because this position will change the emphasis of the lift and require the spinal erectors to act as the prime movers to raise the load.

To return to the starting position, the hips should be extended by a forceful action to unload the hamstrings from their stretched position, causing both the hips to extend and the knees to flex as the hamstrings forcefully contract (a function of the stretch reflex). The trunk will return to the upright starting position, and the legs will return to the slightly flexed position.

This variation of the movement arguably places less emphasis on the concentric action in the hamstrings, but by developing a more natural action–contraction pattern in the muscles around the hip and knee joint, it can be considered more functional, especially because the real strength benefits in this lift come from the eccentric loading phase. In addition, this variation is a good exercise for athletes who cannot disassociate between hip, knee and lumbar spine actions in movement.

Another example of incorporating the stretch reflex into a lifting action that more effectively transfers into sporting movements can be seen in the pulling phases of clean and snatch movements. Indeed, the two overhead lifts (with the jerk following the clean) that have been contested in weightlifting since 1972 are of particular interest to the practitioner seeking to improve the rate of force development in sport performers who have a good basic movement and strength-training education.

These complex total-body movements not only challenge the body to produce high power outputs in a short time but also, like most explosive sporting actions (running, kicking and throwing), rely on the reflex and elastic properties of the muscle–tendon complex to express power, even from a static starting position. This reflex is elicited through rapid coordinated flexion of the hips, knees and ankles (eccentric portion) followed by a rapid coordinated extension of the hips and knees and plantarflexion (concentric portion). For more complete technical guidance on how to execute this movement in full, see Brewer and Favre (2016),[4] but the following paragraphs illustrate how establishing correct joint position (the correct technique) can elicit more functional execution in a complex movement that athletes often perform incorrectly.

The amortization phase between the eccentric and concentric muscle actions should be as short or rapid as possible. This ability is fully trainable in athletes who are exposed to appropriate training methods and coaching processes. Strength-training actions that use the stretch-shortening properties of muscle will enable power outputs far in excess of more traditional strength (force production) exercises that do not fully use these elastic properties.

As figure 10.6 illustrates, the first pull is the first movement performed in the snatch and its derivative exercises. The first pull straddles the period between the weight disks leaving the floor (the moment of separation) and the lifter and bar complex moving upwards and backwards (in terms of weight distribution through the stationary feet) until the bar is above the knees. At this point, note that the bar doesn't stop; it continues moving through the subsequent phase of the lift (the transition), but the classification of movement phases is helpful from an analysis and teaching perspective.

The first pull phase of the movement is crucial to the overall success of the lift. First, it represents the slowest phase of the lift, because the lifter must overcome inertia from the static position and impart momentum into the bar. What is more important is that during the movement, the position from which the subsequent stretch-reflex action occurs is established. Without establishing the correct position, the effectiveness of the athletic movement is severely diminished.

Besides achieving a biomechanically efficient position, this movement pattern serves to reduce mechanical disadvantage within the athlete's lever system.[5] Reducing mechanical

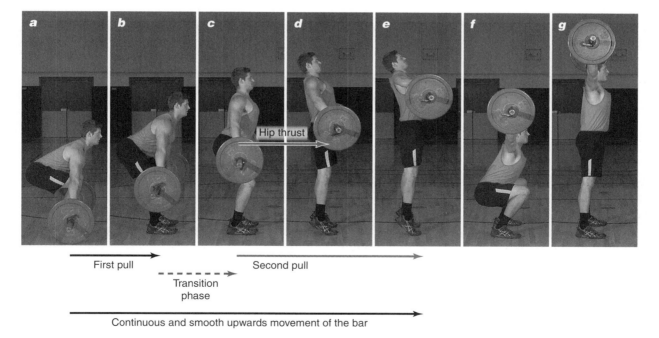

**Figure 10.6** Snatch: *(a)* starting position; *(b)* end of first pull with bar above the knees; *(c)* jump position with bar at inguinal crease; *(d)* end of second pull; *(e)* drop under bar; *(f)* receiving the bar in the overhead squat position; *(g)* recover to standing and finish.

disadvantage allows the lifter to execute the movement without expending a disproportionate amount of energy. This technique reduces the tension (force requirements) through the lower back because the athlete is able to establish and maintain an optimal combined centre of gravity (COG).[6] Achieving this position is of paramount importance, because maintaining balance depends on the relationship between the centre of mass (COM) and the base of support (the lifter's feet). Thus, in the snatch (or equally the clean or other derivative training movements) the success of a given lift is largely determined by precise and consistent execution of the correct first-pull mechanics.

The stretch-reflex action that the first pull prepares for is executed during the subsequent transition phase, which potentiates for the second pull. The second pull is the phase of the lift when both peak power output and maximal bar velocity occur as all the extensors of the lower limb contract to push explosively into the ground, creating a triple extension of the hip and knee extension and ankle plantarflexion. For this action to occur effectively, a smooth transition from first to second pull is vital. The second pull movement completes the pull phase of the lift, as the athlete pushes into the floor to cause the bar to rise vertically.[6] The internationally recognized terminology is ironic in that it is obviously a push into the floor that lifts the bar, not a pull of the weight.

With the correct execution of the first pull, tension in the hamstrings increases as the bar rises past the knees. As the bar continues to rise and the hips extend upwards, this tension 'unloads', or decreases. With the hips stabilized and the hamstrings stretched, the subsequent unloading initiates a reflex contraction for the hamstrings to perform their main function, which is to flex the knees forward under the bar. This action is a reflex that arises from the loaded stretch to the hamstrings, but it is a reflex that has been deliberately contrived in the taught action, in the same manner as in a depth or drop jump (see chapter 9). This action is deliberately taught in athletes who have been appropriately coached to move through the key positions in the lift, not a phenomenon that coaches should expect athletes to create accidentally.

As with all stretch-shortening cycles, the faster the hamstrings are stretched, the faster the myotatic reflex is and the more powerful the subsequent contraction is. Therefore, developing a faster transition phase is a key objective of the athlete development programme.

Analysis of bar velocities during the various stages of the lift consistently shows that the vertical velocity of the bar slows during the transition phase (figure 10.7). Accompanying this loss of bar velocity is an unweighting moment at which force production drops significantly as the athlete's body positions itself to generate high vertical forces (figure 10.8). There is no evidence that a momentary drop in velocity impairs subsequent performance; the drop in velocity corresponds to the transition phase in which the lifter is moving into a more advantageous position for subsequent force production and RFD. In fact, the final velocity can be higher as a result of the transition phase.[7]

Although identified as the jump (or power) position (figure 10.6), this position is moved through rapidly. The knee rebending action in the transition phase, coupled with the beginning hip extension action in the glutes, means that the quadriceps and gastrocsoleus muscles will now be rapidly stretched, optimizing them to produce a more forceful concentric action as the athlete's thigh makes contact with the bar. This contact is the signal for the athlete to jump or push into the floor as rapidly and powerfully as possible, initiating the movement from the hips.

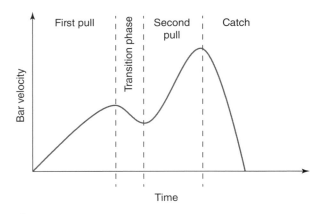

**Figure 10.7** Bar velocity decreases during the transition phase of the clean to enable acceleration in the second pull.

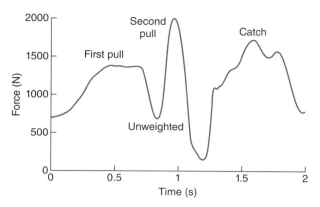

**Figure 10.8** Force production decreases in the transition phase of a clean in preparation for high force production during the second pull.

Reprinted, by permission, from A.L. Souza, S.D. Shimada, and A. Koontz, 2002, "Ground reaction forces during the power clean," *Journal of Strength and Conditioning Research* 16(3): 423-427.

During the second pull, peak force, rate of force development, power and bar velocity are at their highest values (figures 10.7 and 10.8), following the optimized physio-mechanical positioning of the athlete's joints at and before the power position. The duration of the second pull lasts from the end of the transition phase (power position) to full extension of the hips and knees, plantar flexion of the ankles and elevation of shoulders (the shrug). This action is often referred to as the triple extension.

By ensuring appropriate joint positioning and the sequential development of movement actions within a strength-training movement, the athlete appropriately develops eccentric and concentric muscle actions and stretch-shortening cycles. The exercise becomes much more functional in the sense that the athlete is using the control and power-producing mechanisms that evolution has developed for powerful performance and injury reduction within the training movements.

## Principle 5: Develop Functional Programming Through a Broad Spectrum of Movement and Load Challenges

Sport performance is based on a combination of efficient movement and sport-specific skills such as running, jumping, throwing, landing, changing direction and rotating. Although many total-body actions occur in one plane (e.g., when sprinting, all motion is in the sagittal plane), in many instances the sequential involvement of different body segments requires movement control in multiple planes of motion. Similarly, the body will be subject to a range of loading patterns, from collisions to multiples of body weight when landing to unloading in flight or in the specific phases of movement. Therefore, strength training in an athletic development programme should incorporate a broad spectrum of movement and loading challenges.

These challenges typically begin with bodyweight exercises, although this preparation is not always essential. A full range of pulling, pushing and squatting movements, overhead activities, and rotational actions should be employed to ensure that the neuromuscular system and musculoskeletal structures are significantly overloaded to achieve learning and therefore training adaptation. A balance also needs to be struck between posterior and anterior chain movements, a factor often overlooked in strength training; many programmes use a regime of higher loading or different repetition ranges to facilitate overload. Undoubtedly, this important part of the strength-training process cannot be underestimated, but it should not be the sole focus of the training programme. Although a suitably periodized programme of loading and unloading of resisted load is essential and will promote strength development, most loaded exercises challenge only sagittal plane movement, leaving the athlete deficient in other movement ranges, compromising performance and probably increasing the chances of injury during multidirectional sport performance.

A balance needs to be achieved between strength training with load and strength training through adaptive movement challenges that incorporate single-leg and single-arm actions, unilateral movements and multiplanar movements into the athlete's routine. This approach challenges the full spectrum of the neuromuscular system appropriately and uses the full range of myofascial slings that are crucial to transferring forces along the kinetic chain.

An exercise can be made functionally more difficult in many ways before adding additional load. As illustrated in the sidebar Manipulating Exercise Difficulty: The Press-Up, variation in the movement challenge of most body-weight exercises (in this example, a press-up) can be provided by altering the position of the centre of mass, the position of the working joints, the length of the lever arm, the number of points of support and the speed of the movement before adding external load.

An important principle throughout these progressions is that the key coaching points of the movement do not deviate because of the change in exercise difficulty. Typical compensations include reducing the range of movement through which the shoulders adduct and the elbows flex, and raising the hips, which reduces the challenge on the working muscles by shortening the lever arm of the body.

# Manipulating Exercise Difficulty: The Press-Up

Figure 10.9 shows the standard press-up. Note the straight-line body position through the ankles, knees, hips and shoulders. Hands are shoulder-width apart and thumbs are facing forwards so that the shoulders can be fully retracted.

Manipulating joint position changes the involved muscle actions. Bringing the hands closer together (figure 10.10a) means that the triceps brachii have greater involvement in the movement. Moving the hands wider apart (figure 10.10b) increases the action of the glenohumeral joint and reduces the emphasis on elbow extension; therefore, the pectoral muscles are required more and the triceps brachii less.

Putting the knees on the floor (figure 10.11) reduces the length of the lever arm. The weight of the lower leg is also effectively removed from the movement, which will slightly raise the centre of mass. The reduced leverage reduces the requirement for force production during the exercise, so this variation is less of a strength challenge than the standard press-up.

Raising or lowering the centre of mass relative to the working joints (the shoulder, elbow and wrist) changes the difficulty of the exercise significantly. With the trunk raised relative to the centre of mass (figure 10.12a), the load going through the upper body is reduced through a full range of movement, making the exercise easier. Increasing the height of

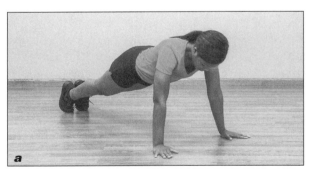

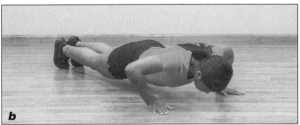

**Figure 10.9**  Press-up: (a) top position; (b) bottom position.

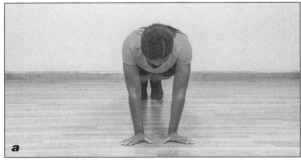

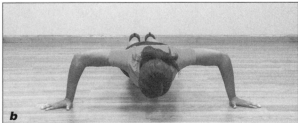

**Figure 10.10**  Changing hand positions in the press-up: (a) hands closer together; (b) hands wider apart.

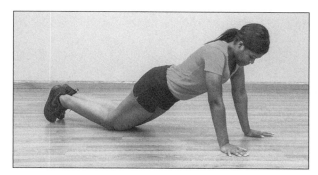

**Figure 10.11**  Press-up with knees on the floor.

the feet (figure 10.12b) moves the centre of mass above the chest and arms, which increases the load through the joints as they flex and extend. The height that the feet are raised can be progressively increased. This variation also changes the focus on the pectoralis major; the higher the incline is, the more emphasis is placed on the superior portion on the muscle. When a handstand position is reached (figure 10.12c), the movement becomes predominantly shoulder flexion and extension. At this point, the line of force of the centre of mass is directly above the arms, the only base of support, making this exercise extremely challenging. Performing the handstand press-up without a wall support is an extreme postural challenge in terms of strength to maintain a balanced and stable position.

A one-handed press-up (figure 10.13) significantly reduces (by 50 per cent) the base of support; hence, the wide feet position is generally adopted to enable balance to be maintained. The load going through the working arm is now doubled. Simultaneously, the postural challenge to keep the shoulders level with one shoulder unsupported is increased. A less-dramatic challenge is for the athlete to reduce the base of support at the feet by lifting one foot off the floor. This action raises the centre of mass slightly but requires the athlete to work harder to maintain a level hip position throughout the movement.

Powering into a side plank (figure 10.14) from the bottom position requires increased acceleration from the bottom position followed by a controlled deceleration around the shoulder at the top of the side plank to maintain position without overbalancing. As the athlete moves from the side plank back into the press-up for the next repetition, the velocity of movement increases because the centre of mass moves through a greater range on the second repetition. This movement needs to be controlled for in the subsequently explosive press-up action.

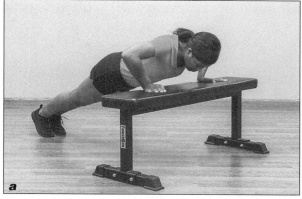

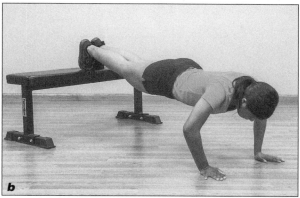

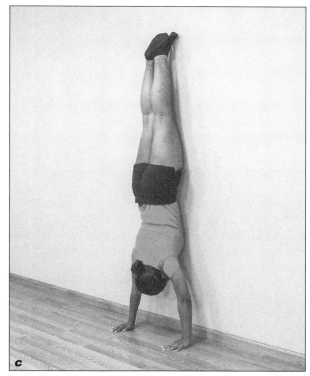

**Figure 10.12**  Press-up variations in which the centre of mass is raised or lowered relative to the working joints: (a) trunk raised; (b) feet raised; (c) handstand press-up.

*(continued)*

## Manipulating Exercise Difficulty: The Press Up *(continued)*

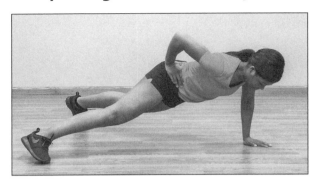

**Figure 10.13** One-handed press-up.

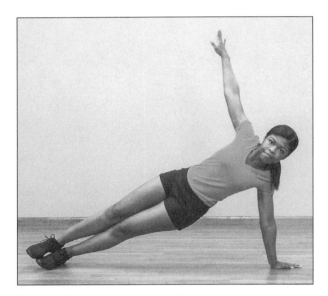

**Figure 10.14** Press-up into side plank.

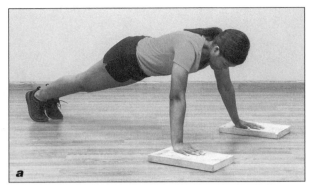

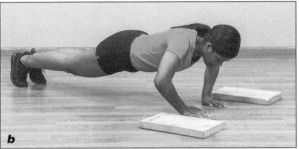

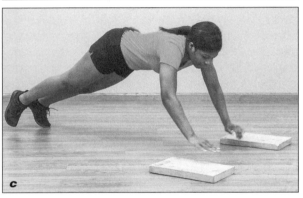

**Figure 10.15** Clap press-up with hands on blocks: *(a)* starting position; *(b)* hands between block; *(c)* press-up and clap.

A clap press-up (figure 10.15) or other ballistic variation significantly increases the velocity of the action and the force required to accelerate the centre of mass through a greater range against gravity. The clap ensures that the wrists remain extended in preparation for landing in subsequent actions. Athletes often lose the straight-line body position in this exercise because they attempt to gain additional leverage by lifting the hips first. Be warned: If the athlete isn't strong enough to cope with the additional load caused by gravitational acceleration of the centre of mass as it moves through a greater range, he or she can injure the face by performing this exercise. The ballistic nature of the exercise can be increased by starting the exercise with the hands on blocks to increase the range through which the centre of mass will accelerate (gravity assisted) and the height through which the

athlete must rapidly raise the centre of mass (gravity resisted).

Similarly, starting the press-up in an extended prone bridge position—with the longest leverage going through an extended kinetic chain (figure 10.16)—places great emphasis on postural stability in the shoulders. To drop from this position into a press-up and then return requires eccentric strength in force control on landing, concentric strength in accelerating the body vertically and postural strength in rapidly achieving a secured shoulder position.

The addition of an external load (figure 10.17) increases the force requirement as the load acting

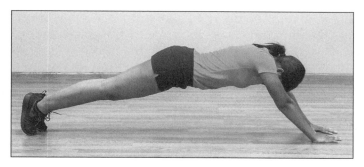

**Figure 10.16** Press-up from extended prone bridge position.

through the centre of mass is increased. Typically, external load is provided by adding a vest to the athlete's trunk, placing weighted disks across the athlete's upper back or using a resistance band that becomes stretched as the athlete extends the elbows. This variation may be a more functional means for overloading the shoulder and arm extensors whilst maintaining scapular stability and postural control than more traditional supine exercises such as the bench press.

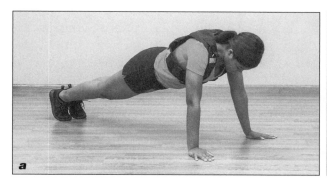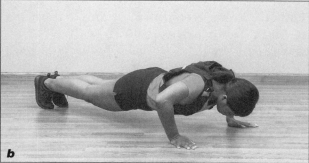

**Figure 10.17** Press-up with external load: *(a)* starting position; *(b)* bottom position.

# Principle 6: Make Strength Accessible Rather Than Specific

The aim of the athletic development practitioner is to provide the tools that the athlete needs to execute movement solutions to the relevant sport-specific problems. As the athlete advances in his or her career, the training needs to become more specialized to reflect the more specific demands of both the sport and the athlete's position. The importance of a generalized approach to athletic development and movement education was highlighted in the early chapters of this book, and the development of a curriculum was widely covered in chapter 7.

Specificity is often regarded (wrongly in many instances) as the most important training principle for coaches to consider. Taken at face value, this notion would suggest that all training needs to relate directly to the movements for the particular event. Many practitioners misrepresent the specialist end of the continuum in attempting to replicate sport-specific skills in strength-training modalities. This philosophy of coaching is commonly justified by referral to the mechanical demands that characterize event-specific or activity-specific actions. It implies that strength training is not needed outside movement ranges that typify action in a particular sporting context, but analysis of many sport actions suggests that this approach would limit training to small ranges of movement of the hips, knees and trunk.

Although sporting actions such as a runner using a sprint start from the blocks or a defensive lineman exploding from a three-point start at the line of scrimmage clearly occur in much larger ranges of movement, the execution of the most common sporting skills suggests that any strength-training movement that progresses below a quarter squat is not relevant to performance. Similarly, this action-based analysis also implies that strength training should largely focus on single-leg activities, because most actions in sport occur either in a unilateral stance or on a single limb. The simplest solution is to achieve event-specific strength training through competitive efforts (sprints, jumps, throws) in practice. But this method is problematic if it is viewed as the only source of specific strength conditioning and is limited if the practitioner is to understand specificity and the ability of the athlete to transfer trained strength gains into athletic performance. Indeed, functionality is about providing the strength tools to underpin the movement solutions, not replication of sport-specific skills.

When considering functionality in relation to strength as expressed through movement, remember that strength isn't a singular quality but a product of both force and velocity. Newton's laws dictate that force is required to change the state of an object (i.e., to cause motion), but the velocity of movement dictates the period over which force (strength) can be applied. This concept is illustrated by comparing the jump heights of drop jumps and depth jumps (chapter 9). In the drop jump, in which the objective of the training movement is to develop explosive forces in short contact times, the athlete has little time to apply force into the ground. In the depth jump, in which the objective is to achieve greater height, the ground contact time is longer, which results in greater forces being exerted against the ground and subsequently an increase in impulse ($F \times t$) and thus acceleration of the whole body upwards against gravity.

Functional programming (i.e., the spectrum of strength inputs to which the athlete is subject) needs to reflect a range of force and velocity inputs; therefore, both types of jumps are required in the athletic development curriculum. The same applies to all forms of strength training. Strength inputs with a force objective develop more force (i.e., the force–velocity curve moves upwards), and velocity inputs move the force–velocity curve upwards and towards the left. The sport-specific requirements of strength are met; that is, periods for the application of strength are minimal (as described in chapter 4), and those forces that take longer to generate than the given period in contact (with the ground, racket, opponent and so on) remain inaccessible to the performer.

But it is not only the periods for action that require consideration. The range and extent of muscle actions that occur in sport, and conversely in strength training, need to be considered. Also, the practitioner needs to consider how to develop the muscles required to execute the identified joint actions. For example, many exercises recommended for strengthening the gluteus maximus for its role as the prime hip extensor require hip movements much deeper than those required in sport movements.

The ability of muscles to develop force rapidly through a full range of joint action is essential in both performance and injury prevention. In the sporting environment, the practitioner needs to provide an appropriate stimulus that will result in specific adaptations to improve sporting performance. Therefore, the coach must consider the specificity of force and power characteristics as well as ranges of movement in the sport before prescribing a particular exercise technique. Also, the practitioner must remember that joint motion will determine muscle recruitment.

This principle can be illustrated through further analysis of the squat (figure 10.18). The squat can be performed through various movement ranges, resulting in different muscle activation patterns and force–velocity characteristics. The two issues of recent debate are the depth to which the squat should be performed and the extent to which the knees might go beyond the toes at the base of the movement.

Squat depth has provoked significant debate recently, but opinion needs to be informed by the research on the relationship of hip positioning on muscular activation, especially in relation to the powerful hip extensor muscles of the gluteals and the hamstrings, because in most dynamic sporting activities, hip extension is central to explosive movement. The minimum depth at which the downward movement of the full squat should be deemed sufficient is where the centre point of the hip joint passes below the midpoint of the knee (figure 10.18). Past this point, the hips can continue for as low as the athlete is able to maintain the correct lumbar–pelvic alignment. But beyond this minimum depth, a point of diminished return is reached in terms of achieving higher levels of training performance. The anatomical

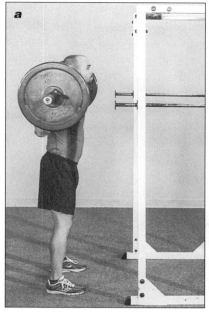

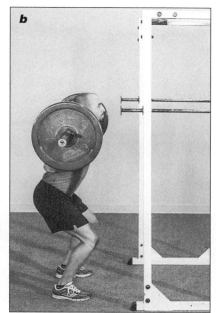

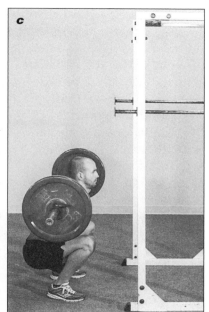

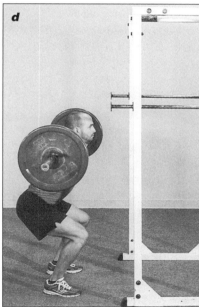

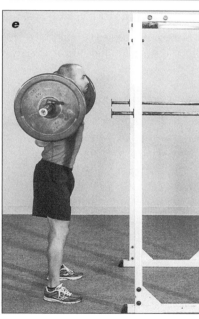

**Figure 10.18** Maximal high-bar back squat: *(a)* starting position; *(b)* controlled descent; *(c)* bottom position; *(d)* explosive ascent through the sticking point; *(e)* finish position.

landmark of the centre of the joint has been found to be a more consistent landmark than other popular terms of reference, such as the thigh breaking parallel.

Achieving this depth means that the knees will flex past 90 degrees. Because most sport movement patterns depend on powerful and coordinated actions in the hamstrings and glutes to facilitate powerful extension movements around the hip joint, this depth is crucial. During a full-range back squat, the gluteus

maximus, a powerful hip extensor, becomes increasingly more active the deeper the squat is performed.[8] This relationship highlights the importance of performing the movement through its full range if improvement of specific force and power characteristics is desired.

Coaches often prescribe partial squats, the rationale being that the knee angle is specific to the angle that occurs during running. Force and power characteristics, however, are often neglected, and the load required in the partial squat to overload sprinting or jumping is substantial. Similarly, in the upper ranges of the movement, the quadriceps are the prime mover. Although this action is expected, coaches who prescribe only partial squats are in danger of exacerbating a problem that typifies the motor programmes of many young athletes—quadriceps dominance, underactivation of the glutes and tightness in the hamstrings. Variations in squat depth have a role in a programme, but these variations should be considered progressive options from the athlete being able to perform a full movement. Prescribing partial squats should be carefully considered through analysis of the athlete's training history, his or her ability to load through the spine and the power and force characteristics of the event or sport. These considerations will establish an understanding of the partial squat load, which is required to give an appropriate training overload for a particular event. Such a load will need to be considered in relation to the athlete's ability to perform the exercise effectively and thus produce a positive transfer of training effect whilst avoiding injury.

In the bottom position, the knees will track along the line of the toes, but they may be in front of the toes. For an athlete with no history of knee injuries, there is no evidence to suggest that this positioning is a problem, providing the athlete has followed the appropriate lowering pattern and the weight is distributed towards the heels in the bottom position (as detailed in chapter 6). If the two criteria defined here are met, chances are that the knee position is because of the athlete's anthropometry, and there is little that a coach can do about it!

Many think movement range is about the amount of flexion or extension achievable within a joint or range of joints. Some realize that range is also a dynamic quality, in that it is limited within time constraints if performance without injuries is to occur. Few relate range to the acceleration path required for the object (implement or athlete) because of the action. The athlete may need to give an object momentum (i.e., impart impulse, such as in throwing a ball) or accelerate a mass over a surface (e.g., run) or upwards against a constant resistance such as gravity (e.g., when performing a slam dunk in basketball). Decelerations of external objects such as in tackling an opponent in American football or checking an opponent in ice hockey also should be considered when looking at the active movement ranges that the athlete requires. The functional training programme will have a spectrum of activities with differential acceleration paths as part of the range-of-movement considerations. This notion may seem common sense, but it is often not common practice.

The resultant movement action is not the only issue. The intended movement action is also essential. Newton's second law states that after mass is established, maximally accelerating the object will enable maximum force to be established. So in a dynamic movement such as a maximal squat, gravity will accelerate the bar to the floor in the descent and will decelerate the load through the ascent. The key coaching points in terms of movement speed are to control the descent, maintain technique and posture under form, and to explode on the ascent.

The squat was identified as a fundamental strength movement in chapter 6, where key technique points were discussed. As figure 10.18 shows, a sticking point occurs during the lift when the relative load of the mass is at its most difficult to move, because of the length, velocity and tension relationships in the muscles and the limb leverage occurring in that particular position. In the squat, this point occurs in the lowest third of the ascent phase. A number of compensations might be observed as athletes attempt to move through this sticking point with near maximal loads.

The forward lean moves the load forward of the hip joint, enabling the hip to extend, which extends the lever arm of the trunk and stresses the back extensors to return the trunk to the upright starting position. This strategy should not be actively encouraged because it may overload the capacity of the spinal extensors in a mechanically disadvantageous position. Instead, the load should be reduced until the athlete can lift it whilst maintaining postural integrity in the torso.

Through hip adduction, the athlete moves the knees inwards as the adductor magnus is recruited to act as a hip extensor (a fourth hamstring muscle). The resistive mass is overcome (i.e., the strength deficit is bridged) whilst the athlete maintains postural integrity in the back. In chapter 6, inward rotation of the knees during descent was regarded as poor movement patterning that should be corrected; the load should be reduced to avoid an injury through collapsing inwards at the knee. This same movement on the ascent is not so potentially injurious, and reduction of the load will not allow strength to be overloaded. Experienced practitioners will regard this compensation as a mistake, but one that can be worked through rather than corrected.

With a heavy load (a relative term for any athlete), the key to achieving a successful lift is the intent to lift the load maximally. Maximal activation of motor units is required within the neuromuscular system, which requires maximum volitional effort as well as a heavy load. The neuromuscular response to the heavy axial load activates a large number of motor units through the lowering phase of the lift. An explosive and deliberate acceleration 'out of the hole' (the position at the base of the squat at which the knees are below the hips) and through the sticking point enables the bar to accelerate maximally and gain momentum. The effort can be reduced somewhat in the final phase of the lift to prevent driving the bar off the shoulders.

This principle can be similarly applied to ballistic actions, in which a body or a projectile is launched because of a strength action. Whether this is a body running or jumping or a ball or implement being thrown, the purpose is to launch the object (which has a known and constant mass) with maximal velocity. The athlete should accelerate forcefully and fully throughout the range of movement so that force is transferred through the kinetic chain to set the object or body in flight with maximal impulse.

The same should be thought of with semiballistic actions such as the clean, jerk or snatch, in which the bar is accelerated to a position where it is thrown vertically with maximal acceleration but not actually released from the hands. Because the movement of the bar up the trunk is vertical, gravity will act directly on the load and rapidly decelerate it, so the arms are not required to decelerate the bar actively unless the movement is being performed with a submaximal load.

In designing functional strength-training programmes, practitioners should incorporate the full range of nonballistic, semiballistic and ballistic actions at appropriate points to develop the force–velocity characteristics of movement and the various acceleration patterns within the body segments. These movements may be similar in nature but differ in load, intent and release actions.

# Principle 7: Use Functional Methods That Are Objective Driven and Evidence Based

A logical hypothesis is that strong structures are built on solid foundations. Indeed, a common saying states that you cannot fire a cannon from a canoe, reflecting the inverse relationship between stability and mobility. Something that generates massive forces in one direction requires a sound structure to resist those forces in the other direction (Newton's second law). The same applies to strength training; for the posture to be trained to develop and express forces, it needs to be anchored on a stable surface.

Forces are transferred through the kinetic chain from the ground up; a solid base is needed from which to transfer these ground reaction forces. Strength training needs to be done on a solid surface. This guidance differs from a popular trend in the 'training industry' that is based on unstable surfaces, such as Swiss or stability balls, bosu balls or inflatable cushions. Athletes use these tools as a surface from which to perform an exercise by standing or kneeling on them, rather than using them as an aid to performing a ground-based exercise such as a squat with the ball behind the athlete. Exercises on unstable surfaces may have a place in training progression, especially during rehabilitation when joint proprioception and muscle activation to stabilize may be an important part of the process. But in terms of transferring and generating forces (i.e., strength training), the physics do not underpin the methodology. Recent research[9] clearly demonstrates that the electromyographical (EMG) activity in muscle groups (a reflection of the motor unit stimulation) is vastly higher in exercises that are performed with higher loads on stable surfaces than with lower loads on unstable surfaces.

The common justification for the use of unstable surfaces is that sport is played in a dynamic environment where the surface may change, particularly if it is grass. This hypothesis doesn't have face validity because even a 200-kilogram athlete jumping up and down on most playing surfaces wouldn't distort the surface one bit; it would remain intact and stable. Even on a trampoline, on which the canvas stretches as the athlete lands, the athlete is still required to push into the stretched (taut) canvas to get a reactionary force that will launch him or her vertically into the next skill.

The reality is that grass may be slippery at times, especially in muddy or wet conditions. The athlete may require elements of athleticism (such as proprioception) to help redress balance, but this shouldn't affect the strength-training regimen. If balance, not strength, is the desired outcome of training, then the practitioner should design exercise progressions to enhance balance. Objectives determine methods, and if the objective is to get stronger, the application and transference of force must be the primary objective when designing and delivering strength progressions.

Training with unstable implements is not the same as training on unstable surfaces. With unstable implements, such as large barrels partly filled with water, the load is constantly moving within the athlete's grasp. Therefore, the distribution of mass is dynamic, which causes perturbations (small disturbances) in the load. The neuromuscular system supporting the load must accommodate these perturbations to execute the movement. Such methods may be effective in collision sports, in which the athlete has to exert or resist forces into dynamic objects such as moving opponents.

The key to this principle is that practitioners can easily become distracted from the central objective in designing an exercise to make it more functional. The question needs to be whether the adaptation in some way challenges or overloads the athlete towards achieving the objective or whether it detracts from the objective. To illustrate this concept further, let's consider the combination of two exercises: the walking lunge and the single-arm upturned kettlebell carry.

The walking lunge has many variations and progressions that are explored in detail later in this chapter. It is a unilateral leg exercise that is axial loaded (i.e., the load is typically supported directly through the axial skeleton, the spine) and can be adapted to focus strength development within the posterior or anterior kinetic chain, depending on the identified objective. The key actions in any lunge variation are hip and knee flexions and extensions with the trunk held erect throughout the movement.

The single-arm upturned kettlebell carry is a single-arm walking exercise that is designed to strengthen the rotator cuff muscles (infraspinatus, subscapularis, supraspinatus, teres minor) isometrically. This exercise is used in late-stage rehabilitation protocols or in preparation or warm-up for a training session. It is designed to teach the athlete to use the scapulohumeral muscles to hold the shoulder girdle stable whilst walking. The asymmetrically loaded walking action provides small perturbations that challenge the integrity of the joint position as the athlete moves.

Although the lunge has a number of variations that can provide differential challenges to the neuromuscular system, as a dynamic total-body lift, the objective of each variation is to challenge the trunk positioning whilst the athlete executes loaded hip and knee flexions and extensions. (A common compensation is to lean forward at the trunk when moving out of the bottom position.) The single-arm upturned kettlebell carry uses a much lower load to challenge the relatively small muscles in the subscapular region to act isometrically to fix the shoulder girdle whilst the wrist and forearm act isometrically to control the loaded wrist position. The lower load is important in this activity because of the functional requirement of the muscles being challenged whilst the arm is fixed in the scapular plane.

Combining these exercises would not sufficiently challenge the loading through the axis of the body to facilitate overload in the athlete, and the slower lunging action would cause less perturbations through the kinetic chain, meaning that the shoulder girdle and forearm wouldn't be challenged to the same extent. Therefore, the objective of neither activity is achieved and any potential benefit of variation is compromised.

Repetitions and work volume also are important considerations related to functionality in strength work. Strength, by definition, is about force production. To produce high forces by using dynamic strength movements such as the squat, bench press or overhead press, the neuromuscular system must be relatively unfatigued. Athletes typically work in sets (i.e., work groups) that consist of 1 to 5 repetitions to increase strength. Work sets may extend to 10 repetitions at the early stages of a fully periodized programme.

Ballistic and semiballistic exercises are highly suited to developing power, which requires high-quality movements. Such exercises are best considered fatigue unresistant; that is, the movement quality quickly degrades because of neuromuscular fatigue. As table 10.2 illustrates, the power created in the highly complex movements of the clean, snatch and jerk, especially in the second pull phase of the lift, is the defining quality of these movements and the reason that these lifts are incorporated into training programmes for a variety of sports.

These lifts are deemed complex because they involve rapid and explosive multijoint actions that require coordination throughout the entire kinetic chain. Coaches and researchers have recognized for many years the clear and inverse relationship between fatigue levels and the ability to perform complex skill movements. This knowledge has led many coaches to assume that a reasonable approach is to practise the execution of complex skills under fatigue so that the athlete is ready to perform these skills under fatigue in the sporting arena. Although this premise may be viable, it doesn't clearly link with high-power sport movements. Indeed, under no circumstances are such high-force, high-velocity movements required in sport under fatigue. Even in a weightlifting contest, competitors have a break of 2 minutes at the top end of competition, so the work-to-rest ratio is approximately 1:120.

As discussed in chapter 8 with regards to speed endurance, the aim of training that produces high force and high power is to increase the maximum execution of either the force- or speed-producing components of

**Table 10.2** Power Outputs of Various Exercises

| | ABSOLUTE POWER (WATTS) | |
| --- | --- | --- |
| Exercise | 100 kg male | 75 kg female |
| Bench press | 300 | |
| Squat | 1,100 | |
| Deadlift | 1,100 | |
| Snatch* | 3,000 | 1,750 |
| Snatch second pull** | 5,500 | 2,900 |
| Clean* | 2,950 | 1,750 |
| Clean second pull** | 5,500 | 2,650 |
| Jerk | 5,400 | 2,600 |

*Total pull sequence. Lift off until maximum bar velocity.

**Second pull. Transition until maximum vertical velocity.

the movement. This training in turn makes submaximal efforts more efficient at higher absolute levels (e.g., if an athlete weighs 100 kilograms and can squat 150 kilograms, the movement of body weight becomes more efficient when maximal squat capability is increased to 160 kilograms). Similarly, if 150 kilograms represents a one-repetition maximal effort, then a reasonable expectation is that 130 kilograms will be a five-repetition maximal effort or a relatively easy (85 per cent capacity) lift for a single effort.

Training for strength and power endurance then becomes a relative concept. By using strength and power training to increase maximum capabilities and using appropriate training of the bioenergetic system to develop aerobic and anaerobic metabolic qualities, strength endurance becomes trainable. What isn't advisable is using high-force, high-velocity exercises for multiple repetitions to enhance strength endurance. First, by combining distinct and opposing objectives, the training benefits are liable to be lost, certainly in terms of the ability to influence strength or power development significantly, the real reason these lifts would be chosen in the first place. In fact, little recognized scientific or training methodology literature supports the efficacy of such high-repetition exercise prescription, especially in terms of the transfer of training benefits to sport. Despite this, some fitness training cultures are beginning to explore this concept with little researched basis for generic fitness gains.

Second, and more practically, the execution of the skill in terms of the quality of movement has an increased chance of being compromised with the reduced loads necessary to execute the movements repetitively. The athletic capacities required to perform a snatch (the highest velocity loaded movement in the resistance-training exercise range) for 1 to 5 maximal repetitions are very different from those required to perform the movement for 30 repetitions with submaximal loads. This practice often leads to incorrect sequencing or coordination of the movements, incorrect bar paths and other errors, and can increase the injury risk from such loaded activities.

Functionality in training is related not only to the choice of movements and the execution of the specific technique, but also to the way that the movements are programmed. How many repetitions? How many sets? How much rest between movements? Exercise sequencing is also important. Exercises critical to a programme (for example, those with higher neuromuscular demand or those that are more fatigue unresistant) should be sequenced before assistance exercises, which might be considered less demanding or which potentially contribute less towards achieving the session objective.

A number of factors should be considered to ensure that an exercise, or more appropriately a scheme of strength work, can be considered functional:

- The ability to develop and express force is the central theme that runs through the strength programme. Variation in the loading and movement regime are required to challenge the spectrum of the force–velocity curve.

- The strength challenge should be through as much of the kinetic chain as possible. Few isolated joint actions occur in sport, yet the ability to maintain dynamic postural integrity is fundamental to every sporting situation.

- Even if the resultant movement is controlled in only one plane, the body must be able to move in more than one plane. Resistive loads should challenge the athlete to control them in more than one plane.

- Muscle sequencing is important. The forces should be generated through large-muscle actions and transferred through the kinetic chain from the ground (base) upwards and through small muscles to the extremities.

- Eccentric muscle actions should link with concentric muscle actions so that stretch-shortening cycles increase the force production capabilities within the movement. Where dynamic rather than ballistic actions aren't quick enough to enable this to happen, concentric movements will benefit from the elastic energy stored in the eccentric movement component.

- To enhance strength and power, the focus should be on high-quality movements (quality is a percentage of perfect!) that demand high neuromuscular involvement, require precision in execution and enhance coordination and timing.

- Strength movement challenges can be achieved through variation, not simply linked with increased resistive loads. Progressive and linked movements should all be clearly defined by an objective that can be explained and justified as being linked to enhancing postural strength and control rather than variation to provide entertainment.

# Movement Curriculum Based on Individual Needs

Given the many considerations for classifying training movements as being more or less functional, what should be delivered to athletes? Many texts and resources provide a multitude of loaded and unloaded movements that can develop strength. The aim of this book is to challenge the practitioner not just to engage specific techniques but also to apply these techniques to different contexts and regress or progress the difficulty of exercises to provide benefits to the athlete.

Remember the concept of competency with regards to movement execution. Is the athlete able to execute the movement consistently without compensation for the required number of repetitions? Does the movement still present a challenge for the athlete, or has the athlete already adapted to the exercise demands? Does the athlete therefore need a further challenge? Answering these questions will form a basis for determining when to present a more stimulating challenge or load to the athlete.

Functional strength movements can be explored and categorized in many ways. The remainder of this chapter examines a series of progressions, beginning with basic strength movement games for young children. From this starting point, a series of progressions

and options is presented with guidance for decision making to help develop strength and power through a number of key sporting requirements:

- Ground-based bipedal axial-loaded exercises
- Unilateral stances
- Single-leg actions
- Overhead movements
- Horizontal trunk strength
- Rotational trunk strength
- Pulling actions

This list isn't all encompassing; it misses some major strength exercises, such as the bench press and its variations, that many consider fundamental to a strength programme. The aim of this text, however, isn't to provide a comprehensive guide for every strength exercise. In considering functional strength, practitioners should explore various exercise movement principles and critique exercises against these principles in the examples provided. Cornerstone exercises such as the bench press may naturally follow some of the movements previously described, such as the loaded press-up (figure 10.17). But the bench press doesn't entirely replace press-up variations in a programme, because these exercises bring different functional qualities than simply increased force production in the glenohumeral joint abductors and the elbow extensors (for which the bench press is undoubtedly a core exercise).

Following this, basic programming considerations are identified. The text demonstrates how sequencing a series of exercises based on achieving competencies can lead to teaching progressions for complex exercises such as the snatch and clean.

# Developmental Considerations to Strength Programming

Unlike endurance training, strength training has few developmental contraindications. This statement needs some clarification. As discussed in chapter 3, before the onset of puberty, children do not produce the enzyme phosphofructokinase (PFK). PFK is rate limiting in terms of the breakdown of glucose towards ATP, the body's energy currency. Without PFK, anaerobic glycolysis (the energetic pathway that produces ATP under high-intensity exercise conditions, when demand exceeds the ability to produce ATP using oxygen) cannot be undertaken.

In contrast, neural development, skeletal development and muscular development are all positively stimulated by strength challenges and external load, as long as the load challenge does not exceed the structural capabilities of the child's posture. Indeed, the neural system develops rapidly and early within childhood and responds well to strength stimuli, especially in the form of relative loads. In 2013, an international consensus statement supported by many agencies worldwide advocated the use of properly structured and supervised resistance training in youths.[10]

With appropriate practices, demonstrable improvements in strength can occur before puberty. These improvements occur primarily because of neural development within the motor unit as opposed to any morphological changes in the muscle fibres. Any activity that provides a positive stressor to the musculoskeletal system will improve strength and connective tissue structure, as well as encourage appropriate posture. The identified principle of using few repetitions for strength work still applies, because repetitive stress from high work volumes can damage the epiphysis of the bone.

Young children engage best with exercise movements that are part of an interesting and engaging game. Children also relate well to the examples they see in nature; therefore, animal movements provide great opportunities to engage children in strength-developing activities at an early age. But the animal walk exercises and their many variations are not only for young children; they are total-body movement control exercises that can be used in preparation activities or as remedial exercises for athletes at many levels. Indeed, as with any skilled activity, as competency is achieved at a particular level of difficulty, the exercise moves from being a challenge to being a practice to being a warm-up for practice. Therefore, using these activities with more advanced athletes is appropriate, as long as they can maintain the required movement control.

All athletes, especially younger children, respond well to goal setting for exercises or having challenges to aim for. Variation in the animal walk challenges can be time based (how many can you do? How far can you go in 30 seconds?), distance based (How few jumps do you need to cover 20 metres?) or repetition based (Can you do two more than last time?).

Practitioners using the movements with young children or with athletes who have a lower training age can use questions to develop the athletes' understanding of how the body interacts differently with the ground or how posture can be adapted by changing things such as hand position, feet position, feet width and so on.

## LIZARD ON HOT SAND

The athlete starts in a four-point stance with the toes and hands touching the ground but the knees off the ground (figure 10.19a). The hips and shoulders should be level and the back flat. The hip, back and shoulders should remain this way throughout the movement.

The athlete lifts the right hand and left foot off the ground (figure 10.19b) and holds the position for a count of 3 to 5. The athlete should not tip or dip at either the hip or shoulder, mimicking a lizard standing on sand that is too hot. The movement is small and subtle but challenging nonetheless. As silently as possible, the athlete returns the arm and leg to the ground and repeats the movement on the other side. Again, the emphasis is on maintaining control of the body position. The athlete performs 5 to 10 repetitions on each side.

As the athlete improves, the movement range can be increased to make the challenge more difficult. Lifting the arm in front of the body or extending the leg behind the body increases the coordination challenge and extends the lever arm of the limb.

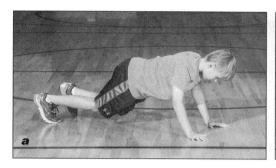 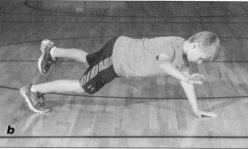

**Figure 10.19**    Lizard on hot sand: *(a)* starting position; *(b)* right hand and left foot lifted.

# BEAR CRAWL

The bear crawl is a moving progression from the lizard on hot sand. The bear crawl adds another dimension of control because the athlete moves in different directions.

The athlete starts in a four-point stance with the toes and hands touching the ground but the knees off the ground. The wrists are turned out sideways so that the thumbs face forwards, putting the shoulders into a naturally stronger position (figure 10.20*a*). The feet point forwards throughout the movement. The hips and shoulders should be level and the back flat. The hip, back and shoulders should remain this way throughout the movement.

The athlete lifts the left hand and right foot off the ground and moves them forwards simultaneously (figure 10.20*b*). The athlete must not tip or dip at either the hip or shoulder. The athlete should experiment with how far he or she can move the arms and legs forwards whilst maintaining posture and control of the movement. The athlete will find that optimal control comes when the forward-travelling knee comes level with the supporting arm. The hand and foot should land silently at the same time. The athlete repeats the forwards movement on the other side. Again, the emphasis is on maintaining control of the body position. The athlete performs 5 to 10 repetitions on each side. The exercise can be repeated with a backwards movement using the same opposite arm, opposite leg pattern or with a sideways movement.

As the athlete improves, the movement speed can be increased to add difficulty.

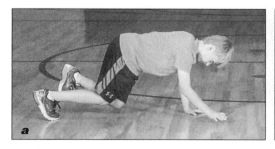 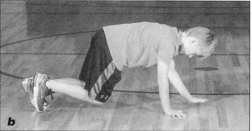

**Figure 10.20**    Bear crawl: *(a)* starting position; *(b)* left hand and right foot raised as the athlete moves forwards.

# WALKING ALLIGATOR

Depending on the athlete's competency, he or she can start either in a shortened lever position with six points of support or in a four-point plank position. The athlete aims to keep a straight line through the shoulders, hips, knees and ankles throughout the movement.

Keeping the hips and shoulders level, the athlete moves the right arm and leg forwards at the same time (figure 10.21a). Then the athlete moves the left arm and left foot forwards (figure 10.21b). The movement continues for a specified number of repetitions (usually 10). The movement can be reversed so that the athlete moves backwards; the athlete should maintain the straight-line body position and not raise the hips. The movement also can be performed sideways.

As the athlete improves, the movement speed can be increased to add difficulty.

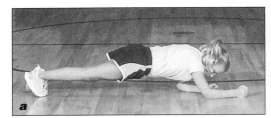 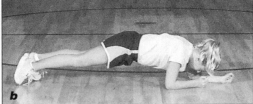

**Figure 10.21**  Walking alligator: *(a)* right arm and right leg forwards; *(b)* left arm and left leg forwards.

# CHIMPANZEE

The athlete starts in a low and wide squat with the knees fully bent, hips fully flexed and weight back on the heels (figure 10.22). The trunk should be upright. The athlete reaches the hands forwards and downwards so that they contact the ground with the hand farthest from the direction of travel just outside the leading foot (i.e., if moving to the left, the right hand is placed just outside the left foot). The athlete should be encouraged to experiment with hand positions and find the optimum for both stability and mobility. Leaning forwards and transferring the weight to the arms, the athlete pushes through the feet so that the lower body is lifted off the ground and moves laterally in the direction of travel. At midpoint the feet enter a flight phase, and the upper body briefly supports all body weight. The athlete lands with the feet widely spaced and outside the hands. The landing should be controlled and as silent as possible. The weight is transferred from the hands to the legs as the athlete sits back into a balanced squat position with the trunk upright. The movement can be reversed for four repetitions (one repetition is left movement followed by right movement), or the athlete can perform a number of repetitions to the left followed by the same number back to the right.

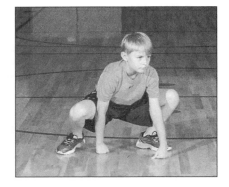

**Figure 10.22**  Chimpanzee.

# CATERPILLAR

The athlete starts in an inverted V position with the hands and feet on the ground (figure 10.23a). The weight should be distributed more towards the hands than the feet.

Keeping the feet in place, the athlete walks the arms forward (figure 10.23b). This movement increases the weight moving through the hands, which should stay in front of the athlete as the athlete moves forward. The movement continues as far forward as possible, as long as the athlete can maintain his or her body weight off the ground and be supported by the hands and feet. Shoulder strength and mobility at the extremity of movement is almost certainly going to be the factor that limits the extent of the movement.

After holding the bottom position for 0.5 seconds, the athlete walks the feet in towards the hands (figure 10.23c), continuing as far as posterior chain mobility allows. This movement can be continued forwards for a number of repetitions or can be reversed (i.e., the feet walk away from the hands).

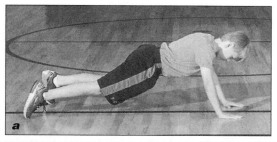

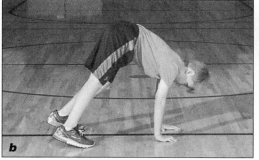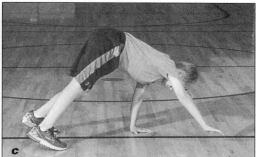

**Figure 10.23** Caterpillar: (a) starting position; (b) athlete walks hands forwards; (c) athlete walks feet towards hands.

# SPRINGBOK

The athlete lies on the ground with the knees bent to 90 degrees and the feet flat on the ground. The feet are restrained by a partner sitting on them, who also may hold the athlete's calf muscles for support (figure 10.24a). The athlete performs a powerful sit-up, engaging the braced abdominal muscles to move the trunk forwards (figure 10.24b). As the athlete moves to the top of the sit-up, he or she engages the hip extensors (glutes and hamstrings) to drive up to a standing position (figure 10.24c), using the partner's support as little as possible. Hip and then knee extension continues until the athlete is standing upright. The athlete reverses the movement under control.

*(continued)*

### Springbok *(continued)*

Using the arms to aid the action makes it easier and provides an opportunity for the athlete to progress. Arms can be used to aid the push from the ground (easiest version), the arms can lead the movement by being in front of the body, or they can be held across the chest so that they play no part in the movement. Holding the arms straight above the head is the hardest version because this position raises the centre of mass. Further progression can be achieved by removing the sit-up and starting the movement with the athlete in the sit-up position. This variation reduces momentum of the centre of mass, meaning that only the hip extensors, which are in a mechanically disadvantaged position, can be used to overcome inertia and raise the centre of mass.

The athlete performs up to 10 repetitions. Emphasis is always on control throughout the movement.

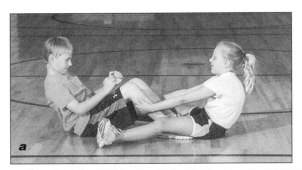

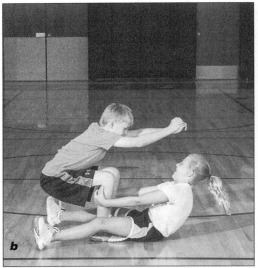 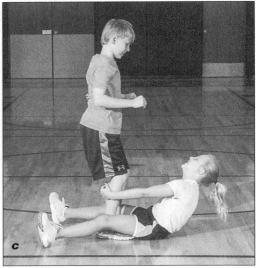

**Figure 10.24** Springbok: *(a)* starting position; *(b)* drive to standing; *(c)* finish in standing.

## Double-Foot Axial-Loaded Exercises

Lifting objects from a low position to a high position has been a fundamental human movement since prehistoric times. Indeed, the human hip anatomy developed to enable the hips to drop to a low position where the person can rest, interact with objects at ground level or forcefully pick something up from the ground. In a squat, the weight is on the feet and the knees are flexed to various depths. Culturally, it is a position that may replace sitting or standing in social interaction.[11] Over time the squat and deadlift have been recognized as the gold-standard exercises for developing total-body strength.

At first glance, these exercises look mechanically similar (see figures 10.25 and 10.26) because both involve forceful hip and knee extensions from a fully flexed knee position with the hips flexed and the trunk upright. But the similarity ends there. The term *deadlift* (figure 10.25) refers to the lifting of a weight lying on the ground that is therefore 'dead', or without momentum. The action of lifting from the floor means that the lift is essentially performed using concentric muscle actions only. This movement is in contrast to the majority of sporting movements, in which eccentric (lowering or braking) actions precede concentric ones. The deadlift is largely done without muscles benefitting from stored elastic energy or stretch-shortening cycles.

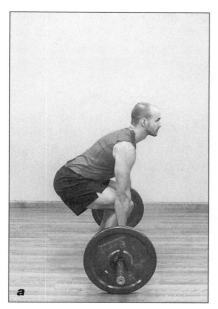
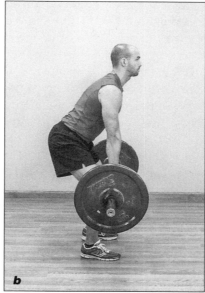
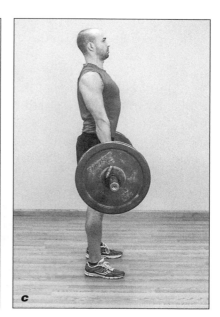

**Figure 10.25**   Deadlift: *(a)* starting position; *(b)* midpull; *(c)* top position.

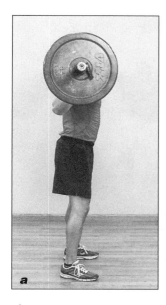
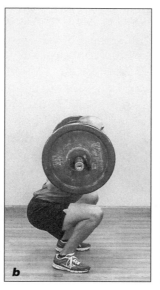
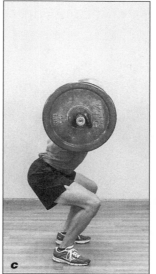
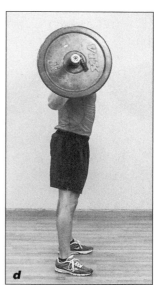

**Figure 10.26**   Squat: *(a)* starting position; *(b)* bottom position; *(c)* midascent; *(d)* finish.

In contrast, the squat (figure 10.26) can be regarded as a structural exercise,[12] because the spine is directly loaded throughout the movement. This attribute is reflected in the technical checklist for the movement in chapter 6. The ability to perform a basic squatting pattern regardless of load is reflective of an athlete's general movement and dynamic postural control abilities. The squat has many variations (i.e., it is adaptable to suit the training or performance objectives required). Powerlifting squats, sumo squats and box squats are all variations that coaches and athletes will come across in different contexts. In terms of an exercise to develop the strength, posture and flexibility requirements of most athletes (and transfer the training benefits to sport), however, the full high-bar back squat is generally considered the most appropriate variation.

The practitioner needs to be confident the athlete can execute the correct movement pattern under various constraints before a relatively heavy load is applied through the spine.

This point is illustrated well in figure 10.27, which presents a series of progressive variations, starting with body mass supported by a wall as the athlete moves through a full range of motion. With the feet anterior to the line of force (through the centre of mass), this movement is more dominated by knee extension (and therefore knee extensor action) than hip extension, but the athlete is getting used to a full range of movement and an upright trunk. Reducing the size of the Swiss ball (for example, progressing towards a medicine ball) enables this variation to be progressively addressed.

The body-weight squat with the arms in front of the body enables the athlete to experience the full range of motion and appreciate the balance challenge that comes from dropping the centre of mass downwards between the base of support whilst maintaining an upright torso. The addition of a relatively small anterior load with a medicine ball or similar implement enables the athlete to experience overload in terms of mass for the first time.

The movement may be progressed in a number of ways. One is to introduce the front squat, a barbell exercise in which the bar rests on the upper front deltoids during the movement. A shelf is created by moving the elbows upwards and forwards to a position at which the upper arms are parallel to the floor. The wrists are fully extended, and the bar rests in the athlete's fingertips with the hands slightly wider than shoulder-width. The athlete maintains this position throughout the lift.

An athlete with limited mobility through the spine commonly compromises the movement by lowering the elbows during descent. This error should be avoided, because it moves the weight towards the front rather than the rear of the feet, increasing the shearing forces through the knees and compromising the trunk position.

The major benefit of the front squat is that by locating the bar anteriorly, the athlete must maintain an upright torso throughout the movement. If the trunk moves forward (common in novice athletes), the bar will fall forward, providing instantaneous feedback to the athlete about body position. The anterior location of the mass also facilitates more anterior chain muscle action than what occurs in other squat variations, but that is more a training consideration than a learning consideration.

The front squat has other versions, the most common of which is having the arms crossed in front of the bar to hold it in position across the deltoid. This position is often considered more useful for those who need to front squat but lack the flexibility in the shoulders to execute the more conventional racking position. This position can be challenged in a number of ways for an athlete with no pathology in the upper limb or shoulder. First, because the bar is supported squarely on the anterior deltoid by the glenohumeral joint, if the upper arms remain parallel to the floor with the elbows high, the fingers do not really need to hold the bar. Indeed, this version can be seen as an additional balance challenge to the athlete who does not have the required flexibility. Anterior shoulder tightness is the most common reason that athletes do not have the required flexibility to achieve the correct front squat movement. Note that crossing the hands across the bar will probably exacerbate this

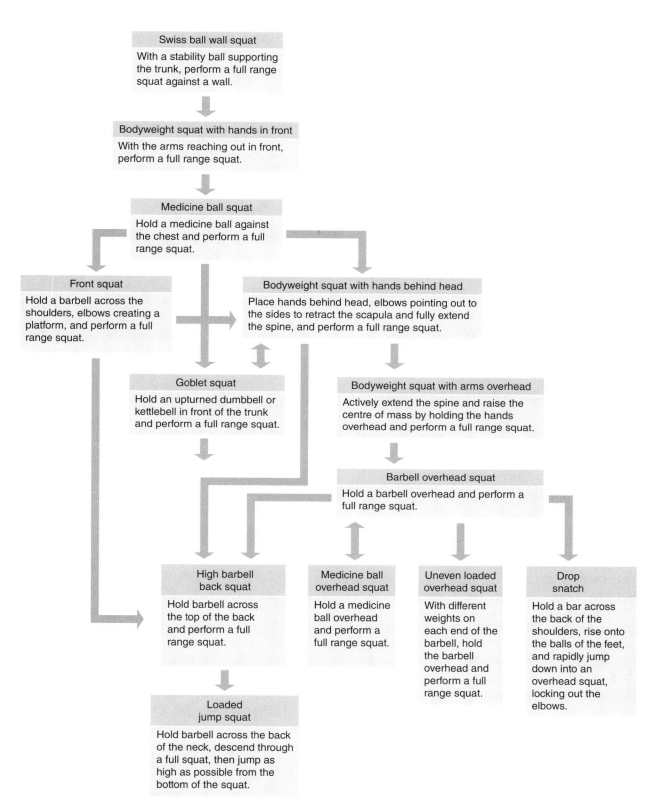

**Figure 10.27** Progression of the squat.

problem rather than remediate it in the long term. Second, if the athlete is ever going to practise the clean movement and receive the bar properly, he or she must first practise the catch position in the front squat.

Some practitioners may want to focus alternatively (or simultaneously!) on challenge to the athlete's posture in the squat by changing the position of the centre of mass. To do this, the length of the kinetic chain must be influenced. The goblet squat is a good exercise to consider for developing postural control through a full range of movement. This exercise places a dumbbell or kettlebell load close to the centre of mass whilst requiring the trunk to remain upright through the full movement range.

Performing a body-weight squat with the hands behind the head is another way to influence the position of the centre of mass, and it represents a significantly greater mobility challenge than the body-weight squat with the hands in front of the body. The challenge can be further enhanced by raising the arms above the head to elevate the centre of mass farther, and it can be progressed to a barbell overhead squat. (The barbell alone can weigh 5 to 20 kilograms.) The barbell overhead squat can be performed with a dowel instead, if desired.

The overhead squat (any variation) is an excellent conditioning movement for all sports because it places the loaded bar as far away from the base of support as possible. This exercise both raises the athlete's centre of mass relative to the base of support and challenges postural integrity with the kinetic chain fully extended. Therefore, it is considered one of the best exercises for developing trunk strength throughout a full range of movement.

The overhead position of the load means that the athlete needs to work extremely hard through the shoulder girdle to maintain the bar position above the back of the head. In this position, the athlete gets immediate feedback if the upper body leans too far forward, another reason to consider this exercise a progressive stage towards teaching an upright posture through a full range of movement in the back squat. This lift is also considered a

vital component of the teaching progression towards the snatch, because the overhead squat is the receiving position for the bar in the snatch.

In the most basic version of the overhead squat, the bar is held in a wide grip slightly to the rear of the crown; the athlete takes as wide a grip as is comfortable. After the hands are in place, they should pull apart from each other without moving on the bar to facilitate isometric actions within the shoulder muscles, thus maintaining stability within the shoulder girdle with the arms straight.

After the athlete masters the overhead squat and can perform it competently and consistently, other options are available to develop the exercise further:

- The overhead squat can be done under increasing loads to develop force-producing capabilities.
- The hand spacing can be narrowed (e.g., by gripping the medicine ball), which will significantly increase the flexibility challenge.
- The athlete can be challenged to maintain postural integrity under an asymmetrical load (e.g., a 2.5- to 10-kilogram disparity between the load on one end of the bar and the load on the other end). This load asymmetry forces the shoulder and trunk muscles to work hard to prevent rotations in the bar and keep one side from dipping. Note that this variation is not suitable for the back squat, in which the asymmetrical load would be in direct contact with the cervical vertebrae. With the kinetic chain fully extended, only a small offset in the load could cause a disturbance in postural balance, making this an effective variant in the overhead lifts.
- Velocity can be added to the movement with the introduction of the drop snatch. In this movement, the athlete drops into the overhead squat from a standing position without the barbell rising from its starting point. This movement requires braking strength in the hip extensors to decelerate the downwards velocity of the movement as the athlete jumps under the

bar (powerful concentric actions in the hamstrings), as well as courage, balance and coordination to stick the landing position.

When the athlete can execute a full bodyweight squat, the programme can take him or her straight to the high-bar barbell back squat and from there develop the overhead and front squats. After the back squat can be done with sufficient load and the athlete's strength increases, the option of loaded jump squats is available. The 'need to do' exercises are the front, back and overhead squats (and single-leg variations discussed later); the 'nice to do' progressions are not introduced until the athlete has had significant training experience with the major lifts.

Progression and variation are essential to develop learning as learning occurs. They should not be used as means of athlete entertainment before skills are mastered. To incorporate advanced exercises such as the drop snatch or asymmetrical loading into a programme before an athlete has sufficient training history with the core lift is at best inadvisable and potentially negligent. These lifts, however, do provide alternative means of challenging the athlete's movement competency.

Fewer potential variations in the movement are required to pick up a load from the floor.

The major progressions tend to be limited to the load lifted or the range of movement. (The starting height of the load can be altered so that the athlete does not necessarily have to lift from the ground in the early phases.) But this variation changes the mechanics of the lift significantly and therefore may not always be a good choice.

Figures 10.28 and 10.29 show different means of lifting dead weight from the floor. These exercises vary in load positioning and movement velocity. For example, the deadlift is a high-force, low-velocity movement typically done with relatively heavy loads. The clean pull is a high-power movement that involves a push into the floor by the leg extensors. Consideration of how (or if) each variation may be incorporated into a strength development programme can be further explored after the relative merits of each movement have been presented.

The trap bar (or hex bar) deadlift (figure 10.30) locates the weight on either side of the athlete's body after he or she has settled into the starting position. The load is more evenly distributed between the anterior and posterior kinetic chains. After the athlete is in the starting position and has 'taken the slack' from the bar, he or she is less likely to lose the upright trunk posture and the straight-back position,

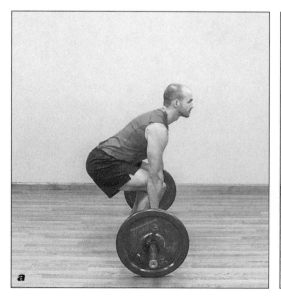 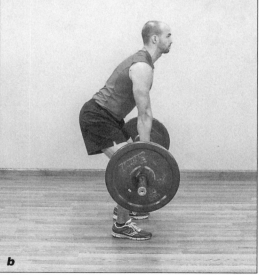

**Figure 10.28** Barbell deadlift: *(a)* starting position; *(b)* midpoint.

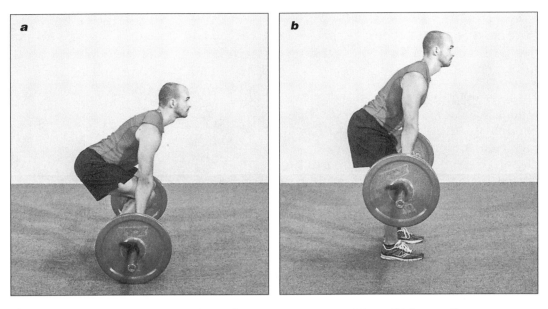

**Figure 10.29** Clean grip pull from floor: *(a)* starting position; *(b)* first pull.

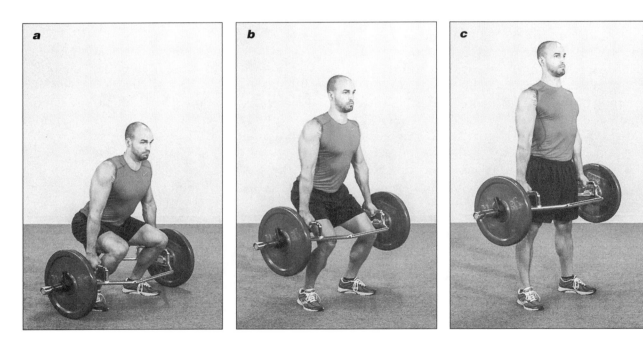

**Figure 10.30** Trap bar deadlift: *(a)* starting position; *(b)* midpoint; *(c)* final position.

one of the common faults of the regular dead-lift, in which the weight has to be pulled up and slightly backwards as the hips and knees extend simultaneously, because the weight is out in front of the athlete.

In both deadlifts, the weight is distributed towards the heel throughout the lift (hence, many lifters prefer to perform the deadlift without shoes, because the barefoot position puts the feet flatter on the floor). Pushing through the heels in this movement causes the weight to rise with simultaneous hip and knee extension until the load has been lifted and the athlete is standing. Because the athlete can let go of the weight at any time during the movement (unlike in a squat exercise), this lift is relatively easy and the athlete gets used to moving heavy loads with high forces. The critical coaching point that will lead progression is the maintenance of the tight back posture. This technique point also is important in deadlift activities that do not involve a barbell or a pair of dumbbells, including activities such as tyre flipping, commonly used in training programmes to provide variety.

Contrast the simultaneous hip and knee extension of the deadlift with the clean pull from the floor, in which the movement is led with a knee extension to facilitate the stretch-shortening actions in the subsequent phases of the lift. This lift is designed not for maximum force production, but for maximum power production, so bar velocity can be maximized and the bar gains as much momentum as possible in the second pull phase. The joint action means that the bar path is different from the floor to the thigh than it is in the deadlift. In addition, the extension mechanics are somewhat different.

Each technique has been adapted to achieve the identified objectives. The movements are both different and similar. The athlete development specialist has to determine whether they are different enough to be coached simultaneously or whether learning one action (for example, the deadlift) will interfere with learning the clean or snatch pull. The decision comes down to how the athlete learns; coaching programmes may need to adapt teaching strategies with different athletes. For example, using the trap bar in the deadlift may feel different enough to the athlete that the first pull sequence of the clean can be taught at the same time.

## Contralateral Stances

Many major sporting actions are performed with the legs in a split stance or a single-leg stance. In the split stance, the athlete needs to be able to maintain a stable posture, keeping the hips and shoulders level whilst managing the forwards and backwards distribution of the base of support (figure 10.31). With the forwards–backwards weight distribution, the width of the base of support is usually narrowed in the transverse plane compared with the double-foot base of support, which may add to the balance challenge in such movements.

In the split step, the athlete looks to maintain a position with the knees tracking the line of the second metatarsal of the foot and the shin of the lead leg nearly vertical. This position distributes weight evenly through the middle to rear of the front foot and keeps the knee from coming forward of the toes, which would lead to the action being dominated by knee extensor activity. The trunk should remain upright.

The challenge provided by the narrowed base of support can artificially increase with the incorporation of specialist exercises such as the in-line split squat (in which the feet remain fixed throughout the repetitions) or the lunge, in which the athlete steps into and out of the bottom position with each repetition, narrowing the base of support in the transverse plane. This variation puts additional stress onto the gluteus medius to maintain a stable and balanced position at the hip, pelvis and trunk. With increased depth, this movement also aids the development of mobility in and around the hip joint.

Movement through these exercises typically has three variations in the global patterning or setup. Typically, the athlete begins with exercises that have only a vertical movement pattern through hip and knee extension, meaning that the feet are static throughout the movement. These exercises progress into more dynamic movements in which the athlete transitions into and out of a position with a range of progressive challenges that develop motor control in the contralateral stance. Variation or progression can be provided by changing the transition mechanics between repetitions or by varying the positioning of the load relative to the base of support. These progressions are presented in figure 10.32.

Each of these progressions has common routes by which variation in movement challenge can be achieved. Variation, however, should follow mastery; the decision to progress the strength challenge should be determined not by the desire to entertain but by the need to overload the motor system that has adapted to an imposed challenge.

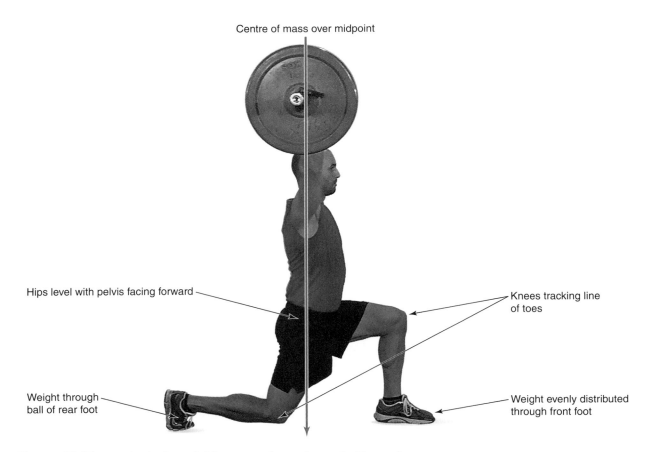

Centre of mass over midpoint

Hips level with pelvis facing forward

Knees tracking line of toes

Weight through ball of rear foot

Weight evenly distributed through front foot

**Figure 10.31** Technical model for contralateral step (split-step) movement.

As figure 10.32 illustrates, from a common starting sequence in which the athlete's feet remain fixed to the floor, the movements progress to incorporate increased vertical forces (stepping onto or off blocks of varying heights so that the athlete lifts the load directly against gravity) and forwards and backwards actions with one foot on the floor acting as a pivot from which the lead leg steps.

The first level of difficulty in terms of altered foot positioning in a lunge sequence is the in-place lunge, which is introduced with body weight only, after which a number of options can be introduced as competency is demonstrated. The athlete steps forwards into the bottom position and then pushes back to the starting position. This type of movement is excellent for developing eccentric control as the athlete lowers into the bottom position after the forward step, as well as powerful knee extension to return to the starting position. As with the split-squat movement, raising the

front foot or the platform onto which the lead leg steps requires the athlete to flex the hip to a greater depth, which increases the involvement of the posterior kinetic chain.

Similar rear kinetic chain benefits can be derived from reverse lunges, a hip-dominated movement in which the athlete steps backwards from the starting position. Moving away from the field of vision automatically challenges the kinaesthetic and proprioceptive mechanisms to produce a controlled movement, and the athlete can drop into a low-hip position that requires eccentric (braking, in descent) and concentric (driving, in returning to the starting position) muscle actions led by the superior portions of the hamstrings and the gluteals. More important, because the front knee is fixed above the ankle throughout the exercise (i.e., knee flexion and extension is passive and a function of the hip moving), this exercise targets the eccentric control and concentric powering actions of the hip flexors

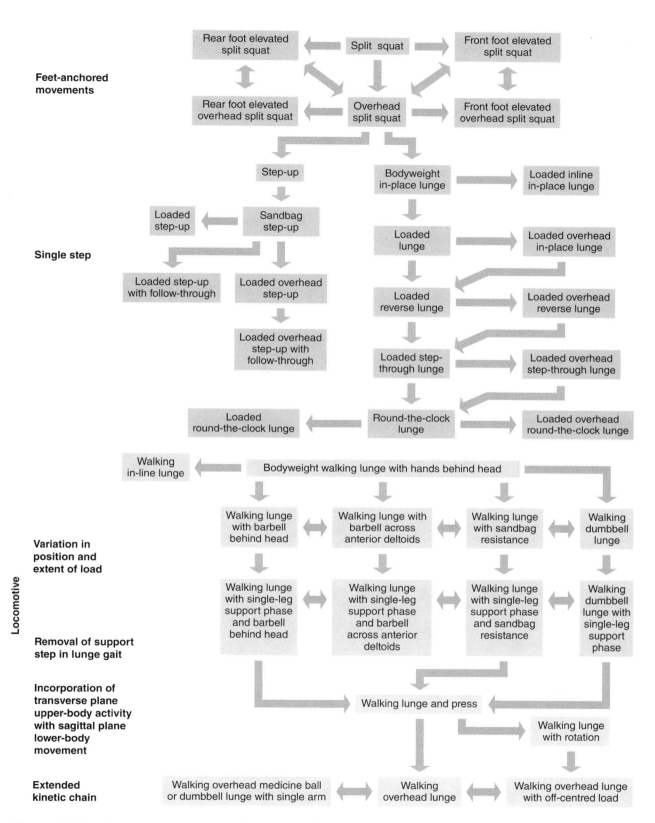

**Figure 10.32** Progression in ground-based contralateral movements.

(high hamstrings, gluteals). For this reason, the reverse lunge is especially attractive for inclusion in many programmes, because the upper hamstring is a region of particular sensitivity when it comes to injuries in many sports.

The forwards–backwards action, after it is mastered in isolation, can be linked in a step-through lunge, in which the athlete steps back into a reverse lunge and then forward through a single-leg stance into a forward or 'in-place' lunge in a cyclical action. This sagittal plane action requires a lot of control to develop a smooth and fluid motion. Transverse plane control is added in the round-the-clock lunge, in which the lead leg moves from a sagittal plane (forwards–backwards) to a lateral plane in sequence. The standing leg anchors the body, and the lumbar–pelvic alignment is challenged to maintain the upright trunk. This movement provides additional challenge to the adductors and abductor of the hip and groin to control the movements.

After mastery of the 'in-place' variations is achieved, whole-body locomotion can be introduced to the lunge, requiring postural control to accommodate the challenge of horizontal momentum as the centre of mass moves forward. Initially, the athlete moves from a contralateral stance to a bilateral stance in which the rear leg is brought level with the lead leg. Removing the bilateral stance requires the athlete to maintain a single-leg stance as the rear leg swings through to become the lead leg. This change not only adds momentum as the leg swings forward but also provides challenge in the frontal plane because the hip and trunk need to maintain a level position with an off-centred base of support.

Loading in such movement progressions always generates an interesting discussion. The obvious means of developing the force-producing capabilities within the neuromuscular system using these exercises is to increase the resistive load being moved. But the positioning of the load also challenges the neuromuscular system because the athlete must maintain postural integrity and proprioceptive control. Dumbbell or kettlebell loads can be incorporated below the centre of mass and close to the base of support, which makes the position

relatively stable, or the centre of mass can be raised by using an overhead load, maximizing the distance between the load and the base of support in an unstable position.

The overhead position is particularly challenging for postural integrity. With the body moving in the sagittal plane and the glenohumeral joint fully extended, the shoulder girdle musculature is challenged to maintain the position of the load directly above the crown of the head. As the body moves forward, the load gains horizontal momentum that must be decelerated if the load is to remain in the same position relative to the trunk throughout the movement.

Lateral stages of progression in the locomotive lunges demonstrate some loading variations unique to this contralateral movement sequence. These variations challenge postural integrity, particularly at the hips and shoulders, through the different dynamic loading patterns. For example, the lunge and press action requires the shoulder joint extensors to generate vertical force whilst the trunk is moving forward in the sagittal plane. Similarly, the off-centred overhead loading (provided through either an unevenly loaded barbell or a resistive load, such as a medicine ball, dumbbell or kettlebell held in one hand) introduces frontal plane control through the hip and shoulder girdle because the athlete is required to resist the rotations caused by off-centred loads.

Transverse plane rotations in the upper body are easily introduced with a medicine ball or similar load. The athlete holds the relatively low resistive load at arms' length to increase the leverage throughout the action and twists it over the knee of the lead leg. Movement compensations may occur in response to such a challenge. Common compensations are forward leaning of the trunk (which brings the weight towards the toes of the lead leg as the centre of mass moves forward) and the inward rotation of the knee in the lead leg as a movement in opposition to the outward rotation of the trunk. The athlete must avoid the valgus knee movement; the hip and lumbar–pelvic region should effectively manage the transverse plane forces.

Contralateral actions also can be used to accelerate a load directly against gravity so that the transition movement is vertical rather than horizontal. Step-up variations enable loads to be placed directly over the axial spine or held overhead to challenge the kinetic chain to load knee and hip extensor activity through different ranges of movement, as determined by the height of the block. The higher the step is, the greater the glute activation (i.e., reliance of hip extension) versus quadriceps activation (reliance on knee extension) needed to complete the movement is (figure 10.33).

The foot on the floor in the starting position can be balanced on the toes or on the heel. Either position is acceptable, but the athlete who starts with a flat foot may be tempted to initiate the step-up by pushing off through the calf muscle complex of the rear leg (i.e., it becomes a loaded ankle extension exercise) rather than using knee–hip extension in the front leg. This method may be acceptable, depending on the desired movement outcome and its place in the programme. Starting the movement with the rear leg already in full ankle plantarflexion prevents this action from

occurring, although athletes often shift their weight back onto the rear leg in an attempt to gain some push through the ankle. This action can be countered by beginning the movement with the rear toe elevated and the ankle fully dorsiflexed, although this significantly increases the exercise difficulty because the athlete can move through an active push only with the front leg.

The importance of a velocity continuum has also been highlighted in this chapter. As figure 10.34 shows, step-up actions can also be plyometric. Note that in starting, the front foot is forcibly raised off the block. This rapid action initiates a stretch reflex through the hamstrings and gluteals that assists the explosive hip extension movement through the rest of the sequence.

As figure 10.35 illustrates, athletes who have sufficient motor control and have advanced through a range of progressions can experience additional challenge by complexing a lunge with the step-up. A reverse lunge into a step-up provides both a sagittal plane and progressive vertical challenge with the need to control posture through a complex movement.

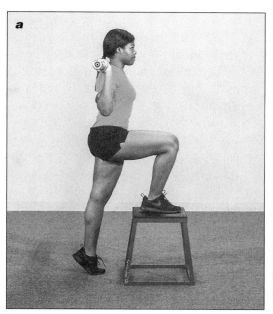 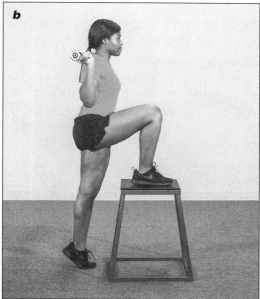

**Figure 10.33** Outcomes of step-up variations: *(a)* A lower box places equal emphasis on hip and knee extension; *(b)* a higher box places the hip joint below the knee, requiring the athlete to initiate movement through hip extension, increasing glute and hamstring involvement.

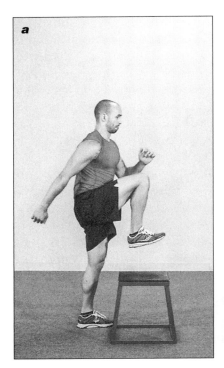
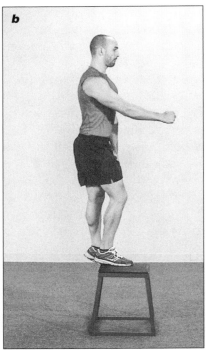
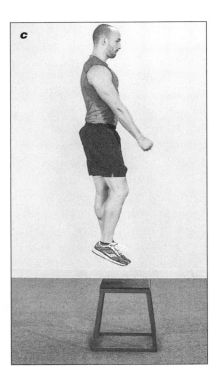

**Figure 10.34** Plyometric step-up: *(a)* starting position with front foot off step; *(b)* drive; *(c)* top position.

## Unilateral Actions

Many sport actions require force production through a single-leg stance. At a basic level of motor control, single-leg squats are extremely challenging movements. The base of support is off-centred relative to the centre of mass, which means that the neuromuscular system is faced with a dynamic balance challenge from the outset. The load is also doubled compared with the normal squat, moving through a single limb, so that even without external load a significant force challenge is presented.

The mechanical actions are the same as in the squat. The practitioner should look for the weight distribution moving towards the rear of the foot as the athlete descends, the knee tracking the line of the toes and the trunk remaining upright with the natural lumbar curve maintained throughout the action. A common movement compensation is to initiate the action by knee flexion, increasing the quadriceps involvement. Often this compensation is accompanied by a forward lean of the trunk. Both of these actions serve to move the line of force forwards rather than rearwards.

The easiest way to start the movement is to decrease the balance challenge by supporting the trunk. The large surface area of a wall plus the large surface area of a physio ball (figure 10.36) enables the athlete to achieve the single-leg squat whilst maintaining an upright trunk. The athlete can more ably work through a full range of movement with the centre of mass behind the supporting leg and a wide base of support (distance between the foot and the wall). The hips have a lot of room to drop into the supported squat position. Support can be reduced over time by replacing the physio ball with a smaller medicine ball. The Swiss ball single-leg wall squat is a somewhat artificial position, because the standing leg is anchored in front of the body and the lack of need to achieve a balanced position somewhat alters the aspect of the trunk relative to the lower limb. But the exercise does familiarize the athlete with the movement and loading challenge and enables the practitioner to identify potential movement dysfunctions such as inward knee tracking.

Progressions are related to movement range or incorporation of external loading. The use of

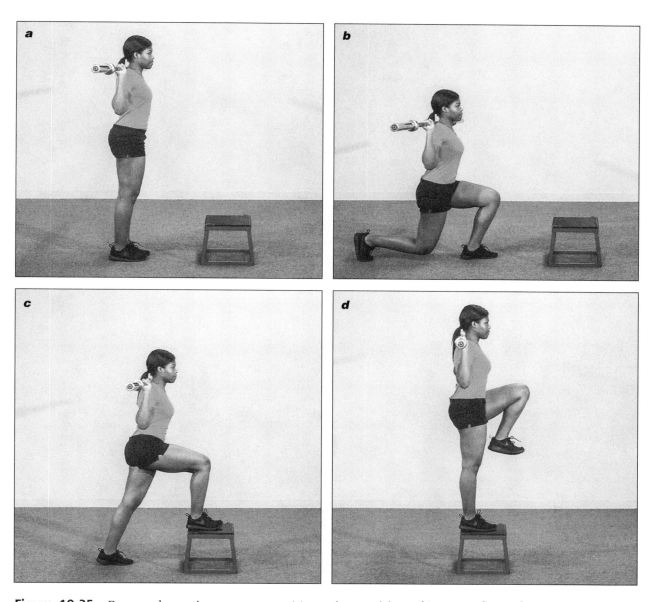

**Figure 10.35** Reverse lunge into a step-up: *(a)* starting position; *(b)* reverse lunge bottom position; *(c)* step-up; *(d)* finish position.

a box in a squatting movement is potentially controversial; done incorrectly, a single-leg box squat can lead to abhorrent spinal loading patterns during lifting, which should be avoided at all times. Like any exercise, however, if coached properly, this movement can be useful in developing force production capabilities and promoting confidence in a controlled descent. The instructions to the athlete should be to lower under control until the buttocks just touches the front of the box, at which point the athlete should forcefully squeeze the buttocks to drive back up to a single-leg stance. The practitioner must ensure that the athlete does not sit down on the box; sitting takes the tension away from the muscles and allows the athlete to relax his or her posture before returning to standing. The height of the box can be gradually reduced over time, because there is little point in developing a heavily loaded movement with limited hip and knee flexion and extension at the sacrifice of movement range. Load can be applied after the depth of movement has increased sufficiently.

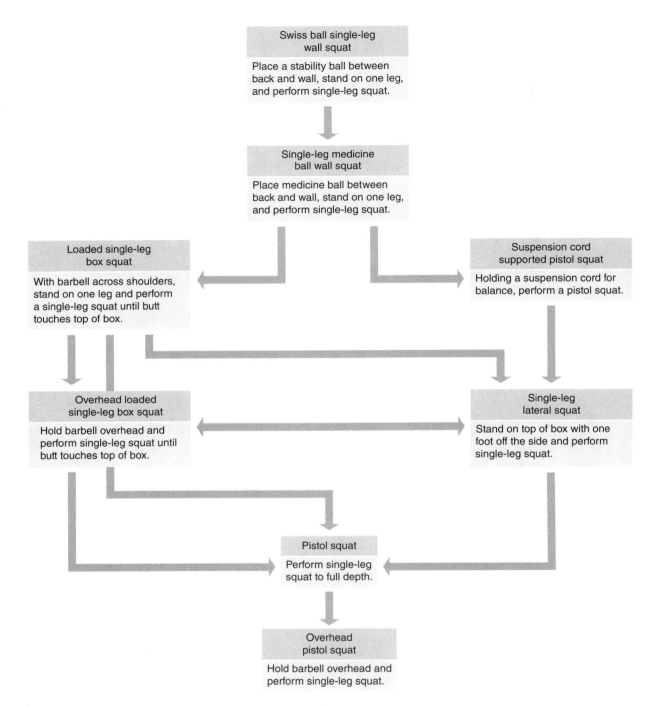

**Figure 10.36**    Example progression for the single-leg squat.

Extending the kinetic chain using an overhead lift is also a useful means of progression.

The use of a single-arm suspension cable is another means of developing confidence and addressing the balance challenge presented by the single-leg squat. Using the front support of the arm opposite the standing leg (which helps keep the hips and trunk square), the athlete can naturally sit back into the squat. In the bottom position, the arms should be fully extended so that the athlete is supported without pulling the trunk (and therefore weight distribution) forward. The practitioner should take time to set up the equipment so that the length of the cable is appropriate for the athlete.

Single-leg lateral squats encourage the athlete to maintain a level hip and shoulder position with an upright trunk. Observation from the side will enable the practitioner to identify whether the athlete distributes weight correctly (towards the heel) during the descent and whether the movement is correctly initiated with the simultaneous hip and knee action. As the athlete achieves mastery of the movement, the height of the box or step can be increased to advance the movement challenge. In addition, external loading through dumbbells can be incorporated to increase the resistive mass being moved through the range.

The pistol squat is one of the hardest movements for many athletes. This exercise represents a considerable balance and strength challenge for the gluteal complex and much of the musculature around the hips and groin. The athlete must move body weight through a full range of movement (i.e., a relatively large distance) using a single limb. The hardest point of the movement comes as the thigh reaches parallel to the floor, when the lever arm of the femur is at its longest. As the athlete passes this position, coaches may observe the athlete tucking under the pelvis (posterior pelvic tilt), usually accompanied by a forward lean (sometimes flexion) in the spine.

Although this position would be regarded as dysfunctional in any movement in which the spinal axis is loaded (because of compressive forces acting through the spine), in an unloaded pistol squat such compressive forces (other than gravity) do not occur. Indeed, such movements help to bring the athlete into a position of balance in the pistol squat, and rarely is this movement executed without some form of compensatory action in the lumbar–pelvic or thoracic–lumbar regions. As part of the balance challenge, the knee will move a long way forward of the toes to enable the athlete to achieve depth. To do this whilst maintaining flat foot contact with the floor requires significant

range of movement in the ankle. Without this flexibility, the full-depth squat position cannot be achieved.

## Horizontal Trunk Strength

Posture relates to the relative alignment of the parts of the body. The ability to generate internal forces to maintain a strong positioning of the axial and appendicular skeletons should be focused on throughout all athletic development programmes. Many exercise variations emphasize this ability whilst the athlete is standing. Some exercise progressions focus on maintaining strength in the postural muscles that maintain shoulder girdle position and lumbar–pelvic alignments.

The prescription and coaching of these exercises within the programme needs to be carefully considered. As with any strength exercise, the key to achieving success lies in correct execution of the technique. But common execution errors in these techniques often go uncorrected and lead to compensatory strength gains rather than those that are the desired objective.

As figure 10.37 illustrates, the alignment of the hips and shoulders largely determines the muscles involved to support the athlete's position. If the hips are not in neutral position, the hip flexors and rectus abdominis are recruited to support the lumbar–pelvic

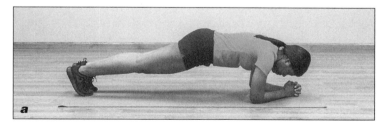

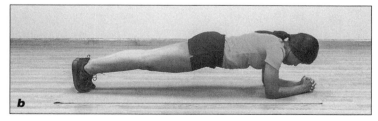

**Figure 10.37**  Joint position determines muscle function. When a plank isn't a plank: *(a)* incorrect position of the pelvis; *(b)* correct position of the pelvis.

position. Uncorrected, this malalignment can lead to tight hip flexors and the inability to maintain correct pelvic position through isometric (but not isolated) contractions of the multifidus or transversus abdominis muscles. A neutral pelvis (thighs maintaining a straight line with the line of the trunk; keeping the lines on shorts horizontal is a useful guide) means that the athlete's neuromuscular recruitment to maintain the body positioning is much more appropriate.

As figures 10.38 and 10.39 illustrate, a number of exercise progressions can be incorporated into an athletic development programme. These have been differentiated into primary (figure 10.38) and advanced (figure 10.39) movements for ease of communication. The distinguishing features between the two levels are simply that the primary exercises involve less motor control and force exertion than the more advanced exercises. That said, practitioners may wish to intertwine some of the starting versions of exercises in figure 10.38 with some of the more advanced progressions in figure 10.39.

The core technical consideration for all these exercises is the maintenance of neutral pelvic and shoulder girdle alignments to achieve straight body positions. Even in relatively simple movements such as the bridge, athletes can achieve a position that resembles the desired one through the lumbar spine rather than by squeezing the gluteals to raise the hips to a level position. In early stages of learning, athletes should always focus on the quality of movement rather than achieving a prescription of sets and repetitions, and this focus should be reinforced through the programme supervision (instruction, observation, corrective reinforcement) that the athlete receives.

Besides the addition of an external load, such as a loaded barbell across the hips to resist the bridge movement, progression in the primary exercises can be achieved through manipulation of the base of support or the position of the centre of mass. For example, progressing a bridge to a single-leg support position can be extremely challenging. Similarly, the length of the lever arm and the relative positioning of the centre of mass can increase the movement

challenge significantly. For example, in the superman exercise series, maintaining shoulder and hip alignment when raising an arm is easier than when raising a leg because the arm is typically shorter and has less mass than the leg. Maintaining a two-point balance position in the superman exercise is also significantly more difficult when the arm and leg on the same side of the body are raised, compared with when a contralateral support position is achieved. With the arm and leg on the same side raised and fully extended, the combined leverage, together with an off-centred base of support, makes the desired balance position extremely challenging to attain.

The basic plank position is achieved with the knees on the floor, thus reducing the lever arm and putting less stress on the lumbar–pelvic region when compared with the more typical plank position in which the toes and forearms support the athlete. Prone, supine (reverse plank) and frontal plane (lateral plank) positions should be developed simultaneously within a programme to maximize the benefits on postural strength. Progressions within each of these variations are achieved through incorporating movement (walking plank, stir the pot) or altering the base of support by reducing either the number of points of support (for example, by raising a foot) or the size of the base. (For example, compare the support position for lateral plank versus star plank). In the lateral plank with limbs in the transverse plane, adding a separate plane of movement by bringing the arm or leg across in front of the body requires the postural control muscles to work extremely hard, because the centre of mass is now moved lateral to the base of support.

Candlesticks and rollouts similarly progress; the lever arm and the base of support are the major means of exercise progression. These exercises emphasize postural integrity by fully challenging the eccentric control abilities of the pelvic and shoulder girdles. Therefore, they are reasonably advanced exercises that should be approached with caution. The longer the length of the lever arm is, the more demanding the exercise will be, at both the shoulder girdle and the pelvis. A common error associated

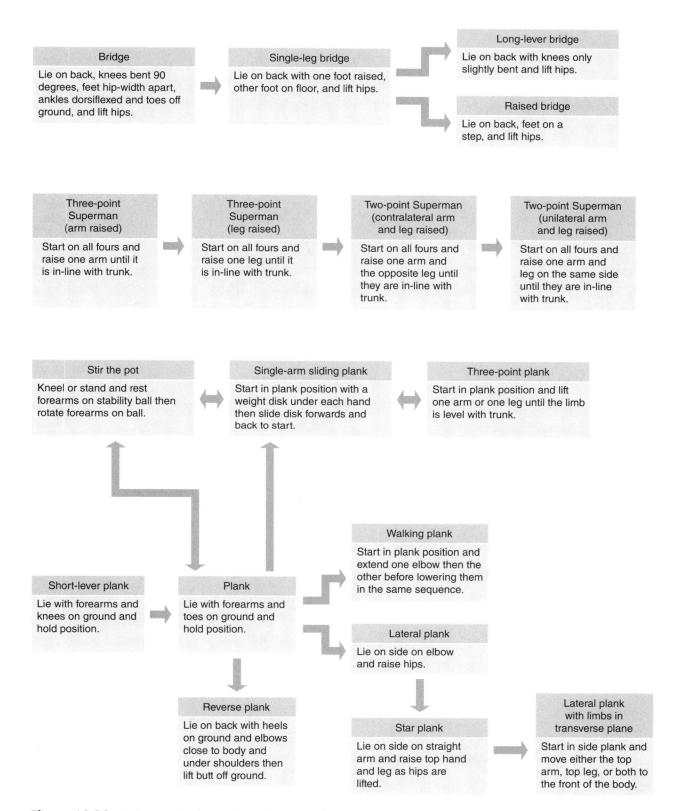

**Figure 10.38** Primary horizontal trunk strength exercises.

**Short-lever**
**rollout**

Kneel next to barbell on the ground, hands shoulder-width apart on barbell and arms straight. Roll barbell away from the body.

**Caterpillar**
**(walking rollout)**

Stand with feet and hands on ground. Walk hands away from body as far as possible.

**Long-lever**
**rollout**

Stand next to barbell on the ground, hands shoulder-width apart on barbell and arms straight. Roll barbell away from the body.

**Dumbbell**
**rollout**

Stand next to dumbbells on the ground, arms straight, hands on dumbbells. Roll dumbbells away from body.

**Single-arm**
**rollout**

Stand next to single dumbbell on the ground, arms straight, hands on dumbbell. Roll dumbbell away from body.

**Short-lever**
**lowering candlestick**

Lie on a bench and grip the bench behind the head. Bend the knees 90 degrees and lift the body vertically off the bench. Lower the trunk towards the bench under control.

**Long-lever**
**lowering candlestick**

Lie on a bench and grip the bench behind the head. Legs straight, lift the body vertically off the bench. Lower the trunk towards the bench under control.

**Short-lever candlestick**
**lowering and raising**

Lie on a bench and grip the bench behind the head. Bend the knees 90 degrees and lift the body vertically off the bench. Lower the trunk towards the bench under control then lift the body again before the trunk contacts the bench.

**Long-lever candlestick**
**lowering and raising**

Lie on a bench and grip the bench behind the head. Legs straight, lift the body vertically off the bench. Lower the trunk towards the bench under control then lift the body again before the trunk contacts the bench.

**Lowering and raising**
**with a twist**

Lie on a bench and grip the bench behind the head. Legs straight, lift the body vertically off the bench, rotating the hips. Lower the trunk towards the bench under control, rotating the hips in the other direction, then lift the body again before the trunk contacts the bench.

**End-of-bench**
**candlestick**

Lie on a bench with the shoulders at the end of the bench and grip the bench behind the head. Legs straight, lift the body vertically off the bench. Lower the trunk towards the bench under control.

**Figure 10.39** Advanced horizontal trunk strength exercises.

with rollout exercises is leading the movement with the shoulders. If the shoulders extend too far outside the body before the hips fully extend, shoulder strength will limit the range of movement possible.

As a check, assuming that the athlete is starting with knees on the floor (limited lever arm), the hips should be in neutral position (straight line through knee, hip and glenohumeral joint) before the arms begin to move the bar outside the line of action of the shoulders. The athlete might also experiment with the interrelationship between the base of support and the lever arm. For example, when the athlete achieves mastery of the full rollout on toes with the barbell, going straight to working with a dumbbell may be a step too far. Shortening the lever arm and returning to a kneeling position may produce a more achievable exercise.

Similarly, an athlete attempting to progress candlesticks beyond his or her level of competence may extend the lumbar spine too far, creating unnecessary strain. This movement should be slow and controlled, especially in the later stages of the lowering phase. Although predominantly a sagittal plane movement, the addition of a twist brings in transverse plane control as well as an added coordination challenge.

The added complexity in moving the exercise from one end of the bench to the other should not be underestimated. This change significantly reduces the amount of shoulder and upper back that forms the base of support for the movement, and it enables the athlete to descend through a greater movement range as he or she adapts to the reduced base of support. The end of the bench away from the athlete must be loaded; otherwise, the athlete may cause the bench to tip forwards.

## Rotational Control

Rotations are essential components of sporting actions. The ability to generate torque forcefully through the trunk is vital in many sport-specific actions (throwing, hitting, grappling). Rotational control should be recognized as part of the athlete's overall strength development programme.

Rotations require developed coordination between the anterior (rectus abdominis, external obliques, internal obliques, transversus abdominis) and posterior muscles. The posterior muscles can be divided into two major groups because of function. Deeper, transversospinalis muscles (multifidus, rotatores, semispinalis) are responsible for contralateral rotations in the spine (i.e., the muscles on the right rotate the trunk to the left). The more superficial muscles (erector spinae, splenius capitis, splenius cervicis) are ipsilateral rotators, meaning that the muscles on the right contract to turn the trunk to the right.

Exercises that develop trunk rotations typically are based on a fixed trunk with lower-limb rotations or a standing position in which the upper body rotates around a fixated lower-body base of support. This relationship between the upper- and lower-body components reflects typical sporting demands; rarely does the upper body twist in one direction whilst the lower body turns in the other. Indeed, under loading (even from simple gravitational forces) such a movement may place extreme stress on the spine and the associated trunk musculature.

Also, athletes who typically perform large volumes of sagittal plane work may trend towards hypomobility (reduced ranges of movement) around the hips and the thoracolumbar regions. Active rotational exercises that isolate this region provide additional mobilization and strength to address this particular problem. In half-kneeling diagonal cable woodchoppers (figure 10.40), the athlete's hips are anchored so that rotation can occur only through the trunk as the load is moved through the range; the arms stay long so that forces can effectively be transferred. The exercise starts with the athlete moving the head and cervical spine away from the weight stack and then extending the trunk whilst rotating in the same direction. This exercise can be done as either a low-to-high movement, finishing with the arms raised overhead, or a high-to-low movement, finishing with the hands level with the waist.

Changing to a standing position (figure 10.41), which allows the exercise to be

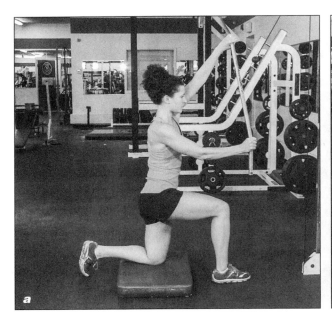 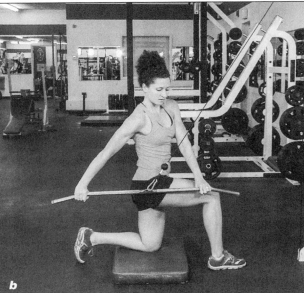

**Figure 10.40** Half-kneeling diagonal cable woodchopper, low-to-high movement: *(a)* start position; *(b)* finish position.

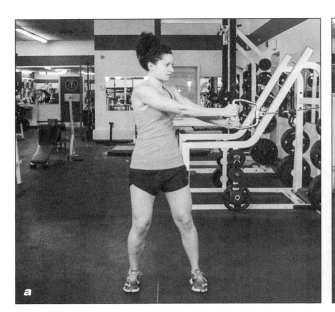 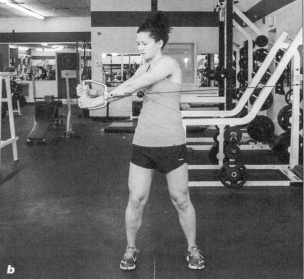

**Figure 10.41** Standing lateral cable woodchopper: *(a)* start position; *(b)* finish position.

performed with diagonal or lateral movement patterns by adjusting the height of the cable, forces the athlete to control the hip position so that it remains neutral and facing forward (i.e., the hips do not rotate). Maintaining a neutral hip position requires activation of the gluteal muscles and isometric actions in the pelvic and groin regions. The athlete must enable transverse plane movements only through the trunk whilst pulling the load across in front of the body. Common progressions between the seated and standing extremes include tall-kneeling and half-kneeling (kneeling on one knee with the other bent) positions, which are extremely transferable to sports.

Increasing the resistive load too much risks introducing compensatory movements from the hip to initiate the movement, rather than enabling the trunk to perform the rotation. At the sport-specific end of the training progression (i.e., after the athlete has done a lot of generic development work), this type of heavy rotational work, initiated from the hip, may be introduced because power needs to be produced from the hip and transferred through the kinetic chain in ground-based movements.

Cable machines that enable the height of the resistive load to be adjusted are extremely useful. Exercises can be designed that enable rotational forces to be resisted. In many contact sports, this component of strength is important. The resisted cable rotation press (figure 10.42) (often referred to as Palloff press) is such an exercise. The athlete must maintain a static trunk position and perform arm extension movements in the sagittal plane whilst resisting transverse plane forces.

The reverse corkscrew (figure 10.43) is a unilateral rotational strength exercise that encourages a contralateral transfer of force from the lower limb through the trunk to the upper body. Correct execution requires the athlete to maintain knee, hip, trunk and shoulder integrity as forces are transferred from the core to the extremity. Hip and knee flexion in the unsupported leg allows the trunk to extend and rotate from a flexed position; the action is initiated by leg extension. The force generated by the leg should transfer from the extending leg through the rotating pelvis and trunk into the extending back and through to the opposite shoulder. As it does so, the cable should move away from the body, following the line of the thoracolumbar fascial sling.

Rotations also can be developed by anchoring the upper body rather than the lower body. Such exercises obviously are not useful in aiding thoracic mobility, but they can develop rotational strength. In windscreen wipers (figure 10.44), the upper body remains fixed to the floor and the length of the legs provides a resistive load that moves from left to right with the hips flexed to 90 degrees throughout. As the athlete's postural strength develops, this exercise can be made increasingly more functional by removing the ground support and requiring direct musculature action to fix the upper body. This advanced exercise (suspended windscreen wipers; figure 10.45) requires a high level of isometric strength to hold the trunk in a horizontal position from where the legs can rotate through the side-to-side action.

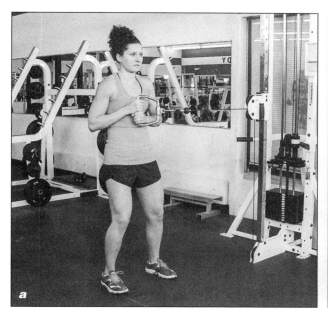 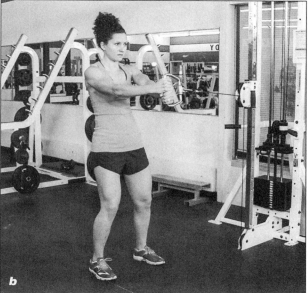

**Figure 10.42**    Resisted cable rotation press: *(a)* start position; *(b)* finish position.

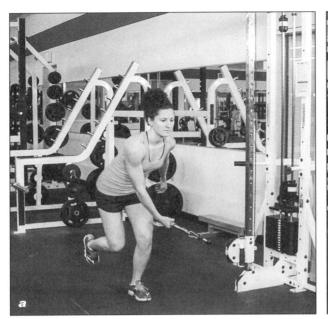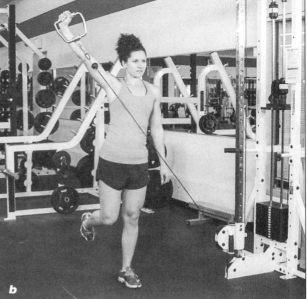

**Figure 10.43**  Reverse corkscrew: *(a)* start position; *(b)* finish position.

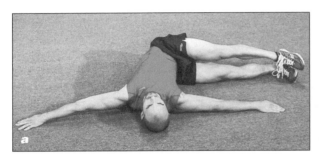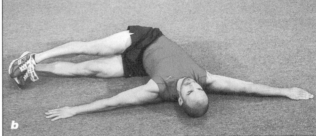

**Figure 10.44**  Windscreen wipers: *(a)* start position; *(b)* finish position.

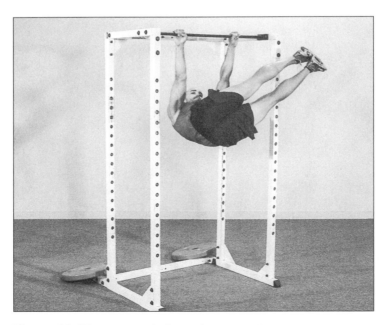

**Figure 10.45**  Suspended windscreen wipers.

## Overhead Strength

This chapter ignores many traditional strength movements that may be important to developing global strength in order to prioritize functional strength exercises that are directly linked to athletic movement skills and postural control. Many readers may question the focus on developing overhead strength when many sporting movements do not directly require this skill. The answer is twofold. First, any overhead load provides a direct challenge to the athlete's extended kinetic chain and therefore significantly challenges the athlete to maintain postural integrity. Second, in working overhead, the athlete applies load in direct opposition to gravity, and it is through the execution of overhead movements that athletic strength and power can ultimately be best expressed.

The best overhead movements, both pushing and pulling, often begin with the athlete performing basic gymnastics movements of the overhead pull (for example, by climbing rope) and the handstand. Both of these movements involve coordinated actions of the upper and lower body and, especially in the handstand, involve significant midsection isometric strength to hold the body upright.

The handstand is a challenging gymnastic movement that requires the athlete to hold the centre of mass directly above a very narrow base of support. The handstand is significantly more challenging than the headstand, which has a wider base of support and a lower centre of gravity. Achieving the most basic level of this exercise is relatively easy for an athlete who has access to a wall, which reduces significantly the sagittal plane challenge of the movement. Although many will be tempted to place their hands next to the wall and kick up their feet, this approach often puts the athlete in an overbalanced position with the feet on the wall but not directly over the centre of mass or base of support (i.e., the hands). Incidentally, without the wall, many athletes are not strong enough to kick their legs up into the handstand position. The reality is that this movement doesn't take much relative power. The normal cause is that the athlete worries about overbalancing at the top, and the lack of kick is a confidence factor.

A more practical way to learn the handstand is to place the feet on the wall and walk the hands backwards whilst moving the feet vertically up the wall (figure 10.46). This movement results in the head and hands coming very close to the wall and the body ending up in a

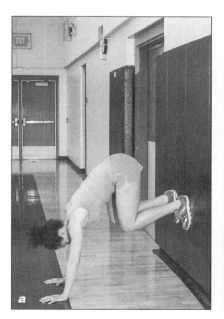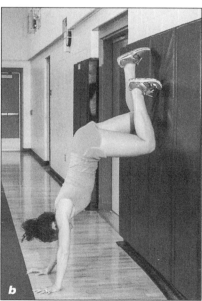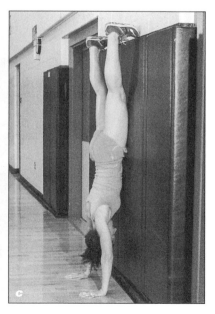

**Figure 10.46**  Walking up the wall into the handstand puts the athlete into a balanced position: *(a)* start position, press-up with feet on wall; *(b)* midpoint, walk hands backwards and feet upwards; *(c)* balance point, handstand with head facing wall.

vertical position. While holding this position, the athlete learns to provide sufficient force to support his or her body weight on a fully flexed glenohumeral joint, with full thoracic and arm extension.

The handstand can progress significantly by reducing the amount of support (i.e., using a spotter to support the feet only) or by maintaining an unsupported handstand position. The position is an inversion of the overhead pressing movement; ground reaction is through the hands instead of the feet. The load, however, is fully through the arms and shoulders, and an athlete will need time to progress to overhead pressing his or her body weight. Indeed, the handstand can be turned into a pressing action through the introduction of a press-up movement (figure 10.47). This variation requires significant shoulder and arm strength as well as postural control.

Rope climbing has traditionally been a staple component of junior physical education programmes, but it has fallen out of favour in recent years. Rope climbing is a challenging exercise for anyone who can be encouraged to climb the rope as far or as fast as possible. This skill can progress from the total-body movement that involves the athlete pushing with the legs and pulling with the arms to achieve a higher position on the rope to an advanced version in which the athlete climbs using the arms only.

The pull-up (figure 10.48) also has evolved through many variations over the years. In its most basic form, the athlete takes an overgrasp grip and hangs from the bar. The overgrasp grip is the most common form of carrying grip in sport and everyday activity. In this exercise, the grip emphasizes the back musculature, especially the latissimus dorsi and the teres major, and at the top of the movement, the rhomboids and trapezius.[3] A lot of arm flexor (biceps brachii, brachialis and brachioradialis) work is also involved in the movement, and this emphasis can be increased by reversing the grip to an undergrasp movement. Typically, the undergrasp grip pull-up is easier for the athlete to perform.

The overhead pulling action makes the pull-up an attractive exercise for fundamental and functional strength. The pull-up is a basic movement that can be increased easily at an individual level, because the athlete is totally in control of his or her body weight throughout the movement. For example, the athlete can perform the pull-up at a high velocity in the lifting phase and a slow eccentric descent, or increase the load by adding a weight belt. Often, athletes compensate by swinging to generate momentum to the centre of mass, but this error is easily corrected through coaching the correct form.

As figure 10.47 illustrates, three basic overhead movements with external loads result in a fully extended trunk, in which the load is supported by locked arms in a position over the rear of the head as the athlete faces forwards. The load is directly above the base of support, which minimizes anteroposterior torque that challenges the equilibrium of the position. For this reason, these lifts often start with the bar resting on the athlete's upper back on the shelf created by the shoulders and the upper trapezius. The bar is held in an overgrasp grip slightly wider than shoulder-width. Pushing upwards from this position moves the bar directly and vertically to the natural overhead finish point, whereas lifting from the front requires the bar to be brought vertically and rearwards to reach the same location. The movements can also be done with dumbbells, which requires a lot more isolated control in each arm and shoulder, The movement is more challenging, so less external load usually is lifted.

Subtle differences are associated with the use of the legs in the overhead press, push press and push jerk. Indeed, to push a load powerfully overhead in a sporting context, the athlete naturally uses the largest driving muscles in the body, the hip and knee extensors, to overcome inertia in the load and generate momentum that the arms then maintain to guide the load into a safe receiving position.

The overhead press removes the legs from the equation. After the athlete is in a balanced standing position with the feet wide (maximal base of support) and the trunk braced, the shoulders and elbows extend to move the bar upwards. It is a total-body movement in the

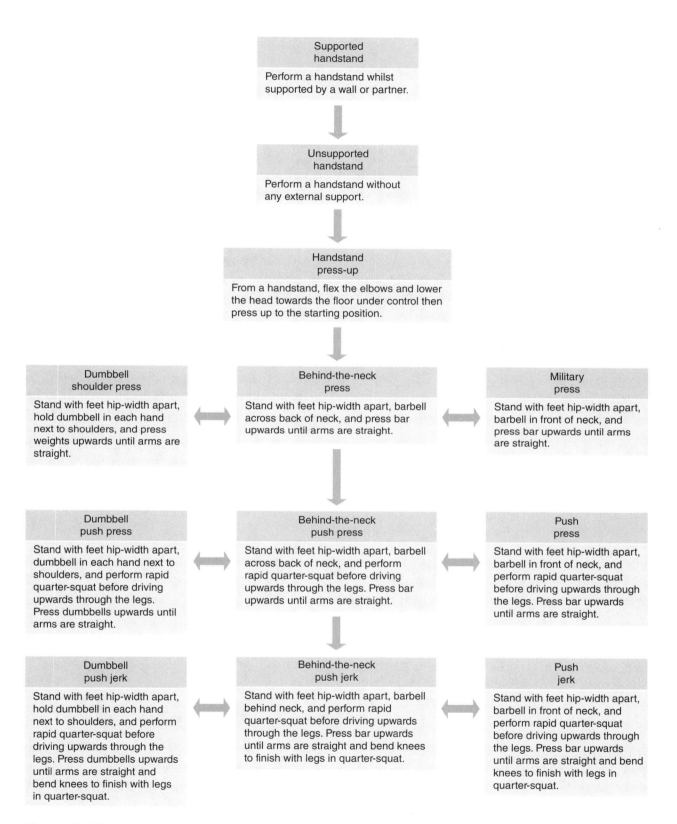

**Figure 10.47** Progression from handstand to push jerk.

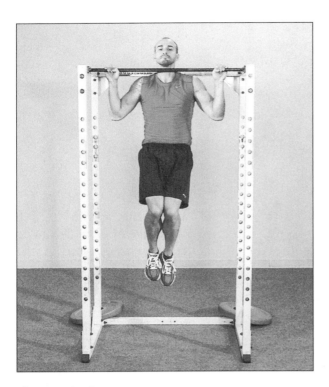

**Figure 10.48** Pull-up.

sense that many muscles work as synergists to support the frame, but the prime movers are all upper body. Contrast this with the push press, which begins with a countermovement of the hips and knees. This dip-and-drive motion uses the stretch reflex to increase the lower-body force output, generating momentum into the bar that the arms simply continue.

The jerk movement (many are familiar with the split-stance position demonstrated by the majority of athletes in international weightlifting) is a higher velocity movement in which the athlete drives the bar vertically in the same manner as the push press. But after the bar leaves the athlete's shoulders and the vertical drive from the legs ceases to accelerate the bar vertically, the athlete explosively rebends the hips and knees and jumps back under the bar to receive it in the overhead position. Less vertical displacement of the bar occurs, and the arms have minimal pressing in the action. Receiving the bar and controlling the catch, however, significantly challenge the arms and shoulders as the athlete extends the hips and knees to stand upright with the bar overhead.

The split stance provides additional stability by widening the base of support in the sagittal plane. The athlete moves into the split-stance catching position following full extension of the hips, knees and ankles as the bar leaves the shoulders. This split action should be performed about an imaginary cross (it can be drawn on the floor if it helps; see figure 10.49). The front leg (which can alternate with each repetition) should move forwards and be planted flat on the floor, with the centre of pressure towards the heel. Simultaneously, the back foot moves backwards into the opposite quadrant of the cross, and the athlete lands on the ball of the foot. The width of the split depends on the resistive load; the heavier the load is, the less height will be achieved and the wider the split needs to be. The athlete's centre of mass should be immediately above the centre of the cross (i.e., it should not have moved from the start position of the jerk).

After the split position is achieved and the athlete stabilizes his or her position with the weight locked out overhead, the feet should move back to shoulder-width apart. The front foot moves backwards towards the midline, and then the rear foot moves forwards. The lift is completed when both feet are level and the bar is fully extended overhead.

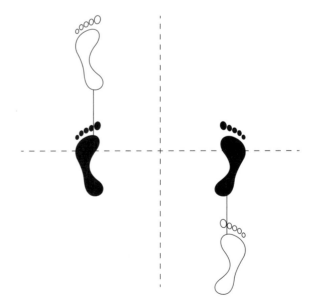

**Figure 10.49** Achieving an effective split stance in the jerk catch position.

# Exercise Sequencing and Programming

This chapter analysed the concept of functionality in strength training and its importance when developing the athleticism of the athlete and translating training into sporting performance. Many texts address other aspects of strength training and programming it at various stages of the athlete's career. The key consideration of this chapter is how strength training is integrated within the overall training programme to achieve balanced prescription aligned to the generic and sport-specific needs of the person at the time.

Some key principles are inherent within any programme design. The first is that strength exercise prescription should be differentiated so that the challenge is appropriate for the athlete's competence, a theme in keeping with all aspects of athletic development coaching. The second is that volume load considerations are appropriate. The sets, repetitions, sessions and intensity (for example, the loading) are carefully assessed to ensure that the athlete is being trained appropriately. The major consideration with strength and power work is that quality work is what keeps the athlete fresh with relatively low volume loads.

When learning movements, volume is high to increase repetition and practice, but this approach may mean performing large numbers of one to three movements with plenty of coaching in between. Even well-trained athletes looking at advanced exercise prescription for strength or power objectives rarely use sets of repetitions that exceed the one to five range. Beyond this, the challenge to the neuromuscular system is significantly reduced through fatigue. In contrast, athletes looking at rehabilitation training (re-educating the neuromuscular system) may look at performing more repetitions (10 to 15) to establish the neural patterning of the movement, but this will be done with significantly reduced loads compared with a training or performance objective.

# Summary

The ability to access strength (force-producing capabilities) is a critical component that underpins an athlete's success in executing a wide range of movement skills. The crucial consideration is not how strong the athlete needs to be, but how much strength he or she can access during the execution of movement skills to make these skills as forceful and effective as possible.

The concept of functionality within strength training is related to a range of considerations within the athlete's training programme. At the heart are issues relating to how the strength stimulus challenges the athlete's motor system. Postural integrity, neuromuscular demand and rate of force development are all important determinants of the functionality of an exercise within the overall programme.

Achieving overload within a strength programme should be considered simply a function of increasing the resistive load that the athlete is required to move. By relating movement complexity to considerations of lever length, position of the centre of mass, extent or ranges of movement or the size or position of the base of support, a series of progressively more complex or more difficult strength challenges can be presented to develop the athlete's ability to recruit functional strength to underpin sporting performances.

As with most aspects of movement-related training for sport, progressive challenge should be based on the athlete's competency. To learn effectively, athletes need to be stretched beyond their level of comfort, but not to such a degree that it exceeds their ability to achieve a mechanically correct or efficient movement. The aim is to reinforce appropriate motor patterns without incorporating or developing movement compensations that may hinder the athlete's ability to produce force functionally in the long term. Attaining this goal requires the appropriate level of repetition and variation within the strength stimuli throughout the programme over the long term.

# CHAPTER 11

# Applying Principles in Practice

This book examines how the human body works and adapts to physio-mechanical stimuli with respect to enhancing athletic movement skills, and it presents practical exercise progressions so that practitioners can apply these principles in a range of programme contexts. In any analysis of a process designed to aid the athlete to move more efficiently and effectively, the most appropriate means of critiquing understanding is to present a programme that explains how these factors come together to achieve predetermined objectives.

In developing a training programme, any practitioner (be it athlete, sport coach, scientist or athletic development coach) needs to realize that there isn't one right way to develop a programme. A desired outcome can be achieved in many ways, as long as it is underpinned by the principles that govern movement and human physical development. The aim of this chapter is to present some case studies and provide the programmes that might be used to achieve the specific objectives identified for the athlete.

The rationale behind each programme can be found within the previous chapters. Take a critical approach to the analysis of each programme and try to understand why decisions have been made. In trying to communicate these applications and progressions, I have worked on the principal of simplicity, for both session structure and exercise selection. In reality, I may typically have more variation in both of these than it is easy to communicate in

text and without having an athlete in front of me to coach. After all, a vast range of exercise progressions is available to the practitioner. The essential that I wish you to think about is based on principles of progression and using objectives to determine methods. Therefore, in reading this chapter, evaluate how you would have approached the situation. Would you have used the same drills and similar progressions?

Remember that the job isn't to follow a prescribed expectation for athletic development (i.e., strength and conditioning 101 is often misunderstood to be 'Get my athletes to do Olympic lifts, the overhead jerk and so on'), but to provide a value added that will enable athletes to progress in their ability to perform in their sport, with a reduced chance of injury. The transfer of training (learning) benefits to the athlete enables the practitioner to succeed in the long term.

## Case Study 1: Tennis

Stefanie is a 16-year-old tennis player who has been playing the sport seriously for 9 years. She is 180 centimetres tall and weighs 63 kilograms. Stefanie typically practises tennis 2 to 4 hours a day, but her conditioning programme has been limited to cardio routines and some basic weight training undertaken through her school programme and in a local fitness centre. She has a reasonable training age and developed level of physical competence. She aspires to be a professional player and is seeking to play in several national-level events in the near future. Although she is injury free at the start of the training programme, she has a history of ankle injuries (two mild ATFL sprains) in the last year.

The anterior talofibular ligament (ATFL) connects the talus to the fibula and is located on the outside of the ankle. ATFL sprains are the most common type of ankle sprains. Typically, in tennis, an ATFL sprain occurs when a player plants the outside foot to play a forehand cross-court but is not able to control lateral momentum. The centre of mass moves the torso laterally as the ankle lands in a plantarflexed position (a weak position with the toes pointing downwards) and inverted (turned inwards), forcefully causing an overstretch or tear of the ligaments.

Although treatment focused on the symptoms of Stephanie's injury, analysis identified the cause of the injury as occurring higher up the kinetic chain, especially around the hip joint. The injuries are a result of Stefanie's inability to control her posture dynamically, especially when transferring into a single-leg stance, largely because of deficiencies in gluteal muscle activation. This position is important in tennis, because many shots are played from a single-leg or split stance.

Her tennis coach identified that Stefanie has a tendency to use steps that are too small to move between shots and that she plays shots from a very narrow stance, when moving both forwards and backwards. She is weak when she stretches for a ball, and she needs to be able to place her feet so that she has a more stable heel or flat-foot ground contact to provide a stable base from which to play shots and to make transitions between single-leg and double-foot stances.

Unless performing a linear acceleration to reach a drop shot from the back of the court, the tennis athlete typically is required to move differently than any other athlete in the first few steps from standing. When moving laterally or rearwards to intercept an object with a flight path perpendicular to the athlete's pattern of acceleration, a small number of large steps is often more efficient than a large number of small steps (a typical linear acceleration pattern).

Stefanie's programme will develop functional strength that will enable her to transmit rotational forces in the upper body through the postural chain (anchored to the floor) and into racket head speed. At the same time, a series of on-court movement development activities will enable her to transfer this control to tennis-specific agility skills that will optimize her movement around the court. Stefanie will develop the basic physio-mechanical qualities of rotational strength to exert forces whilst controlling upper-body torque in a range of foot positions. The programme includes a focus on single-limb support deceleration and reacceleration in all three movement planes and the ability to position her base of support relative to her centre of mass to enable both stability (shot playing) and mobility (shot reaching).

The following training priorities were identified for a 3-month training period to be integrated with her on-court tennis sessions.

### Functional Strength

1. Develop high force output through the kinetic chain using ground-based exercises, focusing on the lower-limb flexors and extensors, the latissimus dorsi (which, along with superficial connective tissue [thoracolumbar fascia] forms a sling with the glutes to pull the racket back to store elastic energy that can be released in the shot) and the trunk to stabilize the spine and generate torque, which is important in every shot (figure 11.1). The ability to transfer ground reaction forces through the shoulder and into the upper limb (arm) is also important. (Stefanie has previously performed rotator-cuff-specific strengthening work for the shoulder, but these muscles cannot be used in isolation to generate racket head speed).

2. Develop high force outputs in a range of single-leg and unilateral stances.

3. Develop high power output in end-range movements in all three movement planes.

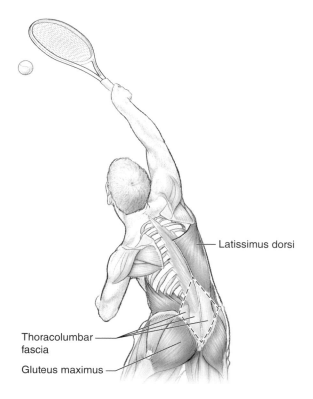

Latissimus dorsi

Thoracolumbar fascia

Gluteus maximus

**Figure 11.1** Global movement of the trunk comes from the interrelationship between the latissimus dorsi, the gluteus maximus and the thoracolumbar fascia.

## Functional Stability

1. Develop double-foot landing mechanics.
2. Develop single-leg landing mechanics and double-leg reactive strength to enable rapid adjustments in the base of support.
3. Dynamically transfer into a wide, low position of support in the lower limbs from which to generate upper-body torques and transition from this position into a movement sequence.

## On-Court Movement

1. From an appropriately stable base, develop specific forwards, backwards and lateral footwork patterns.
2. Increase the complexity of the footwork patterns.
3. Increase the efficiency and speed of the footwork patterns.
4. Apply the footwork patterns to open practices and tennis rallies.

The strength and stability aspects of the programme are performed in the mornings, when Stefanie is relatively fresh. A 3- or 4-hour gap between sessions facilitates recovery. Tennis sessions begin with dynamic warm-ups that progressively incorporate more stability and then lead into on-court movement work. This sequence facilitates a more effective transfer between the movement techniques and the sport-specific skills and enables the tennis coach to work closely with the athletic development specialist to influence Stefanie's on-court movement. Gradually, the movement drills that formed the practice sessions will be migrated into the warm-ups to allow time for progression. As Stefanie becomes more efficient and her postural control and power improve, her racket technique needs to develop to embrace her enhanced physical qualities.

For this block of training, Stefanie's practice weeks are structured as shown in table 11.1, although appropriate restructuring occurs for practice tournaments towards the end of the block. The programme can be adapted for each training block, so that, for example, in block 3, the day 6 conditioning becomes integrated into the tennis session so that the training unit is specific before competition.

**Table 11.1**   Stefanie's Training Week

| Day | 1 | 2 | 3 | 4 | 5 | 6 | 7 |
|---|---|---|---|---|---|---|---|
| AM session | Strength | Stability and conditioning | Stability and strength | Active recovery | Stability and strength | Stability and conditioning | Active recovery |
| PM session | Movement and tennis | Movement and tennis | Tennis | | Movement and tennis | Tennis | |

For more information on cumulative loading strategies and phasic loading strategies such as this, research the contemporary literature on periodization strategies.[1]

The 12-week block is planned as three 4-week blocks. The volume load (volume of work done times the relative intensity of that work) changes each week: Week 1 is a medium-heavy load, week 2 is a heavy load, week 3 is a very heavy load (when planned overreaching will occur), and week 4 is a downloaded (medium) week to facilitate recovery but without reducing training volume. This schedule will enable Stefanie to accommodate to increasing volume loads as the programme progresses. Volume load also varies within the training week, as shown in table 11.2, although the emphasis changes so that greater focus is on the tennis volume load because actualization of the transfer of the training process occurs towards the end of the training block.

Besides variation between weeks, variation also occurs in the volume loading within the week. The training emphasis shifts between the training elements to allow appropriate levels of overload and recovery and adaption. This aspect is important, because although Stefanie has a reasonable training age that can support the training load, training intensity cannot be high in all training elements through the week without causing her to overreach or, potentially, to overtrain in the long term.

# Training Block 1: Weeks 1 Through 4

Weeks 1 through 4 are designed to develop the foundational on-court movement skills and underpinning strength qualities that will enable Stefanie to progress through the exercise progressions and achieve the identified aims. The emphasis is on movement patterning with high-quality neuromuscular system development.

## Strength Sessions

The strength sessions, sets and repetitions for weeks 1 through 4 are shown in table 11.3. Exercises within this programme are presented within the progressions described in chapter 10. They are multijoint, multimuscle exercises that enable the athlete to achieve either high force outputs (for example, squat and deadlift) or high power outputs (for example, clean pull), and the movements are from both single- and double-foot stances.

## Stability Sessions

Stability sessions are designed to achieve several outcomes. Some exercises are aimed at developing gluteal activation to stabilize the hip joint and enhance hip, knee and ankle alignment while moving. Exercises may keep the feet in a static position or be used as a strategy to develop controlled landing techniques

**Table 11.2** Variation of Relative Volume Loads for Each Training Element in the Practice Week

| Day | 1 | 2 | 3 | 4 | 5 | 6 | 7 |
|---|---|---|---|---|---|---|---|
| Strength-training volume load | Heavy | Rest | Light | Active recovery | Medium | Rest | Active recovery |
| Stability-training volume load | Rest | Heavy | Light | | Medium | Rest | |
| Conditioning volume load | Rest | Light | Rest | | Rest | Heavy | |
| Movement-training volume load | Medium | Light | Rest | | Heavy | Rest | |
| Tennis (technical training) volume load | Light | Heavy | Medium | | Light | Medium | |

**Table 11.3** Strength-Training Sessions for Weeks 1 Through 4

| STRENGTH SESSION 1 | | | |
|---|---|---|---|
| **Exercise** | **Sets** | **Reps** | **Description** |
| Deadlift | 4 | 5 | Stand with a barbell in front of the shins. Grasp the barbell in an alternated shoulder-width grip, with chest upright and weight on heels. Extend hips and knees simultaneously and stand upright. |
| Band-assisted overgrasp pull-up | 4 | 8 | Use an overgrasp grip slightly wider than shoulder-width. Hang from the pull-up bar. Using the back muscles, pull yourself up until the chin is above the level of the bar and then lower under control. The band provides support to help you overcome gravity. |
| Single-leg box squat | 4 | 5 each leg | Place a barbell across the back of the shoulders. Stand on one leg and perform a single-leg squat until your butt touches the top of the box. |
| Incline bench press | 4 | 5 | Lie on a bench at a 25- to 35-degree incline. The barbell rests in the rack directly above the upper chest. Grasp the barbell in an overgrasp grip with the hands wider than shoulder-width. Keeping the feet on the floor and the buttocks and shoulders in contact with the bench, lift the bar off the rack and lower it to the midchest. |
| Stir the pot | 3 | 30 sec. | Rest the forearms on a stability ball. Kneel (easy version) or stand (advanced version), maintaining a straight line from the ear through the shoulders, hips, knees, and ankles. Rotate around the ball at the elbows, as if stirring a pot. |

| STRENGTH SESSION 2 | | | |
|---|---|---|---|
| **Exercise** | **Sets** | **Reps** | **Description** |
| Front foot elevated split squat | 4 | 5 each leg | Perform a split squat with the front foot elevated to load the posterior chain in the front leg. |
| Suspension cord supported pistol squat | 4 | 8 each leg | Hold a suspension cord for balance. Perform a pistol squat to full depth and return to standing. |
| Stiff-legged deadlift | 4 | 8 | Hold a barbell in a clean grip against the thigh. Stand with the feet hip-width apart, knees slightly flexed and weight through the midfoot. Initiating movement with an upwards and backwards movement of the hips, lean the trunk forwards as the bar moves down the legs. |
| Handstand (partner supported) | 4 | 30 sec. hold | Perform a handstand whilst supported by a partner. The feet should come directly above the head. |
| Resisted cable rotation push | 3 | 5 each side | Set the cable level with the chest. Stand at a 90-degree angle to the cable machine, with the trunk upright, knees flexed and feet hip- to shoulder-width apart. Start with the arms locked so that there is a lateral pull from the cable. Facing forward and resisting the lateral pull, bend the arms and pull the handle to the chest. |

| STRENGTH SESSION 3 | | | |
|---|---|---|---|
| **Exercise** | **Sets** | **Reps** | **Description** |
| Clean pull from thigh | 4 | 5 | Start on the second pull position of the clean (feet hip-width apart, knees flexed, trunk upright, barbell at midthigh) with the weight through the midfoot. Perform a clean second pull by violently extending the hips, knees and ankles so that the bar rises rapidly and the weight moves to the toes. At the top of the movement, shrug violently. The bar should rise up the front of the body. |
| Barbell overhead squat | 4 | 5 | Hold a barbell above the head. Perform a full-range squat, keeping the trunk upright and maintaining lumbar–sacral alignment. |
| In-place inline lunge with barbell behind the neck | 4 | 10 | Hold a barbell across the back of the shoulders. Lunge forward into a narrowed base, moving the front leg in front of the rear leg so that the front knee aligns with the toes of the front foot and the knee of the rear foot comes to the heel of the front foot. |
| Rope climb | 4 | 1 | Use an alternating overgrasp grip to climb the rope, reaching with the arms, securing the hands onto the rope, pulling with the arms and locking the feet to the rope to anchor the body and enable the next pull. |
| Lateral cable woodchopper | 2 | 6 each side | Stand with feet hip-width apart and hips at a 90-degree angle to the cable machine. Set the cable at midtrunk height. Hold the handle with the arms straight. Move the head and cervical spine away from the weight stack and rotate the trunk in the same direction, pulling the straight arms and cable away from the stack. |

from dynamic movements. Other exercises, especially those on unstable surfaces, are designed to enhance the proprioceptive qualities around the ankles whilst other joints are moving. Besides focusing on the legs, some exercises that focus on shoulder joint integrity and stability during total-body movements are included within the sessions to aid Stefanie's functional control around the shoulder. The stability sessions including sets and repetitions for weeks 1 through 4 are shown in table 11.4.

**Table 11.4** Functional Stability Sessions for Weeks 1 Through 4

| STABILITY SESSION 1 | | | |
|---|---|---|---|
| **Exercise** | **Sets** | **Reps** | **Description** |
| Double-foot drop and hold from 20- to 30-centimetre box | 3–5 | 5 | Step off a box with the trunk upright and ankles dorsiflexed in preparation for ground contact. Stick a two-footed landing, stabilizing the knees in alignment with the toes and distributing weight through the midfoot. |
| 10-meter hop and hold | 4–6 | 1 each leg | Perform single-leg hops for 10 metres. Make sure that each landing is stable (hips and shoulders level, knees aligned with toes, weight through the midfoot) before the next hop. |
| Jump onto 20- to 30-centimetre box | 3–5 | 6 | Perform a two-footed take-off and land two-footed in the middle of the box in a stable position with good hip, knee and ankle alignment. |
| Step-through lunge | 3–5 | 8–10 each leg | Perform a reverse lunge and then transition from the bottom position to a forward lunge on the same leg. Do not pause between the forwards and backwards movements for the duration of the set. |
| STABILITY SESSION 2 | | | |
| **Exercise** | **Sets** | **Reps** | **Description** |
| Star excursion | 3 | 10 each leg | Stand on one leg. The lifted leg remains fixed throughout the movement. Keeping the hips and shoulders square, reach forward with the lifted leg and touch the ground as far in front of the body as possible. With the lifted leg, reach backwards at a 45-degree angle to the left side of the body and touch the floor as far away as possible. Reach at a 45-degree angle to the right side of the body and again touch the floor as far away as possible. |
| Four-way step with resistance band | 3 | 10 each direction | Stand on a single leg with a resistance band around the midshin of the standing foot. Pull laterally. Step forwards, touch the ground and return. Step to the left, right, and backwards or perform a randomized sequence. Repeat with the resistance coming from the front, back and both sides. |
| Single-leg stance tennis ball throw and catch | 3–5 | 8–10 catches each leg | Stand on one leg. Catch a tennis ball thrown by a partner or bounced off a wall at various heights and speeds. Maintain balance. |
| Double-leg glute bridge | 3–5 | 10 | Lie on your back with knees bent 90 degrees, feet hip-width apart and ankles dorsiflexed so that the toes are off the floor. Squeeze the glutes and lift the hips until there is a straight line from knees to hips and shoulders. |

| STABILITY SESSION 3 | | | |
|---|---|---|---|
| **Exercise** | **Sets** | **Reps** | **Description** |
| Forward lunge onto foam pad | 3 | 10 each leg | Stand, lunge forwards and plant the lead foot onto a cushioning foam pad. Lower until the hips are below the level of the front knee and then return to start. |
| Lateral hop and hold | 3–5 | 5–8 each leg | Hop laterally over a microhurdle. Stabilize the landing on a flat foot with hip, knee and ankle alignment and an upright trunk. |
| Single-leg forward hop and hold through agility ladder | 3–5 | 6–8 each leg | Hop through an agility ladder, placing one foot in each square and sticking each landing. |
| Walking single-arm upturned kettlebell carry | 4–6 | 10 metres with each arm | Hold a kettlebell upside down with the humerus of the arm in the scapular plane. Walk forward for 20 metres. |

## Conditioning Sessions

Note that the conditioning work has not been identified as a priority for this period of training. Even so, some conditioning work is needed in the athlete's overall tennis preparation, and this work should be fully integrated into the overall training structure. Conditioning work also needs to complement the work undertaken to develop other aspects of training, in this case the emphasis on high-quality neuromuscular system development.

Conditioning sessions are based on repeat high-intensity (near maximal) work. The focus is on relatively high-speed, total-body movements or high-power, high-cadence movements in the case of the Watt bike sessions. Conditioning sessions promote anaerobic power and capacity and improve aerobic capacity because the developed oxygen debt is replenished in the work interval. At the same time, the neuromuscular system recruits fast-twitch motor units to perform the work, thus complementing the strength and stability development work that is the priority for this period in the athlete's programme.

### Session 1: Off-Feet Conditioning

Concept 2 rowing ergometer: 10 × 500 metres with 60 seconds of recovery between repetitions or

Wattbike Pro: 10 × 1 kilometre with a 1:2 work-to-recovery ratio

### Session 2

Running: 2 × 8 × 200 metres with a 1:1.5 work-to-rest ratio (target time of 35 to 38 seconds per repetition), 4 minutes of rest between sets

## Movement Skill Sessions

I would like to acknowledge the work of Jez Green, long-time fitness coach for Andy Murray and other senior professionals, whom I have worked with for many years, for his knowledge in developing on-court tennis-specific movement drills that focus on transition to interception mechanics. Variations of these drills are presented here. At the start of the training block, these skills are completely closed and performed in blocked practice sequences with a medicine ball. The drills enable the player to simulate a tennis movement with the upper body whilst exaggerating the lower-body movement patterns that typify a range of shots in tennis. These drills should be performed from the baseline of the court; the player moves towards the net as the drills progress, similar to a rally in the game. Choose four drills from this list.

# TENNIS MOVEMENT PROGRESSIONS DRILL 1

Starting in the centre of the baseline (figure 11.2), initiate the drill with a small jump into a widened stance (the tennis split step). From here, externally rotate the right leg at the hip so that the foot is pointing along the length of the baseline. Then bring the left foot across in a crossover movement and land in a wide lunge. The left foot will be close to the baseline in a narrowed stance. From here, bring the right foot around so that you are in an athletic stance with the feet 45 degrees to the net and on either side of the baseline. Perform adjustment steps and then throw the medicine ball in a forehand action, following through to end up in a lunge position with the right leg forward. Reverse the actions for the backhand.

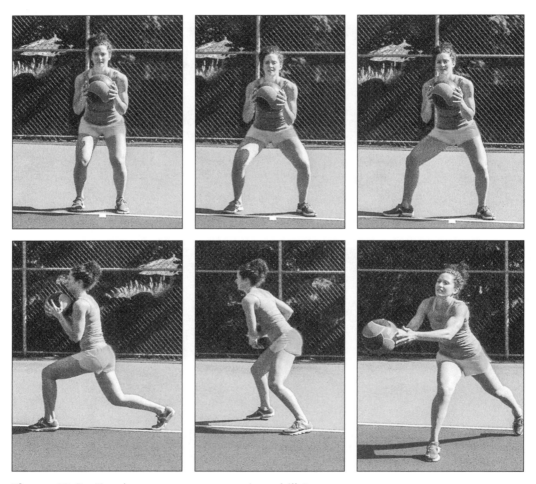

**Figure 11.2** Tennis movement progressions drill 1.

# TENNIS MOVEMENT PROGRESSIONS DRILL 2

Start at the centre of the baseline (figure 11.3). Perform a split step. Bring the left foot inside the baseline and point the toes at a 45-degree angle. Bring the right foot forward so that you are in a deep forward lunge. Now the left foot is aligned so that you are upright and ready to play a forehand shot. Perform adjustment steps and then throw the medicine ball in a forehand action, following through to end up in a lunge position with the right leg forward. Reverse for the backhand action.

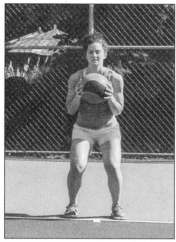
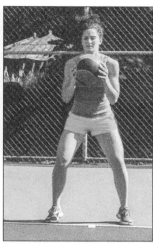
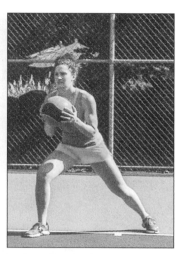
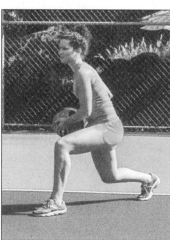
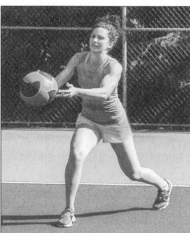

**Figure 11.3**  Tennis movement progressions drill 2.

# TENNIS MOVEMENT PROGRESSIONS DRILL 3

This drill (figure 11.4) mimics an inside-out forehand. Perform a small jump into the split stance. Perform a right foot rearward hip turn with the right leg, pivoting on the left. You will end up perpendicular to the net. Using the right leg as a pivot, bring the left foot forwards, landing on the toes so that you are lined up as if to play a forehand. Perform adjustment steps and then throw the medicine ball in a forehand action, following through to end up in a lunge position with the right leg forward.

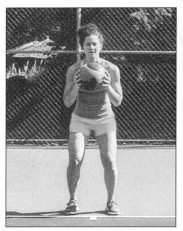
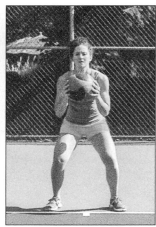
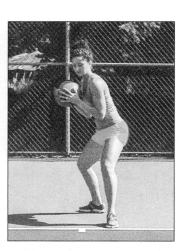

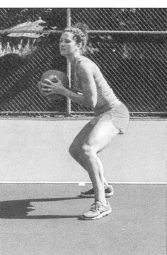
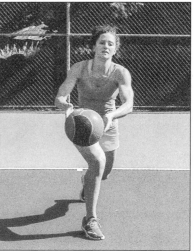

**Figure 11.4**   Tennis movement progressions drill 3.

# TENNIS MOVEMENT PROGRESSIONS DRILL 4

On the baseline, perform a small jump into the split stance (figure 11.5). Perform a crossover jump over the hurdle to catch the thrown medicine ball, landing in a single-foot stance. Bring the other foot to land level with the first foot. You are now perpendicular to the line of the net. Perform adjustment steps and then throw the ball back to the server, mimicking a forehand. Follow through to end up in a lunge position with the right leg forward. Perform adjustments steps to return to the baseline with the feet level. Repeat the drill to the backhand side, reversing the leg actions.

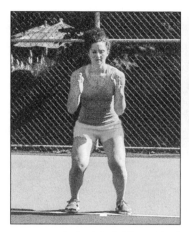
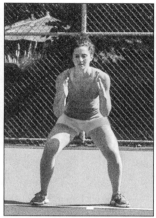
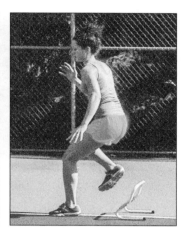

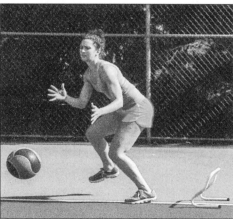
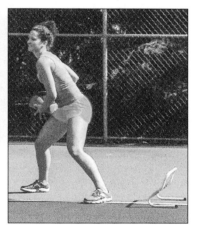

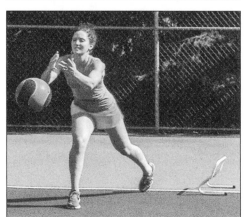

**Figure 11.5** Tennis movement progressions drill 4.

# Training Block 2: Weeks 5 Through 8

The second block of training progresses the complexity and the intensity of the actions. Stefanie should now be familiar with the movements and mechanics, and she can focus on progressing her learning and neuromuscular system development through increased speed of movement or by adding complexities to movement challenges. In the court drills, for example, this comes from making the drills more open, but in the weight room it will be about enhancing the postural challenge to focus Stefanie on the need to maintain control in the dynamic hip, knee and ankle alignment.

## Strength Sessions

The strength sessions, sets and repetitions for weeks 5 through 8 are shown in table 11.5.

**Table 11.5**    Strength-Training Sessions for Weeks 5 Through 8

| STRENGTH SESSION 1 | | | |
|---|---|---|---|
| Exercise | Sets | Reps | Description |
| Deadlift | 4 | 5 | Stand with a barbell in front of the shins. Grasp the barbell in an alternated shoulder-width grip. The chest is upright, and weight is on the heels. Extend the hips and knees simultaneously and stand upright. |
| Pull-up | 4 | 5 | Grip a pull-up bar in an overgrasp grip with hands slightly wider than shoulder-width. Hang from the bar. Using the back muscles, pull yourself up until the chin is above the level of the bar. |
| Single-leg squat with medicine ball support against wall | 4 | 5 each leg | Stand on one leg with a medicine ball between the back and a wall. Perform a single-leg squat through the full range of motion (hips below knee). |
| Incline bench dumbbell press | 4 | 5 | Lie on a bench at a 25- to 35-degree incline. Hold dumbbells directly above the upper chest with arms straight. Grip the dumbbells in an overgrasp grip. Keeping the feet on the floor and the buttocks and shoulders in contact with the bench, lower the dumbbells to midchest and return to start. |
| Plank | 3 | 30 sec. | Lie on the floor, supported on forearms (elbows below shoulders) and toes. Squeeze the trunk off the floor to create a straight line from the ear through shoulders, hips, knees and ankles. Hold the position. |
| STRENGTH SESSION 2 | | | |
| Exercise | Sets | Reps | Description |
| Front foot elevated overhead split squat | 4 | 5 each leg | Stand with the feet staggered and the front foot elevated 20 to 30 centimetres and weight through the heel of the front foot. Perform a split squat while holding a barbell with straight arms directly above the crown of the head. |
| Lateral single-leg squat from box | 4 | 8 each leg | Stand on a box with one foot off the side. Keeping the ankle of the unsupported leg dorsiflexed, perform a single-leg squat, reaching the unsupported heel towards the floor. |
| Stiff-legged deadlift | 4 | 8 | Hold a barbell in a clean grip against the thighs. Stand with feet hip-width apart, knees slightly flexed and weight through the midfoot. Initiate the movement with an upwards and backwards movement of the hips. Lean the trunk forwards and move the bar down the legs. |

| STRENGTH SESSION 2 *(continued)* | | | |
|---|---|---|---|
| **Exercise** | **Sets** | **Reps** | **Description** |
| Behind-the-neck press | 4 | 5 | Stand with feet hip-width apart and the barbell across the back of the neck. Press the bar upwards until the arms are straight. |
| Two-point superman | 3 | 10 each arm and leg combo | Start on all fours with the arms straight, hands directly below shoulders and knees directly below hips. Lift a contralateral arm and leg until they are in line with the trunk. Keep shoulders and hips level. |

| STRENGTH SESSION 3 | | | |
|---|---|---|---|
| **Exercise** | **Sets** | **Reps** | **Description** |
| Clean pull from hang | 4 | 5 | Stand with feet hip-width apart, knees nearly extended, trunk leaning forwards and shoulders in front of the bar, which is above the tops of the knees. Weight is distributed back towards the heels. Extend the hips and bend the knees under the bar, moving through the power position to perform the second pull of the clean, lifting the bar in front of the body. |
| High-bar barbell back squat | 4 | 5 | Hold the bar across the top of the back. Perform a squat. |
| Walking inline lunge with barbell behind neck | 4 | 10 | Hold the bar across the back of the shoulders. Perform an in-line lunge and then step the back foot forward into another in-line lunge. |
| Supine row | 4 | 8–10 | Place the barbell on a rack. Lie under the bar, feet on a platform, and hang from the bar. Keep a straight line from ankles to shoulders with no part of the body in contact with the floor. Pull the trunk up to touch the middle of the chest to the bar. |
| Diagonal cable woodchopper | 1 set high to low, 1 set low to high | 6 each side | Stand with feet hip-width apart and hips 90 degrees to the cable machine. Set the cable above head height. Hold the handle with arms straight. Rotate the trunk away from the weight stack, pulling the cable downwards and across the body. Reverse the direction to go low to high. |

## Stability Sessions

The stability sessions including sets and repetitions for weeks 5 through 8 are shown in table 11.6.

## Conditioning Sessions

Conditioning sessions in this block complement the higher intensity emphasis of the neuromuscular system training. They comprise short interval methods, with near maximal intensity workloads followed by short and incomplete recovery periods that stress the athlete's anaerobic glycolytic power and capacity as well as develop aerobic power through oxygen debt replenishment.

### Session 1: Off-Feet Conditioning

Concept 2 rowing ergometer: $10 \times 300$ metres with 30 seconds of recovery between repetitions or

Wattbike Pro: $10 \times 500$ metres with a 1:2 work-to-recovery ratio

### Session 2:

Running: $2 \times 8 \times 100$ metres with a 1:2 work-to-rest ratio and 3 minutes between sets

## Movement Skill Sessions

The movement skill drills in block 2 are the same as those in training block 1, but they are made more open as Stefanie becomes more

**Table 11.6**  Stability Training Sessions for Weeks 5 Through 8

| STABILITY SESSION 1 | | | |
|---|---|---|---|
| Exercise | Sets | Reps | Description |
| Single-foot drop and hold from 20- to 30-centimetre box | 3–5 | 5 each leg | Step off a box with trunk upright and ankles dorsiflexed in preparation for ground contact. Stick a single-footed landing, stabilizing the knee in alignment with the toes and distributing the weight through the midfoot. |
| Jump onto high box | 3 | 5 | Perform a two-footed take-off, landing two-footed in the middle of the highest box possible, depending on ability. Land in a stable position with sound hip, knee and ankle alignment. |
| Single-leg microhurdle hop and hold | 3–5 | 6 each leg | Perform a single-leg hop over 10 microhurdles, making sure that each landing is stable before the next hop. |
| Reverse lunge with bungee resistance | 3–5 | 6-8 each leg | Perform a deep body-weight reverse lunge. A resistance cord around the waist provides lateral resistance. |

| STABILITY SESSION 2 | | | |
|---|---|---|---|
| Exercise | Sets | Reps | Description |
| Single-leg arabesque with twist | 3 | 8 each leg | Stand on one leg with knee slightly bent but stiff and the ankle of the unsupported leg dorsiflexed. Reach the heel as far back as possible whilst leaning the trunk forwards and hinging at hips until the upper body and raised leg are parallel to the floor. Rotate the trunk and unsupported leg externally. |
| Cable reverse corkscrew | 3 | 8 each leg | Stand on one leg in front of a cable machine. Hold the cable in the hand opposite the standing leg. Pull the cable upwards and away from the machine until the arm is straight. |
| Single-leg stance tennis ball catch on trampet | 3–5 | 8-10 catches each leg | Stand on one leg on a trampet (a dynamic, unstable surface). Catch a tennis ball thrown by a partner or bounced off a wall. |
| Single-leg bridge | 3–5 | 10 each leg | Lie on your back. One knee is bent 90 degrees, and the foot is on the floor. The other leg is lifted. Perform a bridge, keeping the hips level and good alignment of the hip, knee and ankle of the working leg. |

| STABILITY SESSION 3 | | | |
|---|---|---|---|
| Exercise | Sets | Reps | Description |
| Round-the-clock lunge | 3 | 8 each leg | Keeping one foot grounded, perform a lunge forwards and then to the right, backwards, and to the left, returning to the middle position after each lunge. |
| Single-leg hexagon drill | 3 | 5–8 each leg | Mark a hexagon on the floor, approximately 1 metre across. Start in the middle of the hexagon, facing forwards. Hop outside the hexagon and back to the middle around each side in turn, landing correctly each time. |
| Single-leg Icky shuffle through agility ladder | 3–5 | 6–8 each leg | Start on one side of an agility ladder in a single-leg stance. Hop into the first square and then forward and diagonally out to the other side. Hop sideways into the next rung and then forward and diagonally out to the other side. Continue down the ladder. |
| Medicine ball drop-off | 3 | 10 | Get into a press-up position with both hands on top of a medicine ball. Drop both hands off the ball simultaneously, one to each side, and catch yourself on the floor. Immediately decelerate the trunk with no scapular winging or hitching. |

familiar with the movements and needs to be challenged through changing environmental conditions to ensure that learning continues. Stefanie performs the same drills as in block 1, but a ball is delivered to her and she returns the shot. Initially, each shot is performed in isolation so that movements remain as individual events that are not linked or sequenced.

# Training Block 3: Weeks 9 Through 12

Training block 3 is designed to bring together Stefanie's neuromuscular development and movement skills progressions into a mesocycle (4-week block) that will prepare her for tournament play. In such phases, training intensity typically increases and volume decreases, although this change will not be significant in Stefanie's case because learning (not necessarily the performance outcome) is still a key feature of her training. The application of strength and postural control into techniques and the integration of conditioning work into the court sessions are key features of this training block.

### Strength Sessions

Within this mesocycle (4-week block), the emphasis on power increases, as evidenced by the use of velocity-dependent exercises such as the clean pull variations, the single-arm dumbbell snatch and the push jerk exercises. The use of potentiation complexes, in which high force movements are followed by high power output, plyometric exercises, also reflects this change in objective. The strength sessions, sets and repetitions for weeks 9 through 12 are shown in table 11.7.

**Table 11.7**   Strength-Training Sessions for Weeks 9 Through 12

| STRENGTH SESSION 1 | | | |
|---|---|---|---|
| **Exercise** | **Sets** | **Reps** | **Description** |
| Clean pull combo (two clean pulls into clean from thigh is one rep) | 4 | 2 | Perform two clean pulls from the hang position. On the third repetition, perform a clean jerk from the hang position. After catching the bar on the shoulders, descend into a front squat and then return to standing. This sequence is one repetition. |
| Resisted overgrasp pull-up | 4 | 5 | Perform a pull-up with an external load suspended from a belt. |
| Loaded single-leg box squat | 3 | 5 each leg | Hold a barbell across the back of the shoulders. Stand on one leg. Perform a single-leg squat until your butt touches the top of a box. |
| Complex: 1. Alternate arm dumbbell incline bench press | 3 | 3 | Lie on an incline bench. Hold a dumbbell in each hand over the chest. Lower the dumbbells to the chest one at a time. |
| 2. Clap press-up | | 5 | Start in press-up position with hands slightly wider than shoulder-width and thumbs facing forwards. Perform an explosive press-up, pushing the body off the floor and clapping the hands together at the highest point. |
| Single-arm sliding plank | 2 sets each arm | 30 sec. | Start in plank position with weight disks under the hands. Slide one disk forwards and back for 30 seconds. Switch arms. |

*(continued)*

**Table 11.7** *(continued)*

| STRENGTH SESSION 2 | | | |
|---|---|---|---|
| **Exercise** | **Sets** | **Reps** | **Description** |
| Behind-the-neck push jerk | 4 | 5 | Stand with feet hip-width apart and a barbell behind the neck. Perform a rapid quarter squat and then drive up through the legs. As the bar leaves the shoulders, bend the knees. Finish with the arms straight, the bar above the crown of the head and the legs in quarter-squat position. |
| Complex: 1. Barbell loaded step-up | 4 | 4 each leg | Hold a barbell across the back of the neck. Step onto a stable surface and drive up. Bring the rear leg onto the step to join the lead leg. |
| 2. Cycled split-squat jump | | 6 | Start in a split stance. Perform a rapid countermovement and jump as high as possible. In midflight, switch leg positions and land in a split stance. |
| Stiff-legged deadlift | 4 | 5 | Hold a barbell in a clean grip against the thighs. Stand with feet hip-width apart, knees slightly flexed and weight through the midfoot. Initiate movement with the hips. Lean the trunk forwards and move the bar down the legs. |
| Lateral plank | 3 | 30 sec. each side | Lie on one side with the elbow directly under the shoulder and the forearm on the ground perpendicular to the line of the body. Lift the hips from the floor to create a straight line from the nose through the sternum, belly button and midpoint of the knees and ankles, legs together. |
| STRENGTH SESSION 3 | | | |
| **Exercise** | **Sets** | **Reps** | **Description** |
| Single-arm dumbbell snatch | 4 | 4 each arm | Hold a dumbbell in one hand. Stand with the trunk upright, hips and knees flexed and weight through the midfoot. Extend the hips, knees and ankles and pull and shrug. Keep the arm straight. At the top of the shrug, drop to catch the dumbbell in an overhead squat position. |
| Complex: 1. High-bar barbell back squat | 4 | 3 | Hold a bar across the back of the shoulders. Perform a squat. |
| 2. Maximal jump onto box | | 4 | Perform a two-footed take-off and land on two feet in the middle of the highest box possible, according to ability. |
| Single-arm cable row | 4 | 6 each arm | Stand in quarter-squat position at a cable machine with the cable set to shoulder height. Hold the handle in one hand with the arm straight. Pull the cable into the torso and return under control. |
| Reverse barbell lunge | 4 | 5 each leg | Hold a barbell across the back of the shoulders. Stand with feet together. Step one foot back far enough that the hip drops below the level of the front knee. |
| Medicine ball forehand and backhand throw and catch against wall | 3 | 5 each side | Stand 1 metre from a wall. Using a forehand or backhand stance, throw a medicine ball against the wall as hard as possible. Catch the rebound and repeat. |

### Stability Sessions

As table 11.8 reflects, Stefanie's progressive competence and dynamic postural control requires the stability work to focus more on dynamic postural control, in which stabilization is also challenged (and therefore developed) through increasing multidirectional (multiplanar) movements.

**Table 11.8**  Stability Training Sessions for Weeks 9 Through 12

| STABILITY SESSION 1 | | | |
|---|---|---|---|
| Exercise | Sets | Reps | Description |
| 20- to 30-centimetre drop jump into single-leg hold landing | 3 | 5 each leg | Step off the box. Contact the ground with an active flat-foot landing and then jump. Land on one foot and hold. Alternate the landing leg with each repetition. |
| Single-leg four-way microhurdle hop and hold | 3 | 8 each leg | Stand on one leg in the middle of a square of microhurdles. Facing forwards at all times, hop forwards over a hurdle, back to the middle of the square, over the next hurdle and back, continuing around the square. |
| High-box step-up | 3 | 8 each leg | The box should be high enough so that the knee of the lead foot is higher than the hip before the step. Begin with the foot on the box. Without pushing off the grounded foot, push through the heel of the lead foot and step up onto the box. |
| STABILITY SESSION 2 | | | |
| Exercise | Sets | Reps | Description |
| Crossover lunge | 3 | 8 each leg | Begin in athletic stance. Cross the right knee in front of the left knee, putting the foot flat on the ground. Lunge as deeply as possible. Return to standing and repeat to the other side. |
| Single-leg stance tug-of-war | 3 | 10–30 sec. | Stand on one leg holding one end of a rope. A partner holds the other end. The partner's goal is to pull you off balance. |
| Single-leg stance tennis ball throw and catch on bosu on trampet | 3–5 | 8–10 catches each leg | Stand on one leg on a bosu on top of a trampet. Maintaining balance on one leg, catch a tennis ball thrown by a partner or bounced off a wall. |
| STABILITY SESSION 3 | | | |
| Exercise | Sets | Reps | Description |
| Single-leg drop and hold from 20-centimetre box | 3 | 5 each leg | Step off the box and land on one foot. Hold the landing position. |
| Lateral microhurdle hop and hold | 3 | 6–8 each leg | Hop laterally over a microhurdle, stabilizing the landing on a flat foot. |
| Single-leg medicine ball throw and catch against wall | 4 | 5 each leg | Stand on one leg. Throw and catch a medicine ball against a wall. |
| Medicine ball rebounder | 3 | 10 each arm | Start with the arm at 90 degrees and the elbow bent. Internally rotate the humerus without horizontally adducting the shoulder and throw a medicine ball against a wall. Catch the rebound, externally rotating the arm. |

## Conditioning Sessions

The conditioning sessions now need to be tailored to the split demands of high-intensity tennis play. Top-level tennis is highly anaerobic and has low work-to-rest ratios; games may be long but the actual match play typically constitutes less than 25 per cent of overall match time.[2] Therefore, these sessions are designed to be low volume and high intensity. These sessions also typically stress the Type II motor units, thus complementing the work that is undertaken in the strengthening and movement skills components of the programme.

As the player approaches competition, the common practice is to taper the training volume so that the residual fatigue can dissipate before fitness gains are reversed, enabling the athlete to be well prepared for competitions. One means of reducing training volume whilst increasing training intensity towards competitive levels is to incorporate the conditioning into the tennis technical sessions. This approach enables total training volume to be reduced and enables the tennis practices to be of higher intensity. Such practices also allow Stefanie to incorporate all of her training improvements into highly intense and specific practices that begin to stress her newly developed movement skills under fatigue.

### Session 1: High-Intensity Shuttles

Set 1: 10 × 50-metre max pace starting every 30 seconds; 2 minutes of recovery

Set 2: 10 × 5-metre forward sprints, backpedal retreat to start, 10-metre sprint, turn and return to start, 20-metre sprint and return to start; 1:2 work-to-rest ratio; 2 minutes of recovery

Set 3: 20 × 10-metre sprints going every 10 seconds; 2 minutes of recovery

Set 4: 2 × 10 × 20 seconds of continuous maximal 10-metre shuttles, with sharp 180-degree turn at each end; 10 seconds of recovery between repetitions

### Session 2

Integrated into tennis session: 6 × 6 high-intensity rallies for 60 seconds or 15 shots with 20 seconds of recovery between rallies and 90 seconds of recovery after each block of 6 rallies

## Movement Skill Sessions

These sessions are designed to link shot sequences into series of on-court movement patterns that replicate typical patterns of play on different surfaces. Sessions may start with Stefanie linking mental and physical rehearsal as she plays imaginary shots with exaggerated footwork sequences, linking these through a 6- to 10-shot sequence. This sequence can be progressed to a series of fed balls at gradually increasing intensities that enable a more dynamic and reactive response to ball speed and placement whilst continually drilling and refining the particular emphasis of the movement patterns so that these are not lost as sequences become more complex.

These practices are truly sport specific and represent the highest level of integration between the athletic-conditioning and sport-specific aspects of the programme. Such drills and sessions cannot be developed without discussion with the tennis coach. Indeed, the tennis coach, with the involvement of the athletic development professional, typically delivers the sessions. This approach represents interdisciplinary practice and matches specialist skills to the needs of the athlete (athlete-centred coaching).

# Case Study 2: Soccer

Carly is a 19-year-old soccer player. She is in her first year of a full-time professional contract with a leading team in the English Women's Super League. At 177 centimetres tall, she is a central defender. As such, she is required to undertake sprints across the pitch to intercept balls into space or attacking players, run with the ball out of defence, sprint forwards to support attacking moves or intercept balls played into space, and turn and chase back when balls are put into spaces behind the defensive line. She is also expected to outjump attacking players and clear aerial balls hit into the defensive area.

Carly has been playing soccer for 8 years. She also played basketball for her school and played netball for her regional representative team during her school years. She has not had any formal training in terms of functional strength, speed or plyometric work outside the basic work her soccer coaches scheduled within sessions in the last few years. She doesn't have a history of injuries that would indicate particular weaknesses in her kinetic chain. The club has developed a dynamic movement profile on Carly, which included lunge and squat patterning, single-leg squats, repeated tuck jumps and double- and single-leg landings following a sagittal and frontal plane hurdle jump. These tests are reviewed in chapter 6.

Analysis of the profile suggests that Carly has a good level of functional motor control in unloaded body-weight movements, but a lack of strength in her hip and knee extensors may be limiting her movements in more dynamic actions. For example, she struggles to maintain hip and knee alignment during a flat-foot landing. Her landing is heavy and characterized by sinking of the hips because forces are absorbed over a longer period than desirable; she is not able to stick a landing effectively. Also, and a priority to correct, is a knee valgus that occurs from higher drop heights and is obvious on single-leg landings from low heights.

Carly achieved a distance of 1,724 metres in the yo-yo intermittent recovery test for aerobic endurance,[3] which demonstrates that she has a high level of aerobic fitness compared with players of a similar standard and position. In her speed test, she achieved 4.22 seconds for 25 metres, and she achieved a countermovement jump score of 38 centimetres. Her scores indicate that she lacks the basic force-producing capacities to achieve either horizontal or vertical force production, qualities important in achieving the technical requirements for her position, specifically being able to outjump attacking players to headers, achieve high accelerations over short distances and generally be physically robust in collisions.

Carly has a good tactical understanding of her role in the game, which has masked a lack of acceleration that, at the higher levels of performance, will limit her effectiveness. In particular, she is often exposed by balls played behind her (which force her to turn and chase) or when she is required to chase across the pitch to close down an attacker who is running into space following a counterattacking move.

Speed is an important asset to a central defender. Vescovi[4] found that defenders in elite-level female games were required to sprint (speeds in excess of 18 kilometres per hour, or 5 metres per second) for an average distance of 15.3 metres (with a large variation of plus or minus 9.4 metres), with maximum recorded speeds of 6.1 metres per second (21.9 kilometres per hour). In 2012, FIFA produced GPS information on the Women's World Cup, which showed that central defenders at the international level typically covered 10,160 metres in a game, performed three sprints per game in excess of 6.95 metres per second (25 kilometres per hour) and covered an average distance of 16.67 metres in this speed zone.[5] Similarly, they performed 18 sprints between 5.8 and 6.95 metres per second (21 to 25 kilometres per hour) over an average distance of 11.6 metres and 40 sprints between 5 and 5.8 metres per second (18 to 21 kilometres per hour) over an average distance of 8.4 metres. These data indicate that although speed is an important asset, the first few metres of acceleration are essential to the central defender because her high-speed actions occur over distances less than 12 metres. The key physio-mechanical quality that needs to be developed for acceleration is high levels of concentric force production in the hip and knee flexors and extensors. For a female athlete who has lower levels of testosterone bound to muscle receptors, the need to undertake strength training to increase both the neural and hormonal (growth hormone, IGF-1) responses to training to maximize the potential for force production is important.[6] Carly is using an oral contraceptive pill to regulate her monthly menstrual cycle, and therefore her strength training does not need to be manipulated to take this into account.

To obtain greater understanding of the specifics of how Carly moves on the pitch when turning and sprinting, high-speed video analysis was used as Carly performed the pro-agility test (figure 11.6). This test is self-started, so reactive speed isn't measured. The player accelerates 5 metres into a 180-degree turn, performs a 10-metre sprint into another 180-degree turn and then recrosses the start line, where the electronic gate measures the time. In this test, Carly achieved times of 5.4 seconds.

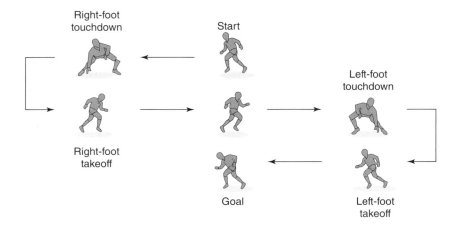

**Figure 11.6**   The pro-agility test measures turning and acceleration speed.

Qualitative analysis of the video sequences demonstrates that Carly has an inefficient turning action in the 180-degree turns, which identifies several areas for technical development. These elements include initiating movement in the desired direction of travel as she moves into the turn, keeping the arms close to the body as the turn begins (which reduces the rotational lever arm, thus decreasing the resistance) and ensuring that there is near full extension of the take-off leg. This action increases the velocity she can achieve in the first few strides by increasing the impulse that is applied over the longer period. Review chapters 4 and 8 for detailed reviews of these concepts.

Reaction and initial movement speed are important considerations in any dynamic acceleration in which players are responding to the game around them. In Carly's case, the coaches identified that her ability to read the play is not necessarily a limiting factor; she makes appropriate decisions based on what she sees in the game. Unfortunately, she is not currently physically adept enough to respond to these decisions rapidly enough at the top level.

Carly's coach is willing to invest in her long-term future as an important member of his plans for the club. He understands that enhancing her strength and postural control will significantly decrease her injury potential, making her more available for team selection in the long run. As a central defender who has skill, vision and ability to read the game, she will be a much more rounded player if she is faster and more agile. Therefore, the coach supports the individualized training designed for Carly. To build foundations in these priority areas, Carly will do less endurance training than her teammates, especially in the early stages of the preseason phase.

## Preparation Phase

As with all individual programmes within a team sport, Carly's athletic development programme for the preseason needs to be fully integrated into the team's preparation programme so that she can participate in all squad sessions with her teammates. As table 11.9 shows, the highest training volume loads can be found in the specific preparation phase, when monitoring of Carly's responses to training need to be carefully considered to prevent overtraining as both training volume and training intensity increase. Because the coach has been fully involved in the development of the physical aspects of the programme, he is aware that Carly may be fatigued and experience delayed onset muscle soreness (DOMS) entering the trial games. He is comfortable with this possibility at this period of the training year, as long as it does not carry over into the competitive season when she will be a key feature of his starting line-up.

**Table 11.9** Basic Phase Plan (Three Mesocycles) for Carly's Development Integrated Into Team Preparation

| Week | 1 | 2 | 3 | 4 | 5 | 6 | 7 | 8 | 9 | 10 |
|---|---|---|---|---|---|---|---|---|---|---|
| **MONTH** | **FEBRUARY** | | | | **MARCH** | | | | | **APRIL** |
| **Games** | Trial game | | | Trial game | | | Trial game | | | League |
| **Objective** | **General preparation** | | | **Specific preparation** | | | **Competition preparation** | | | **Competition** |
| Strength training | Strength conditioning, three sessions per week | | | Maximal force development, three sessions per week | | | Strength–speed development, two sessions per week | | | Strength–speed maintenance, as determined by playing schedule |
| Plyometric training | Landing technique and postural control, two sessions per week | | | Advancing landing technique and concentric vertical jumps, two sessions per week | | | Developing impulse: advancing landing technique and concentric jump into drop jump and repetitive actions, two sessions per week | | | Enhancing vertical impulse without producing DOMS, as determined by playing schedule |
| Speed and agility training | Technique development, linear acceleration mechanics and change-of-direction mechanics, two sessions per week | | | Mechanics development into linear force and acceleration out of change-of-direction, two sessions per week | | | Position-specific speed drills and applied practice scenarios, two sessions per week | | | Position-specific speed drills and applied practice scenarios, one or two sessions per week as determined by playing schedule |
| Endurance training | Extensive interval training, two sessions per week | | | Specific interval training, three sessions per week | | | Game conditioning, three sessions per week (integrated into technical sessions) | | | Maintenance drills within technical sessions |
| Technical training | Basic skills, three sessions per week | | | Individual, position and team technical preparation, three sessions per week | | | Team tactical preparation, four sessions per week and games | | | As determined by playing schedule |

Training in the general preparation phase is aimed at introducing Carly to the basic techniques that will underpin her long-term training for the next few months and years. Although the phase has a dual objective of general physical preparation (typically characterized by a high volume of work in most programmes), the emphasis here is on skill learning and progression. The nature of the workload reflects Carly's relative advanced general training age, whilst taking account of the fact that she has little or no specific training experience in formalized plyometric work and resistance training.

Carly is relatively new to being a fulltime athlete. The temptation is to move towards a training routine that has full training sessions for each aspect of training, but this approach would significantly and quickly increase the potential for overtraining. Therefore, recovery time between sessions is maximized. Training elements are combined so that, with effective planning, all aspects of training can be appropriately targeted. Sessions that are fatigue unresistant are done as early as possible within the training week or as soon after a recovery day as possible. When training sessions are integrated, velocity-dependent work is done at the start of the training session.

This plan is well illustrated in the general preparation phase, in which elements of speed, plyometrics and technical training are integrated into the same session to address specific aspects of work. To enhance long-term learning, the training programme is designed with the principles of random practice distribution (chapter 7) in mind, which can be seen in a typical week from this training block (table 11.10).

### Plyometrics Plus Speed and Agility Technique

The dynamic warm-up series is designed to achieve a number of key outcomes that ultimately prepare the athlete's body to take part in high-intensity activities. This time is also important for reinforcing core principles or patterns for movement mechanics, so it is an important time in which the coaches can establish a learning environment for the session. The speed sessions focus on the areas that Carly needs to improve, such as acceleration mechanics and direction change.

Dynamic warm-up and mobility exercises

Wall drill progressions (see chapter 8): 2 sets × 10 repetitions for each exercise

- Single-leg march
- Single-leg drive
- Two-step

Resisted-partner single-leg march: 4 sets × 10 metres

Jump circuit: perform the exercises in sequence × 3 sets; rest 60 to 90 seconds between sets

- Medicine ball maximum vertical throw × 5 repetitions
- Maximum vertical jump to head ball and stick landing × 8 repetitions
- In-place vertical jump with 180-degree twist midair × 8 repetitions
- Hands-on-hips maximum squat jump × 5 repetitions
- Horizontal jump and stick landing × 5 repetitions

40-metre ladder sprint (figure 11.7): emphasize running technique; 2 × 4; rest 60 seconds between repetitions; rest 2 minutes between sets

### Weights

The weight-training sessions are geared towards developing technique in the basic movements that will enable high force outputs in the hip and knee extensor muscles and those exercises that are important prerequisites for exercises that will be central to later stages of the programme. The weight-training programme (table 11.11) features multijoint, multimuscle compound movements through complete movement ranges, as described in chapter 10.

### Speed and Agility Technique

A specific warm-up (table 11.12) must be done to prepare the neuromuscular and musculoskeletal systems for the following session. Typically, a warm-up begins with low-intensity movement that raises core and muscular temperature and increases blood flow to the working muscles. The warm-up progresses through increasingly higher movement intensity, which includes basic practices such as

**Table 11.10** Typical Training Week for Carly

|  | Monday | Tuesday | Wednesday | Thursday | Friday | Saturday | Sunday |
|---|---|---|---|---|---|---|---|
| Session 1 | Plyometrics plus speed and agility technique | Weights | Recovery | Plyometrics plus weights | Speed and agility technique plus technical session | Weights | Recovery |
| Session 2 | Technical session | Endurance: extensive intervals |  | Technical session | | Endurance: extensive intervals |  |

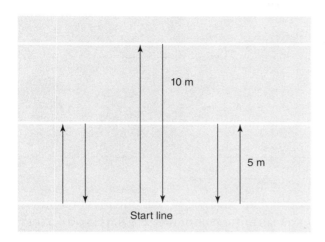

**Figure 11.7** 40-metre ladder sprint.

working through full ranges of movement and incorporating mobilization exercises that stretch muscles and connective tissue throughout the kinetic chain. Activating the neuromuscular system through actions that prepare the body for the following activities is also important. Similarly, incorporating activities that stimulate other sensory mechanisms such as proprioception is also typically beneficial. Each warm-up should finish with some high-speed or explosive actions to potentiate the neuromuscular system for the session to follow.

**Table 11.11** Weight-Training Session

| Exercise | Sets | Reps | Recovery between sets |
|---|---|---|---|
| Clean pull from thigh | 4 | 5 | 3 min. |
| Trap bar deadlift | 4 | 8 | 3 min. |
| Single-leg ball wall squat | 4 | 10 each leg | 2 min. |
| Stiff-legged deadlift | 4 | 10 | 2 min. |
| Stir the pot | 3 | 30 sec. | 60 sec. |

**Table 11.12** Dynamic Warm-Up in Preparation for a Multidirectional Speed and Soccer Session

| Exercise | Description |
|---|---|
| Inside knee boxing | Stand in athletic stance at arm's length from another player. On 'Go', try to slap the inside of your partner's knee whilst moving your feet to prevent your partner from slapping your knee. |
| Walking hamstrings | Step one leg forward with the leg straight and toes dorsiflexed. Keeping the back straight, reach down to touch as close to the ankle of the lead leg as possible. Hold for 0.5 seconds, return to standing and repeat with the other leg. |
| Knee grab | Stand tall. Lift one knee to the chest and reach the arms around the shin. Pull the knee as high and tight to the chest as possible. Hold for 0.5 seconds. Release the leg and repeat on the other leg. |
| Knee grab into kick-out | Perform the knee grab. Instead of releasing from the top position, kick out through the fingers so that the leg goes straight in front of the body. Return to standing and repeat on the other leg. |
| Open the gate | Place the hands behind the head so that the elbows point sideways. Step forward with the right foot. Lift the leg in a forwards rotational movement so that the knee comes up to touch the elbow, which shouldn't drop. Step the left leg in front of the right and repeat. |
| Close the gate | Place the hands behind the head so that the elbows point sideways. Step backward with the right foot. Lift the leg in a backwards rotational movement so that the knee comes up to touch the elbow, which shouldn't drop. Step the left leg behind the right and repeat. |

*(continued)*

**Table 11.12**   *(continued)*

| Exercise | Description |
|---|---|
| Kick-out with raised arms | Stand tall and lift the arms fully above the head. Keeping the knees extended and ankles dorsiflexed, march forwards, kicking the straight leg as high as possible with each step. |
| Squat step | Begin in a half squat. Lift the left foot off the floor and plant it as far away as possible, with the foot facing forwards. Lean onto the foot as much as possible before bringing the right leg in to resume the squat. Alternate sides. |
| Frontal leg swing | Stand on one leg sideways to a wall. Swing the straight leg front to back. |
| Sagittal leg swing | Stand on one leg facing a wall. Swing the straight leg out to the side and back across in front of the body. The foot faces forwards at all times. |
| Trail leg windmill forwards | Stand on one leg sideways to a wall. Bend the knee and rotate the hip to bring the outside foot from back to front, as if lifting the leg over a hurdle. |
| Trail leg windmill backwards | Stand on one leg sideways to a wall. Bend the knee and rotate the hip to bring the outside foot from front to back, as if lifting the leg over a hurdle. |
| Carioca | Stand sideways to the direction of travel. Bring one leg across in front of the body, step to the side, bring the leg behind the body and step to the side. Continue for 20 to 30 centimetres and then reverse direction. |
| Lunge and twist | Perform a forward lunge with hands behind the head. At the bottom of the lunge, rotate the trunk and look over the lead leg. Return to standing and repeat on the other leg |
| Reverse warrior lunge | Perform a wide reverse lunge, reaching the leg back as far as possible without the knee touching the floor. At the bottom of the lunge, reach up with the arms and rotate the trunk toward the forward leg. Hold for 5 seconds, return to the starting position and repeat on the other leg. |
| Scorpion | Lie facedown on the floor with arms outstretched, palms down and legs straight. Reach the left heel over to touch the right hand. Return to the starting position and repeat to the other side. |
| 30-metre build-up | Accelerate from a standing start. Each subsequent build-up should be faster and more maximal. |
| Side slide | Sideways skip for 30 metres with hands swinging across the body. Every two skips, turn into the direction of travel and continue. |
| 30-metre build-up | |
| Mountain climber with rotation | Begin in press-up position. Bring the left foot forward so that it is outside the left hand. Reach the right hand up to the ceiling, rotating through the trunk. Hold for 1 or 2 seconds, return to start and repeat on the other side. |
| 30-metre build-up | |
| Alternating burpees | Begin in press-up position. Bring both feet forward so that the heels land beside the hands. Jump as high as possible. Land and return to the press-up position. Bring both feet forward so that the heels land inside the hands and jump. |
| 30-metre acceleration | |

Following the warm-up, the session moves to simple drills to practice acceleration technique and coordination over a 25-minute period before the technical session based on the concepts of pass and move into space. The basis of these skills is detailed in chapter 8. Complete recovery between repetitions and sets is an important feature of this high-quality work.

Ankling: 4 × 10 metres with walk-back recovery

Double-foot bounce: 4 × 10 metres with walk-back recovery

Single-foot bounce: 4 × 10 metres with walk-back recovery

Single-leg A-skip: 4 × 10 metres each leg with walk-back recovery

Change-of-direction square (figure 11.8): 2 × 4 reps

Rolling accelerations: 5 metres for movement development transition into 10 metres of maximal acceleration: 2 × 6

- Lateral shuffle × 2 each side
- Backpedal × 2

### Extensive Intervals

This session is designed to prepare Carly for high-intensity work and develop an aerobic base through the replenishment of an oxygen debt incurred through near maximal (high-intensity) work in excess of 80 per cent of maximum speed. This session is a precursor for the development of anaerobic work and a basis for maintaining quality work under fatigue. The distances are representative of a length of a typical soccer pitch, and the total distance equates to about 50 per cent of that travelled in a game, although the high-speed running distances will exceed those in a typical game for a central defender. Such work is also complementary to the overall objectives of the programme, as highlighted earlier in the case study. The principle that objectives determine

methods needs to be at the heart of all programme design and delivery.

Dynamic warm-up

Speed technique drills

2 × 40-metre build-up accelerations with walk-back recovery

10 × 60 metres starting every 45 seconds (target time 11 to 13 seconds)

2-minute recovery

10 × 60+40 metres with 60-second walking recovery between reps: 60 metres at 80 per cent, 40 metres at maximal sprint

2-minute recovery

10 × 40 metres at 80 per cent, 30-metre cruise, 30-metre maximal sprint; course must be covered in 20 seconds at most; 60-second slow recovery jog between efforts

2-minute recovery

3 × 60-second efforts (run as far as possible in 60 seconds) with 3 minutes between efforts

Cool-down

## Specific Preparation

During times of heavy volume loading, the need to preserve active recovery time is a priority. Without time for recovery, no adaptation can occur, and gradually the performance potential or training status of the athlete will decrease significantly as overtraining (or underrecovery!) is reached. During such times, little learning is typically achieved, performances can be severely impaired, and the risk of a serious injury or recurrent bouts of less severe injuries increases.

Rather than plan whole training sessions dedicated to specific aspects of performance, the ability to plan training units (small subsections of a whole session) that can be effectively integrated becomes important if all the work required is to be achieved. When undertaking such planning, understanding the physiological requirements for both optimum training status and recovery from training stimuli is important. This speed and power training should be delivered, when possible, before strength sessions, and strength sessions should be delivered before endurance work (table 11.13).

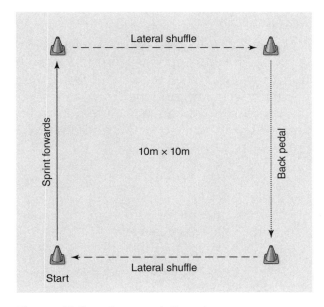

**Figure 11.8**  Change-of-direction square.

**Table 11.13** Microcycle for Specific Preparation Phase

|  | Monday | Tuesday | Wednesday | Thursday | Friday | Saturday | Sunday |
|---|---|---|---|---|---|---|---|
| Session 1 | Plyometrics and weights | Change-of-direction into linear acceleration | Recovery | Plyometrics | Acceleration | Weights | Recovery |
| Session 2 | Technical session | Specific endurance and technical session |  | Weights | Specific endurance and technical session | Endurance |  |

The question might then be asked why, in the week shown in table 11.13, the acceleration sessions are not the first sessions after recovery. Although that sequencing may be ideal, it would leave a scenario in which weight-training sessions occur on simultaneous days. Optimal recovery from demanding neuromuscular and musculoskeletal work takes 24 to 48 hours. Therefore, not doing this work on consecutive days is seen to be beneficial. Equally, the plyometric and weight-training components can be deemed complementary, especially when used as contrast or complex potentiation methods (chapter 9). Therefore, where appropriate, these elements were integrated into the schedule shown in table 11.13.

Similarly, the highest volume running sessions (when the endurance work was integrated into the technical and tactical work) ideally should not be preceded by weight training, because of the potential for structural fatigue loading (damage to the muscles and connective tissue at a microfibre level) on one day to be excessive. With low acceleration work volumes and power production largely through concentric muscle actions, this was deemed a better pairing of training sessions for one day. Compromise is required, however, and the respective time on the feet for each aspect is reduced compared with what might have been planned for any session occurring in isolation.

But this compromise isn't necessarily contraindicated to achievement. Indeed, the strength-training aspects of the training have significant opportunity to potentiate for improvements in plyometric performance.

Although much of the current literature suggests that for this to be wholly successful, training loads need to be within 90 per cent of one-repetition maximum (1RM), which tends to be determined in athletes who are highly experienced in such training modalities.

Similar benefits can possibly be achieved in less experienced athletes working to challenge their neuromuscular systems working within their level of competence. Similarly, maximal vertical jump efforts can also potentiate for enhancements in strength exercises based on powerful hip and knee extension.

### Plyometrics and Weights

The plyometrics and weights exercises, sets, repetitions and recovery durations are shown in table 11.14.

### Directional Change Into Linear Acceleration

This speed-training session encourages Carly to transition into maximal linear acceleration from different directions of movement or foot placement positions. The following is the sample speed-training session in a specific preparation phase. The emphasis is on directional change into linear acceleration.

Dynamic warm-up

Technique drills

- Double-foot bounce 3 × 10-metre course with walk-back recovery
- Single-leg deadleg with A-skip 3 × 20-metre course on each leg with walk-back recovery

**Table 11.14**   Plyometrics and Weights With an Emphasis on Muscular Strength and Neuromuscular Power

| Exercise | Sets | Reps | Recovery between sets | Description |
|---|---|---|---|---|
| Maximal jump onto box | 4 | 3 | 90 sec. | Perform a two-footed take-off and land on two feet in the middle of the highest box possible, according to ability. |
| Clean pull from thigh | 4 | 5 | 3 min. | Stand with feet hip-width apart, knees flexed, trunk upright, bar at mid-thigh and weight distributed midfoot. Perform a clean pull, extending the hips, knees and ankles to lift the bar rapidly and shift weight onto the toes. Shrug at the top of the movement so that the bar rises in front of the body. |
| Complex: 1. High-bar barbell back squat | 4 | 5 | 60 sec. between squat and jump; 3 min. between sets | Hold the bar across the top of the back. Perform a squat. |
| 2. Cycled split-squat jump | | 10 | | Start in a split stance. Perform a rapid countermovement and jump as high as possible. In midflight, switch leg positions. Land in a split stance. |
| Complex: 1. Single-leg barbell box half squat | 3 | 5 each leg | 30 sec. between half squat and push-off; 2 min. between sets | Hold the barbell across the back of the shoulders. Stand on one leg. Perform a single-leg squat until the butt touches the box. The box should be high enough that you are in a half squat at the bottom position. |
| 2. Lateral leg push-off | | 4 each leg | | Start with one foot on a 20- to 30-centimetre box and the other foot on the floor. Push off from the box, jumping sideways across the box. As you land on the other side, push off and return to the other side. |
| Modified razor curl | 4 | 8 | 2 min. | Kneel. Have a partner hold your ankles or place a bar across them to keep your feet still. Place a band around your trunk to support you as you extend the trunk and assist you as you return to the start position. Lower the trunk so that it is parallel to the floor. Extend the hips and push the trunk forward. Keep the shoulders above the hips. |
| Single-arm sliding plank | 2 | 60 sec. (30 sec. each arm) | 60 sec. | Start in plank position with weight disks under the hands. Slide one disk forwards and back for 30 seconds. Switch arms. |

- Straight-leg skip into step-over run 3 × 30-metre course on each leg with walk-back recovery
- Lateral deadleg with high ankle over hurdles × 6 into hip turn and build-up for 20 metres × 3 each leg with walk-back recovery

Partner chase and face, 20-metre course: 2 × 4 with complete recovery between repetitions, 3-minute recovery between sets

Backwards and forwards (figure 11.9): 2 × 4 with complete recovery between repetitions, 3-minute recovery between sets

Lateral ladder and sprint (figure 11.10): 2 × 4 with complete recovery between repetitions, 3-minute recovery between sets

Rolling start (figure 11.11): 1 × 6 with complete recovery between repetitions

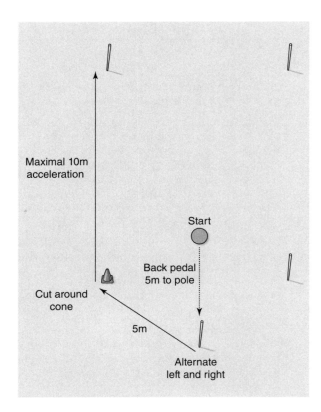

**Figure 11.9** Backwards and forwards.

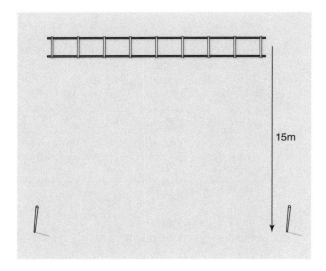

**Figure 11.10** Lateral ladder and sprint.

Agility ladders may be overrated as a tool for developing movement skills; the resultant movement patterns are neither naturally nor typically posturally correct. Even so, they have become popular tools across a range of sports. One purpose of agility ladders that is functional is multidirectional single-foot work. In the

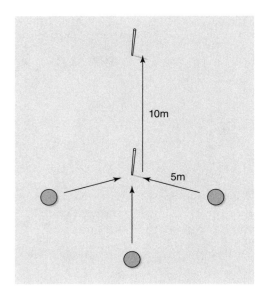

**Figure 11.11** Rolling start.

lateral ladder and sprint drill, Carly must use the side of the foot (inside or outside depending on the foot placement relative to the direction of travel) to produce ground reaction forces to cause lateral movement. At the same time, she is required to maintain a level hip position and hip–knee alignment with each landing and take-off in the single-leg stance.

Carly is still at the associative stages of learning. Therefore, only singular transitions should occur between the direction changes. Highly complex and multivaried changes of direction probably will not enable her to focus on doing the basics well and improve her technique. She should focus on being able to do things on purpose and with purpose. Complex changes of direction also are not specific to the demands of her position, which typically require her to sprint for relatively short distances following a rolling acceleration and with a singular directional change.

For these drills to be successful in enhancing performance, the direction change mechanics need to be well rehearsed and the linear accelerations need to be forceful and executed with maximal speed for the whole distance of the sprint. Video feedback may be useful in aiding understanding of how she performs the techniques relative to the technical model for acceleration (chapter 8). This feedback can be provided to her during rest breaks if the technology is available.

## Acceleration

The emphasis of this session is to maximize the development of acceleration by developing the mechanics of Carly's technique and her ability to apply forces through the technique. Short hill sprints are ideal to incorporate into the week. A gravity-resisted activity, short hill sprints enable the athlete to focus on applying greater forces into the ground in the support phase, appropriately positioning the shin to direct these forces optimally and repositioning the unsupported leg for the next stride more effectively against the rising gradient.

6 × 15-metre accelerations up a 5-degree incline.

1:6 work-to-rest ratio between reps.

3-minute active recovery.

6 × 20-metre accelerations up a 5-degree incline.

3-minute active recovery.

6 × 10-metre accelerations up a 5-degree incline.

3-minute active recovery.

6 × 15-metre accelerations up a 5-degree incline.

## Specific Endurance and Technical Session

This session (figure 11.12) needs to integrate elements of high-intensity (although not maximal) running with some specific technical elements of the game so that endurance work is completed with the player having to demonstrate specific skills under increasing fatigue. This training unit (component of the session) is a 30-minute practice that comes at the end of the training session so that quality work can be undertaken at the start without fatigue.

One repetition is one completion of the entire course. Perform 6 × 4 with a 1:3 work-to-rest ratio.

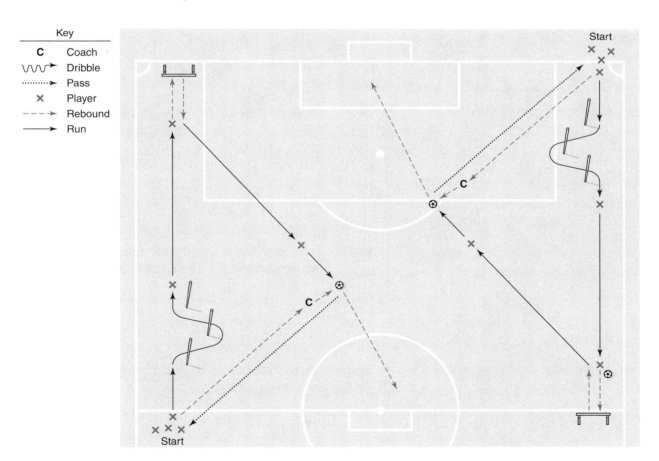

**Figure 11.12**    High-intensity running soccer-specific interval session.

Run 10 metres to collect ball.

Dribble ball through poles.

Turn and pass ball back to start.

Run 30 metres to collect ball.

Play 1-2 against rebound board.

Play long ball to coach at C.

Follow pass.

Collect served ball from coach at X and either head for distance or chip a pass into net.

Run back to start to complete one rep.

## Competition Preparation

During this period (table 11.15), the emphasis for the programme shifts towards prioritizing technical and tactical aspects of training. This shift is reflected not only in the reduced training volume and increased training intensity but also in the order in which training sessions are undertaken. For example, plyometric speed sessions would normally be undertaken when the player was freshest. But in the world of professional team sports, and in a contact sport like soccer, the need for players to be unfatigued for important pitch sessions at times overrides other training elements within the programme.

### Plyometrics and Weights

As can be seen in table 11.16, Carly has progressed in her jumping control to intermediate-level activities. The balance of exercises selected for plyometrics reflects both her needs and the game demand. They include single-leg exercises, double-leg vertical movements and multidirectional jumping and landing. The exercises have been predominantly arranged as complexes, so the explosive exercise set follows the heavy resistance set that has a similar neuromechanical patterning.

The spectrum of exercises covers the full range of the force–velocity curve, and the highest velocity resistance exercise comes first in the session. Carly is still relatively young in resistance-training age, so the session design reflects the basic nature of the work she needs to do. Athletes with greater training age may anticipate doing sets with much higher relative loads (for example, three repetitions) or drop sets (reduce resistive loads in the final set to maximize bar velocity).

More complex exercise sequences may also be considered, such as the reverse lunge into step-up in an advanced athlete. Such exercises, however, do not reflect Carly's needs or capabilities at this time. Such work is possible to plan, but Carly needs to develop the basics of functional strength over a longer term before such strategies become necessary.

### Acceleration

The acceleration session is intense but low in volume, because Carly has a team conditioning session following this session in a couple of hours. The sled drill forces Carly to push maximally through leg extension to overcome the external resistance from the sled. The session uses a complexing system in which unresisted efforts follow resisted ones to potentiate through the neuromuscular system's recruitment of motor units in response to heavier loads.

Dynamic warm-up

Technique drills

- Wall sprint two-step
- Double-foot bounce
- Single-leg deadleg with A-skip
- Single-leg deadlift with single-leg straight-leg skip

**Table 11.15** Training Microcycle for the Competition Preparation Phase

|  | Monday | Tuesday | Wednesday | Thursday | Friday | Saturday | Sunday |
|---|---|---|---|---|---|---|---|
| Session 1 | Technical session | Acceleration | Plyometrics and weights | Recovery | Direction change into linear acceleration and technical session | Trial game | Recovery |
| Session 2 | Plyometrics and weights | Technical session, and game-specific conditioning | Technical session |  |  |  |  |

**Table 11.16** Plyometrics and Weights With an Emphasis on Muscular Strength and Neuromuscular Power

| Exercise | Sets | Reps | Recovery | Description |
|---|---|---|---|---|
| Complex:<br>1. Snatch from thigh | 3 | 5 | 60 sec. between snatch and hexagon drill; 3 min. between sets | Start in jump position at start of second pull. Hold the bar in snatch grip where the legs and trunk meet. Perform an explosive snatch, catching the bar in an overhead squat position. |
| 2. Single-leg hexagon drill | | 5 per leg | | Mark a hexagon on the floor, approximately 1 metre across. Stand in the middle of the hexagon, facing forwards. Hop outside the hexagon and back to the middle around each side. Repeat on the other leg. |
| Complex:<br>1. High-bar barbell back squat | 4 | 5 | 60 sec. between squat and jump; 3 min. between sets | Hold the bar across the top of the back. Perform a squat. |
| 2. Maximal jump onto box | | 3 | | Perform a two-footed take-off and land on two feet in the middle of the highest box possible, according to ability. |
| Complex:<br>1. Barbell step-up with leg drive | 3 | 4 each leg | 30 sec. between step-up and tuck jump; 2 min. between sets | Step up onto a stable surface. Push down through the lead leg to drive upwards. As the rear leg leaves the floor and you drive towards standing, pull the rear leg forward until the knee is parallel to the floor and you balance on one leg. |
| 2. Single-leg tuck jump | | 4 each leg | | Stand on one leg. Perform a rapid quarter squat and then hop as high as possible. Bring knees to the chest in the air and land on one or both feet. |
| Nordic hamstring curl | 4 | 6 | 2 min. | Kneel with a restraint around your ankles (a partner or a bar). Maintaining alignment of the knees, hips and shoulders, lean the trunk forward under control. Continue until you cannot maintain eccentric control. Return to the start position by using the hamstrings to pull yourself back up or press up into the start position. |
| Short-lever roll-out | 2 | 5 to 10 (quality determines reps) | 60 sec. | Kneel and hold a barbell with the hands shoulder-width apart and arms straight. Maintaining a straight line from hips to knees and shoulders, roll the barbell away from the body as far as possible and return to start. |

- Up tall and fall into 5-, 10- and 15-metre acceleration

Sled acceleration: 3 × 4+1 unresisted 15-metre acceleration; complete recovery between repetitions; 3- to 4-minute recovery between sets

Rolling start race (race against partner with 3- to 5-metre rolling start): 3 × 10 metres; 3 × 15 metres; complete recovery between repetitions; 3- to 4-minute recovery between sets

### Technical Session With Game-Specific Conditioning

The conditioning session is specific to soccer. Small-sided games (see figure 11.13) are designed to maximize player involvement. The space is appropriately measured to optimize space and high-intensity movement. Athlete-tracking modalities usually indicate that within match preparation training programmes, players are more likely to produce quality movement patterns at higher intensity levels when involved in small-sided games. These games have the added benefit of integrating technical and tactical skills in a pressured environment, so the session can address a number of key objectives of the specific preparation phase.

### Small-Sided Games (Figure 11.13)

Two teams of eight players start at different cones. On the whistle, they sprint into a 30- by 30-metre grid.

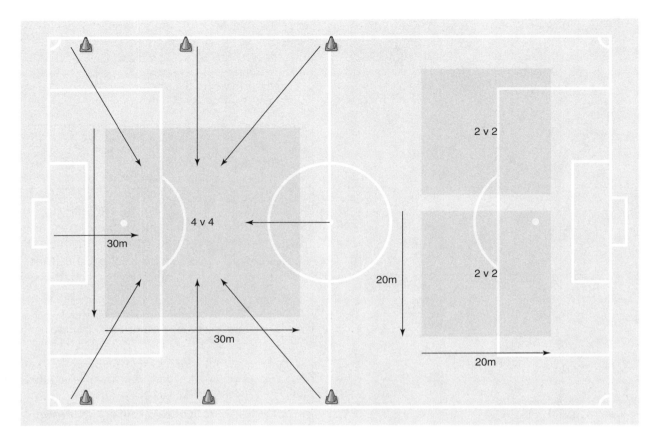

**Figure 11.13** A small-sided games conditioning session provides sport-specific endurance benefits whilst integrating technical and tactical skills.

4v4 game: 4 × 4-minute games with 90-second rest between games, 2-minute rest between sets

2v2 game: 8 × 2-minute games with rotating teams, 90-second rest between games, 2-minute rest between sets

6 × 50-metre sprints going every 30 seconds

Carly will have multiple opportunities to practice change-of-direction and acceleration mechanics during small-sided games, so the games relate to her ongoing training. Small-sided games are also far more enjoyable for players than more traditional forms of endurance training. Therefore, players who have undertaken a foundational period of conditioning can benefit from appropriately planned and conditioned games to refine sport-specific levels of endurance.

### Change of Direction Into Linear Acceleration

This session precedes a technical session and therefore needs to be relatively low volume and high intensity. The session should also prepare Carly for the session to follow. The drills are designed to integrate position-specific movement patterns and skills as much as possible.

Dynamic warm-up

Crazy ball games

- 21s: Throw the ball. Earn 1 point for every bounce. Catch the ball before it rolls. If the ball rolls, all points are lost. First player to 21 points wins.
- Count and catch: Partner throws the ball and calls a number between 1 and 4. Stay close to the bouncing ball and catch it after the called number of bounces.

Turn and burn (figure 11.14): 2 × 6 (alternate sides), complete recovery between repetitions, 3-minute recovery between sets

Clear and close (figure 11.15): 2 × 6, complete recovery between repetitions, 3-minute recovery between sets

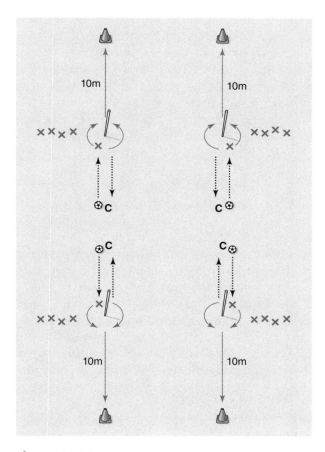

**Figure 11.14**  Turn and burn.

The session commences with crazy ball drills. These partner activities are upbeat and fun. The players play games with a crazy ball to develop foot speed and postural mechanics in response to the stimulus provided by the movement of the ball. Agility drills need to have aspects of reaction and decision making to be considered truly functional, and these competitive tasks are highly appropriate for this task. They also challenge the player to maintain appropriate foot contact with the ground; when constantly changing direction in response to the chaotic bounce of the crazy ball, the athlete must have an appropriate weight distribution through the midfoot whilst having the heel off the floor.

The drills that follow the crazy ball work integrate several aspects Carly has been working on throughout the programme into soccer-specific movement practices that are open and require her to make effective decisions. For example, she times a forward acceleration into a jump to head the ball and then lands, turns and accelerates to intercept a player in response to a fed ball. This drill combines elements of different starting stimuli and positions with directional change and linear acceleration. Controlling or optimizing speed as the player closes the defender is also an element that the clear and close practice (figure 11.15) encourages.

These drills are highly adaptable in nature. For example, the turn and burn practice (figure 11.14) can be altered in how the player moves over the initial 10 metres; for example, side

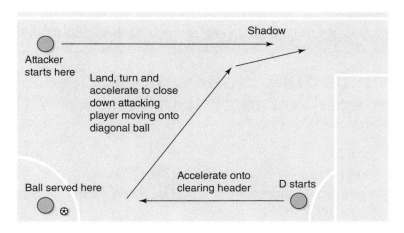

**Figure 11.15**  Clear and close.

shuffle, backpedal, side shuffle into hip turn and sprint can be incorporated into this practice. Similarly, how and when the ball is fed can be altered, and a responsive player can be substituted for the dummy so that the peel and turn move becomes more realistic and pressured by time, space and the need for quality execution.

# Case Study 3: Multisport Academy

For years, Sam has worked as a strength and conditioning coach for many sport teams within a geographical area. He works across a broad spectrum of ages and within a number of sports. Over time, Sam realized he was seeing problems in the athletic abilities of senior players that often were the result of a lack of appropriate development at lower levels in the players' development pathway.

As he observed to a baseball coach,

At adult levels, I should be providing a fitness service that is like the icing on the cake. It should be sophisticated and make the final 5 per cent difference. But in some instances the cake hasn't yet been properly baked. Athletes are at only 60 per cent of their capacity. We need a programme in which the early developmental stages of training and good coaching can have significant effect on helping athletes achieve their potential further along their career pathway.

Sam noted he could see a trend of movement pattern dysfunctions that occurred in later teenage and adult athletes across a spectrum of sporting arenas. He met with a number of senior officials from the basketball, volleyball, soccer, American football, baseball, hockey and track clubs he worked with recently and shared that he saw far too many athletes with habitual movement dysfunctions (typically developed through poor movement mechanics and postural control patterns that were not coached out of the athlete) associated with tightness around the hip, lumbar–pelvic and thoracic regions. These are described in the sidebar Typical Posture Problems Associated With Movement Dysfunction in Teenage Athletes.

Sam presented a compelling and strategic need for a multisport programme (the 'athlete academy') to be a specific component of the regional athlete and player development pathway. This programme would provide a managed and integrated physical curriculum for generic movement and athlete development (running, jumping, conditioning and resistance-training skills and experience) so that players leaving the programme would be suitably prepared for higher performance. Talent and potential could be developed, nurtured and retained within sport. The academy would reduce the high drop rate that typifies many high-performance programmes when athletes' physical competencies do not enable them to maximize their potential or interest for further participation.

# Typical Posture Problems Associated With Movement Dysfunction in Teenage Athletes

Tight Achilles tendon

Tight and dominant hip flexors (poorly developed and tight hamstrings)

Overly strong quadriceps muscles compared with hamstrings

Poorly recruited gluteal muscles (lateral hip control, anterior–posterior pelvic tilt)

Tight thoracic spine

Tight anterior shoulders

To support his proposal to develop this multisport programme, Sam sampled a range of athletes in a simple movement skills analysis day. This assessment day was put together with the aid of an athletic trainer–physiotherapist who assisted with some joint stability and range-of-motion tests such as the star excursion test, modified Thomas test for knee stability, the slump test for range of movement and other joint-specific tests. Standing postural assessment was done with a range of other basic movement screening processes. These evaluations were designed to provide an effective battery of assessment processes that could provide easily interpretable information for the practitioner to feed back to the athlete through a specific action plan. Comprehensive information on screening of this type can be found in chapter 6.

# SQUAT ASSESSMENT

### Start Position
Stand with feet shoulder-width apart and feet facing forward. Initially, place hands to the sides of the head with elbows pointing laterally. Then progress to arms overhead with elbows extended.

### Technique
Lower into a squat position as far as possible while under control.

### Checkpoints
Heels must stay in contact with the floor at all times.

The athlete maintains lumbar lordosis through the full range. Watch for pivoting at the lumbosacral and lumbothoracic junction.

Knees are aligned over second toes. Watch for overpronation, knee moving medially and hip rotating medially.

Ascent and descent should be fluid and continuous.

The player is observed through the following continuum unless competency compromised:
- Squat to parallel (90-degree knee flexion)
- Full squat (hips below the level of the knee)
- Squat to parallel (90-degree knee flexion) with arms overhead
- Full squat with arms overhead

# IN-LINE LUNGE ASSESSMENT

### Start Position
Stand.

### Technique
Place the hands beside the head with elbows flexed and pointing laterally. Step forward with the lead thigh parallel to the floor. Keeping the head and chest up, place the lead foot on the floor with the front knee over the front foot. The back knee touches the ground immediately behind the heel of the front foot. Hold for 2 seconds and then push back to standing. Repeat on the other leg.

*(continued)*

### In-Line Lunge Assessment *(continued)*

#### Checkpoints

Knee remains in line with second toe, and hips are square. The trunk retains lumbar and thoracic integrity.

The player is observed through the following continuum unless competency compromised:

- Front leg to 90 degrees and back knee to ground
- Front leg to 90 degrees, back knee to ground and return to standing
- Level 2 plus rotation over front leg

---

# LINEAR AND LATERAL JUMP OR HOP OVER SMALL HURDLE ASSESSMENT

### Start position

Stand with feet hip-width apart and arms relaxed by sides.

### Technique

Jump or hop in the prescribed direction over four minihurdles and stick the landings.

### Checkpoints

The athlete maintains hip, knee and ankle alignment on landing. Hips are square, and trunk is stable with no loss of lumbar or thoracic integrity. The landing is quiet on a flat foot.

Player is observed through the following continuum unless competency compromised:

- Two-foot jump, two-foot land
- Two-foot jump, one-foot land
- One-foot jump, one-foot land
- One-foot hop with hip drive to 90 degrees, one-foot land

---

# SINGLE-LEG DIP ASSESSMENT

### Start Position

Stand with feet shoulder-width apart before going into a single-leg stand. Arms are relaxed by sides.

### Technique

Maintaining flat-foot contact, perform three single-leg dips under control. Repeat on the other leg.

### Checkpoints

The athlete's knee remains in line with the second toe, and the hips are square.

Spinal alignment is maintained. No drop into anterior pelvic tilt or lumbar spine extension occurs.

Foot position is maintained. No overpronation or early eversion occurs.

Pelvis stays level. No dropping occurs to the left or right.

Shoulders and trunk are in line with the lower body. Control is constant and consistent throughout the movement.

The player achieves the following:

- Dip to 60 degrees
- Dip to 90 degrees
- Dip to 120 degrees
- Full pistol squat

# PRESS-UP ASSESSMENT

## Start Position

See description for each level.

## Technique

Maintain a straight-line position through a full press-up—elbows fully extended to elbows fully flexed, chest to 7.5 centimetres from the floor.

## Checkpoints

Shoulders stay in neutral. No hitching occurs with trapezius.

Scapulae stay in neutral. No winging occurs.

Thoracic and lumbar spine stays in correct alignment.

Pelvis is maintained in neutral throughout the movement. No anterior tilt and no dropping to one side occur.

The player is observed through the following continuum unless competency compromised:

- Wall press with feet placed away from the wall 1.5 times the distance of the tibial tuberosity to the floor, hands shoulder-width apart, forehead dipped to wall
- Inclined press-up on plinth or table
- Inclined push-up on 20-centimetre block
- Floor push-up
- Decline floor push-up (feet on 20-centimetre block)

# FOUR-POINT KNEELING

## Start Position

Begin on all fours with feet hip-width apart and knees under hips. Hands should be shoulder-width apart and aligned under shoulders. Weight should be evenly distributed throughout the four points of contact.

## Technique

Perform the following sequence. The aim is to maintain a level shoulder and hip position, with no change in lumbar–pelvic orientation and no obvious weight redistribution during the movement.

Level 1: Lift one arm until it points forwards and is aligned with the trunk. Hold and return to the start position. Repeat with the other arm.

*(continued)*

## Four-Point Kneeling *(continued)*

Level 2: Lift one leg until it is extended behind the body and the shoulders, hips, knees and ankles are aligned. Hold and return to the start position. Repeat with the other leg.

Level 3: Lift one arm and one leg on opposite sides.

Level 4: Lift one arm and one leg on the same side.

### Checkpoints

Shoulders and hips stay level and in alignment.

No rotation occurs through the trunk.

No extension of the trunk occurs; the athlete does not drop in lumbar or thoracic extension as the limb is lifted.

Pelvis stays level and neutral; no dropping occurs to either side or into anterior tilt.

No hitching or winging of the scapula occurs.

---

Based on their performances in the tests, Sam and the physiotherapist were able to present a profiling document to the athletes that provided feedback and recommendations for progression in terms of future improvements to athletic performance. An example of this feedback is shown in the sidebar.

With the evidence that the programme had a need and could provide valuable benefits to the athletic development of a range of athletes, Sam received the backing of the specific sport programmes to establish his athlete academy and bring his plan to life. His training facility and programming were designed to enable athletes of similar ages and from different sports to come together and improve through achieving a number of objectives displayed clearly within his facility:

### Athlete Academy Objectives

- Develop the athlete's movement competencies through progressive learning practices.

- Develop the athlete's postural control and related functional strength through progressive learning practices.

- Develop a training aptitude in athletes through commitment to a delivered programme in a development environment.

# Sample Athlete Profile

### (Athlete name): Observations and Recommendations

(Athlete) has tightness of his soleus, quads and hamstrings. He should work on both a dynamic and static mobility programme for the muscles around the hips, knees and ankles.

(Athlete) demonstrated poor movement range and control in the squat test and single-knee dip. This deficiency may be correlated with his very tight soleus, quads and hamstrings. He needs to develop, under guidance and with feedback, lumbar spine and knee control during single- and double-leg squatting movements.

He also demonstrated poor eccentric scapula control in the press-up test and lumbar–pelvic control in the four-point kneeling. He should undertake a range of scapula control and rotator cuff strengthening exercises, as well as trunk progressions and gluteus maximus and medius exercises for improved pelvic control.

To ensure the quality of the delivered programme, group sizes were limited to the point where there was one coach per 12 athletes. Any effective athlete development system is built on the foundations laid in previous programmes. Many of the athletes entering the athlete academy at the U14 level will be having their first experience of an organized and well-coached strength and conditioning programme. The academy needs to deliver and build on the key foundation areas relating to neuromuscular, musculoskeletal and bioenergetic system development. The programmes progress from generic, athletic, movement-competence based delivery at the earlier stages to performance-focused stages of the age-related curriculum, which also reflect more sport-specific needs.

Sam is also keen that the programme reflects a progressive philosophy whereby the athlete isn't working to get better simply for the here and now. He wants athletes to be physically prepared for the transitions that await them as they progress through high school and club systems. Therefore, the academy needs to prepare them for high school sports demands when they are still in the final year of elementary school. They will be physically able to cope with the increased training and performance demands when they make the change across the school system.

Note that age ranges are only indicative; athletes who attend the academy can be channelled into higher or lower age-range programmes depending on their competences and experiences. Because the academy serves athletes in multiple sports, all athletes can be suitably challenged and there isn't a social need to retain players within specific year groups.

## Foundations Programme

The aim of the foundations programme is to provide athletes a solid foundation in mobility and stability. This base will enable them to achieve the full ranges of movement around the joints and begin to demonstrate awareness of and the ability to control body positioning in a range of movements. The programme progresses to include aspects of speed mechanics

drills as well as aspects of nonspecific conditioning that enable the athletes to develop the basis for working to and under conditions of fatigue.

Typically, the athletes in this programme are 12 to 14 years old, early in the adolescent stages of development. Female athletes tend to have gone through puberty by this stage, so the training sessions are gender specific. For females, the practices can focus on some of the associated developmental issues, including hip, knee and ankle alignment in dynamic activities as highlighted in chapters 3, 5, 9 and 10. Similarly, the early maturing males will also have gone through puberty. To distinguish the early maturing athletes from those in normal patterns, standing height and sitting height are recorded to monitor progression through periods of accelerated skeletal growth.

Athletes who have gone through puberty and are sufficiently competent in the movement challenges of the programme are quickly advanced to later stages of the progression or moved to the next level to benefit from the increased strength work. This approach enables the athletes to benefit maximally from the high levels of anabolic and androgenic hormones in their bodies. Strength training, however, is prioritized only with appropriate consideration of mobility, stability and postural control.

As discussed in chapter 3, athletes at this stage of development typically experience periods of awkwardness in executing skilled movement because of their accelerated periods of skeletal growth and changes in their neuromuscular systems. Therefore, the focus of this programme is skill mastery using an individualized (differentiated) approach to task setting for each athlete.

Table 11.17 illustrates a typical sequence of eight sessions, identifying the training objective and activities within each session. The programme, which children typically attend once or twice a week for 40-minute sessions, begins with blocked practice that focuses on specific areas of work to ensure early learning of basic positions and skills. This pattern is repeated when new skills (for example, speed mechanics drills) are introduced. Following this, the progressions work on a random distribution of training units designed to foster long-term learning within the young athlete.

The idea of developing a training ethos is further emphasized by giving each athlete simple work-on tasks or homework. These assignments may be simple static stretches that target areas of specific and individualized tightness or exercises with targets that the athlete works towards. These tasks and goals are established by practitioners who monitor the athlete's involvement in and competence at set tasks, using these as an ongoing screening process to supplement the regular screens (three times per year) undertaken with all athletes.

The warm-up is themed so that it uses training movements previously learned to activate and potentiate the neuromuscular system and mobilize joints for the following session. As with all well-structured warm-ups, it begins with low-intensity activities and gradually increases in both intensity and movement complexity through dynamic movements that progress towards the first activity of the session. See the example of session 1.

**Foundations Programme Session 1**

Warm-up (10 minutes)
- Pulse raiser: piggy in the middle (in fours); tennis ball underarm passing, no contact, intercept a pass or change middle person every 10 throws

- Walking on heels and exaggerated toe-offs, both with arms swinging
- 10 × sprint start hamstring stretches
- 10 × single-leg mountain climbers
- Hindu press-up × 10
- Roll-up to roll-out × 10
- Knee to elbow crucifix × 10

Hip mobility (10 minutes)
- Overhead lunge with suspension cable
- Buddha prayer squat
- Hip rotation on all fours: From crab position, elevate hips and externally rotate so that one knee comes down towards the floor laterally and then medially without the feet moving
- Lateral and medial knee patterning from squat: From deep squat position, take one knee backwards and laterally and then bring it forward and medially to touch the floor. Ankle will roll medially as this happens

Double-foot jumps (10 minutes)
- Double-foot jumps with quick ground contact over 10-metre course × 4
- Double-foot jumps off and onto a low step; 5 jumps × 4 reps

Conditioning games: gym assault course (figure 11.16); race in pairs or timed competitions.

**Table 11.17**   Foundations Programme: Eight-Session Block

| Session 1 | Session 2 | Session 3 | Session 4 | Session 5 | Session 6 | Session 7 | Session 8 |
|---|---|---|---|---|---|---|---|
| Warm-up | Warm-up | Warm-up | Warm-up | Warm-up | Warm-up | Warm-up | Warm-up |
| Hip mobility | Ankle mobility and stability | Hip mobility | Thoracic mobility | Ankle, knee, hip, lumbar spine: mobility and movement disassociation tasks | Jump for height and distance | Hip mobility | Thoracic mobility |
| Jump: double-foot ground contact | Running mechanics | Hip and knee extension strength | Jump: landing mechanics | Climbing and upper-body pulling actions | Running: movement speed | Running mechanics | Jump: double-foot ground contact |
| Conditioning games | Postural stability | Change-of-direction mechanics | Total-body power: medicine ball throws | Conditioning circuits | Change-of-direction: evasion games | Postural stability | Conditioning games |

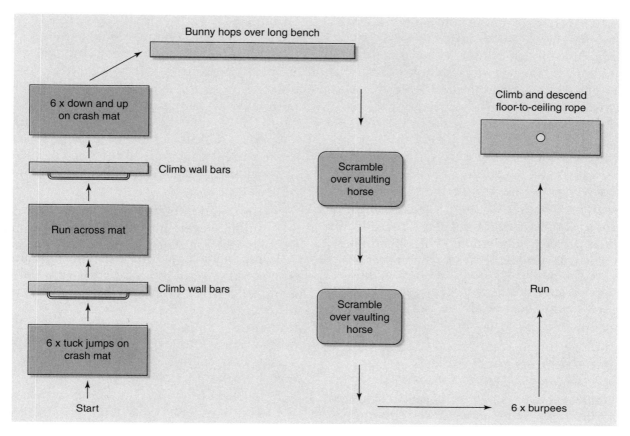

**Figure 11.16**  Gym assault course.

The hip mobility work is based on hands and feet being in contact with the floor and the knee being the focus of the movement. This is possible only with the femur rotating within the ball-and-socket joint at the hip. These movements use a range of active and passive mechanisms to target some of the key areas of mobility that have been identified as high risk among teenage athletes. Some of these activities, such as the overhead lunge, require muscular control as a combination of gravity and a fixation at the hands, and they stretch the athlete's posture. Others require active muscular control to initiate and progress movement (for example, the hip rotation movements in the squat and crab positions). The Buddha stretch, a more passive activity, is a static stretch against resistance.

The jump activities are linear and simplistic, and they focus on achieving an active ground contact with ankle stiffness. They can also take place within a small space, so the equipment

for the conditioning unit within the session can be set up before the session begins. Athletes perform a series of total-body movement challenges that involve a range of actions that are high intensity and typically either high force or high velocity. The overall duration of the work efforts isn't long, and the athlete can choose the rest and recovery intervals between the obstacles. These combined factors mean that prepubertal athletes who are not able to work anaerobically shouldn't have issues of undue stress (see chapter 3).

The competitive element of this activity should be enhanced by the appropriate pairing of athletes to complete the task as a race. Staggered starts can be used so that a number of workstations have athletes progressing through them at the same time. Teamwork is encouraged by having athletes form teams and recording the total time for team completion. Although often controversial, climbing activities over wall bars or up ropes are safe activities when appropriate instruction, supervision and attention to detail are provided. Evidence does not support judging these as high-risk activities, and the inclusion of this equipment in a training facility might be considered advantageous by practitioners.

When the equipment is laid out in formats such as this, the obstacle courses can be turned into games such as off-ground tag for variation. The athletes all run around and can be tagged only when they are in contact with the floor. But they can stay on an obstacle for only a defined (maximum) time, so they need to think strategically about where they will move next. Speed, agility and total-body strength, as well as endurance within these qualities, are required to do well in games such as this. Besides being beneficial, the games are a fun and enjoyable way to end a session.

## Transitions Programme

This programme (table 11.18) aims to build on foundations to prepare the 14-year-old athlete to transition to high school sports. The emphasis remains on movement qualities, but the emphasis on forceful expression within these techniques increases. Similarly, the athlete must master basic functional strength-training movements, some of them under load. With most athletes now being postpubertal, the levels of absolute strength, power and speed between the sexes is growing. Indeed, loading (or exercise performance indicators) is now an increasing consideration. The athlete is encouraged to lift heavier, run faster and jump higher or longer, as long as doing so does not compromise execution of the technique.

The sessions are programmed with fewer training units and more focus on a specific (although typically not exclusive) objective. At this stage, the athlete should be well coordinated and able to demonstrate sound kinetic sequencing during most basic loaded or ballistic movements such as running and jumping. Nevertheless, practitioners are encouraged to emphasise correct joint positioning throughout all movements and not allow movement compensations. The focus is still on postural control and enhancement of the neuromuscular system. Functional hypertrophy is considered a by-product of effective training mechanisms and associated hormonal and genetic influences, rather than a specific aim of the programme at this level. Cellular hypertrophy (discussed in chapter 2) is not a deliberate focus of any work undertaken.

Practitioners deliver movements within the progressive warm-up that were featured as focus exercises in previous training programmes. In the warm-up, the focus is on hip and thoracic mobility with specific activation emphasis on the extensor musculature through the rear kinetic chain. This warm-up leads nicely into the strength technique session, which has the target of developing force through full ranges of movement in the hip extensors whilst maintaining thoracic extension.

**Table 11.18**   Transitions Programme Block

| Session 1 | Session 2 | Session 3 | Session 4 | Session 5 | Session 6 | Session 7 | Session 8 |
|---|---|---|---|---|---|---|---|
| Warm-up | Warm-up | Warm-up | Warm-up | Warm-up | Warm-up | Warm-up | Warm-up |
| Jump: vertical | Running mechanics: linear acceleration | Change-of-direction mechanics | Jump: landing mechanics into drop jumps | Strength technique training | Change-of-direction: evasion technique | Strength-training technique | Jump: low-hurdle plyometric double-foot jump sequences |
| Strength technique training | Conditioning circuits | Strength-training technique | Reaction and decision making into multidirectional acceleration | Conditioning circuits | Lateral jumping and landing technique | Conditioning games | Acceleration into maximal speed |

## Transitions Programme Session 5

Warm-up (10 minutes)

- Pulse raiser: stuck in the mud, a game of tag in which a tagged person has to stand still and be freed by a teammate ducking under the tagged person's outstretched arms
- 10-metre walk on heels into 10-metre exaggerated toe-offs, both with arms swinging
- Reverse Nordics × 10
- Lateral and medial knee rolls from squat × 10: from a deep squat position, take one knee backwards and laterally and then bring it forward and medially to touch the floor. Ankle will roll medially as this happens
- Walking lunge with straight-arm rotation × 10
- Straight-leg hurdle clear with arms raised × 10
- Scorpions × 10

Strength technique and training (25 minutes) with emphasis on hip extensors and maintaining thoracic extension

- Overhead medicine ball walking lunge 1–3 × 8
- Trap bar deadlift 1–3 × 6
- Deep squat into dumbbell push press 1–3 × 5
- Lateral cable woodchopper with split stance 1–3 × 6 each side

Strength–endurance circuit (15 minutes): Work in pairs in which one works and one provides manual resistance or assistance as required. Then swap roles. Transition between the exercises as quickly as possible. Rest for 60 seconds between sets and complete 2 to 4 sets.

- Prowler sled push and sprint × 2
- Partner resisted press-up × 8
- Partner supported supine row × 8
- Springboks × 5
- Round the world × 1

Within this session, each exercise can be easily regressed or progressed depending on the specific limitations or needs of the athlete. For example, if the athlete is not sufficiently mobile through the shoulders to hold a medicine ball overhead when lunging, a dowel can be used or the arms can be held behind the head. If an athlete has known left–right imbalances that may be masked in the trap bar deadlift, then a suitcase deadlift (in which a kettlebell is held in one hand and the other hand is empty as the athlete performs a deadlift movement from the floor to standing and back again, maintaining level hip and shoulder heights) can be prescribed.

The strength unit should be limited to 10 sets of work, the balance of which can be adjusted among the various exercises to achieve the desired balance for an athlete. For example, someone requiring more global strength may do more sets of the deadlift, whereas someone who needs more control through the trunk into overhead movements may do more repetitions of the deep squat into dumbbell overhead press. Obviously, the loads can be adjusted within these movements to match individual abilities. Taking 1 or 2 minutes of rest between the exercises enables the athlete to achieve the appropriate recovery for each exercise and complete the session within the designated time.

The idea behind the conditioning circuits is to follow the strength-training theme by using some total-body strength exercises to develop endurance by performing repetitions under fatigue. Most of the exercises use body weight, so athletes need to be paired with someone of a similar mass and strength. Besides working the athlete under fatigue, with self-paced recoveries, the session requires athletes to work together and communicate when tired to achieve the set task.

As with all sessions, the number of sets and repetitions per exercise can be modified according to individual abilities. The same can be said for the applied resistance For example, a reasonably strong athlete may want resistance during both the lowering and raising phases of the press-up, a less able athlete may want them only during the raising phase (i.e., no eccentric overload), and some may not need any external resistance at all from their partner.

Similarly, in the supine row, the resistive mass pulled through the arms can be adjusted through bending or lengthening the legs to adjust the position of the centre of mass and the relative lever arm of the body. Achieving fun, force development and fatigue in 15 minutes makes this an ideal means of completing the session for children of this age.

## Training Progressions Programme

This programme supplements the increasingly specialized training that athletes are undertaking at this stage of their sporting development. Programmes are multifaceted so that the athlete can tailor training options to suit the nature of his or her preferred sport and individual needs. This programme places greater emphasis on specific and individualized session objectives, rather than integration of training units within sessions.

As outlined in chapter 3, at this stage of development, athletes' aerobic systems can be trained for maximum output. This goal is best attained through multiple ultrashort, high-intensity intervals and game-related activities. This approach ensures that the development of endurance capacities complements the strength, power and speed work undertaken at this time. Developmentally, a normally maturing child at this age will have a fully mature anaerobic system, so a full spectrum of energy system training should be implemented. Therefore, high-intensity training and short- and long-interval training methods should be used.

Practitioners working with athletes in the academy structure must be aware of how to deal with issues relating to weight gain and its effect on body shape. The difference between lean body mass and fat mass needs to be made clear to athletes, and all issues relating to body image must be handled sensitively. This topic may include issues relating to the need for or avoidance of muscular hypertrophy and issues relating to aesthetics, appearance and the balance between an athletic lifestyle and other aspects of social development important to teenagers of both genders.

Twelve to 18 months after the end of the growth spurt for males and at the end of the growth spurt for females, strength training can be optimized to improve overall strength development. The emphasis is on neuromuscular training focussed on high force, high power output, multijoint resistance and jumping activities. For example, athletes will be developing high-quality Olympic weightlifting techniques from the foundations of partial movements learned previously (or continuing to progress from the previous phase if they have not mastered the foundations). They will progress with this training modality as individual development continues.

The young athletes now have their first opportunity to experience emphasis loading within the training progressions. This type of training has been identified as an ideal means of introducing the young athlete to the basics of periodization (i.e., emphasizing specific aspects of the curriculum at different stages of the training cycle). The academy programme becomes increasingly more flexible because athletes in different school sports require different things at different stages of the year. This aspect is reflected in the overall programme descriptors shown in table 11.19.

The athlete and coach identify how the programme can be structured. For example, an athlete may want to spend 8 weeks working on strength development, 4 weeks working on power, 4 weeks working on speed and 4 weeks working on endurance before revisiting strength. Another athlete may want to focus more time on endurance. Besides progressing specific athletic capacities, the athlete is learning important lessons about progressing with a planned programme.

The first of these is that emphasizing a physical quality does not mean focusing exclusively on this component. For example, in focusing on functional strength, it is typically important not to neglect complementary aspects of speed work. After all, strength becomes expressed as speed in many sports, so athletes cannot get too far away from speed at any time.

Second, variation in a training emphasis will lead to enhancements in performance

**Table 11.19** Overall Training Progressions Programme

| | IDENTIFIED TRAINING NEED OR EMPHASIS FOR THE ATHLETE | | | |
|---|---|---|---|---|
| Emphasis | Strength training | Power | Speed | Endurance |
| Strength-training sessions per week | 3–4 | 3 | 2–3 | 2 |
| Speed and agility sessions per week | 0.5 | 1–2 | 2.5 | 1 |
| Plyometric sessions per week | 0 | 1–2 | 1.5 | 1 |
| Conditioning sessions per week | 0.5 | 0.5 | 0 | 3 |

if the appropriate focus is given to a training objective. As identified in chapter 7, achieving a balance between repetition of a stimulus to provide learning and variation in the stimulus to reinforce learning and enable adaption is important. Planned unpredictability within a long-term training and learning programme is important as well.[7]

Third, the athlete comes to realize that certain athletic qualities have prerequisites. To become stronger, the athlete needs to be able to position his or her posture dynamically. To develop power, he or she first has to become stronger. To develop speed, the athlete first needs to be powerful. Remember that within the parameters of the programmed session, the prescription needs to be individualized based on the competencies of the individual athlete.

Although endurance may seem to be given less priority than the other training elements within this scheme of work, many sport-specific training elements will have aspects of endurance within them, as reflected in table 11.20.

Table 11.21 provides more detail for the jumping school session.

Using a menu or modularized approach to training progression in this way enables an exercise theme to be adapted to increasingly individualized needs. Athletes with increased postural control needs can be guided towards appropriate sessions and exercises within the relevant exercise streams (as identified in chapter 10, for example). Similarly, athletes who need to focus on basic landing mechanics

before progressing to more advanced jumping sequences can be appropriately directed to the specific sessions.

# Performance Programme

At 16 years old, many athletes are specialized within sport-specific programmes. This focus may happen much earlier in sports regarded as early specialization sports, such as swimming and gymnastics. The athlete academy programme enables sport-specific programmes to be introduced at this level, following a sound grounding in the basics of athletic movement skills and functional strength development that has progressed through a number of competency stages. This process also allows athletes to revisit exercise progressions to reinforce previous learning of certain movement qualities to ensure that they remain autonomous.

## Steven the Swimmer

Steven is a swimmer who specializes in freestyle. He attends the academy three sessions per week for his land-based conditioning. His major objective is related to the ability to maintain intra- and intermuscular forces in his postural muscles so that he can maintain a horizontal position within the water. Swimming is unusual in this respect; locomotive forces are based not on ground reactions, but on the pull exerted from the arms and the push exerted by the legs against a fluid resistance to enable movement of the streamlined posture through the water.

**Table 11.20**    Training Progressions Programme: Sessions 1 Through 4

| | Session 1 | Session 2 | Session 3 | Session 4 |
|---|---|---|---|---|
| Jumping school: session themes within a training block | Single-leg techniques | Multidirectional jumping | Vertical propulsion: medicine ball and ballistic exercises | Enhancing reactive ground contact |
| Strength training: training multijoint movements, not muscles, across the session themes within a training block | Hang clean 2 × 5<br>Front squat into push press 2 × 5<br>Parallel bar dips 2 × 6<br>Bent-over row 2 × 5<br>Plank progressions<br>Hanging short-lever hip raises | Snatch from thigh 2 × 5<br>Back squat 2 × 5<br>Stiff-legged deadlift 2 × 6<br>Handstand push-up 2 × 5<br>Supine row 2 × 8<br>Candlestick progressions (reverse curl, vertical leg shoots, candlestick variations)<br>Medicine ball rotational throws | Clean grip first pull 2 × 5<br>Single-leg squat 2 × 5 (each leg)<br>Reverse lunge 2 × 5<br>Rope climbs × 4<br>Glute-ham raise progressions<br>Kneeling diagonal plate chops | Snatch and clean grip pulls from thigh 2 × 5<br>Overhead squat 2 × 6<br>Pull-up 2 × 5<br>Standing DB alternating-arm shoulder press 2 × 5<br>Rotational trunk: windscreen wipers progressions<br>Jackknife progressions (short lever, long lever, resisted) |
| Speed and agility: session themes within a training block | Linear acceleration | Chaotic agility: reactions and decision making, acceleration, deceleration, change-of-direction, reacceleration | Maximum velocity mechanics and expression | Chaotic agility: reactions and decision making, acceleration, deceleration, change-of-direction, reacceleration |
| Conditioning: session themes within a training block | Off-feet intervals:<br>Example: rowing 10 × 300 metres maximal efforts with 40 sec. recovery | Running intensive interval training | Conditioning circuits:<br>Example: 10 stations of total-body exercises<br>6 × 30 sec. work, 15 sec. on each station, 1 min. in between | Extensive interval training (running, cycling, rowing) |

**Table 11.21**    Jumping School: Single-Leg and Weight Transfer Session

| Exercise | Sets | Reps | Recovery |
|---|---|---|---|
| Right-leg hop (10% stride length) | 3 | 10 | 2 min. active |
| Left-leg hop (10% stride length) | 3 | 10 | 2 min. active |
| Bound (60–80% maximal bound) | 3 | 10 | 3 min. active |
| Alternate hop and bound (max effort) | 4 | 6 | 4 min. active |

That said, a secondary objective is to be able to generate ground reaction forces so that forceful starts and turns can be executed. Steven needs to maximize these key opportunities to generate horizontal propulsion within a race. Steven's programme is shown in table 11.22.

### Mike the American Football Player

Mike is a promising running back in his high school football programme. He weighs 80 kilograms but needs to work on his strength, acceleration and agility. He has a 7-year training history in American football and has been working in an athletic development programme for the last 3 years, so he is technically competent with most basic techniques.

As a running back, Mike needs to be able to achieve rapid accelerations from a low standing start and change direction efficiently. He also needs to be able to explode into the defender's upper body from a low position when blocking for his teammates. His major objectives in the weight room are related to the need to develop high forces in minimal time and increase his power-to-weight ratio. Mike also needs to be technically competent in a full range of weight-room techniques so that he can execute exercises competently when coaches prescribe them later in his athletic career. His speed and agility work is divided between linear acceleration work, change of direction into three-step acceleration patterns and positional patterning movements.

Mike trains four days a week (see table 11.23) at the athlete academy, working in

**Table 11.22** Performance Programme for Swimming Land-Based Training

| Session 1 | Session 2 | Session 3 |
|---|---|---|
| Clean pull from floor 4 × 4 | Behind-the-neck push press 4 × 5 | Front squat 4 × 5 |
| Overhead squat 4 × 8 | Walking overhead lunge 4 × 10 | Rings: muscle-up to support 4 × 8 (quality determines rep range) |
| Handstand pendulum, 5 sec. hold 4 × 6 (3 each arm) | Weighted pull-up 4 × 5 | Medicine ball slam from isometric glute-ham raise 4 × 15 |
| Bent-over alternate arm cable fly 4 × 5 each arm | Medicine ball medial and lateral rebound throw 4 × 8 each arm | Kneeling cable four-ways 3 × 8 each arm |
| Bench pull 4 × 8 | Weighted hip extension from bridge 4 × 8 | Candlestick 4 × 10 |
| Barbell rollout 4 × 10 | Cable reverse corkscrew 3 × 8 each side | |

**Table 11.23 Performance Programme for Running Back Power Development**

| Monday | Tuesday | Thursday | Friday |
|---|---|---|---|
| Speed: directional change | | Speed: linear acceleration | Speed |
| Dynamic warm-up | | Warm-up: technique drills | Dynamic warm-up |
| Drills<br>Side shuffle into linear sprint 1 × 6<br>Inside-foot cut into linear sprint 1 × 6<br>Outside-foot cut into linear sprint 1 × 6<br>Agility pole weave 1 × 6<br>5-10-5 pro-agility line touch 1 × 6 | | Drills<br>Accelerations with sled for 40 metres, 2 resisted (10 kilograms), 2 unresisted, complete recovery between sets | Drills<br>Patterned running 3 × 10, random variations |
| Strength training<br>Clean 4 × 3<br>Weighted press-up 4 × 5<br>Flow-board side lunge 4 × 6 each side<br>Bent-over row 4 × 5<br>Cable woodchopper 3 × 5 each side<br>Candlestick 3 × 10 | Strength training<br>Split jerk 4 × 4 (alternating lead leg)<br>Back squat 5 × 5<br>Weighted pull-up 4 × 5<br>Stiff-legged deadlift 4 × 5<br>Suspended windscreen wiper 2 × 10 | | Strength training<br>Snatch grip pull from thigh 4 × 4<br>Bench press 4 × 4<br>Complex medicine ball push-up and throw<br>Single-leg pistol squat 4 × 5<br>Straight-leg barbell sleeve lift 4 × 3 each side<br>Landmine 3 × 5 each side |

the weight room for three sessions and doing three speed sessions in a typical week. During the season (August to October) and the play-off and state championship period (October to December), Mike trains four days per week and plays in games on Fridays. The rest of the year he plays a variety of sports as part of his overall athletic development, but he is able to train for his long-term improvement without having to taper training for games. The running drills from Mike's programme are shown in figure 11.17.

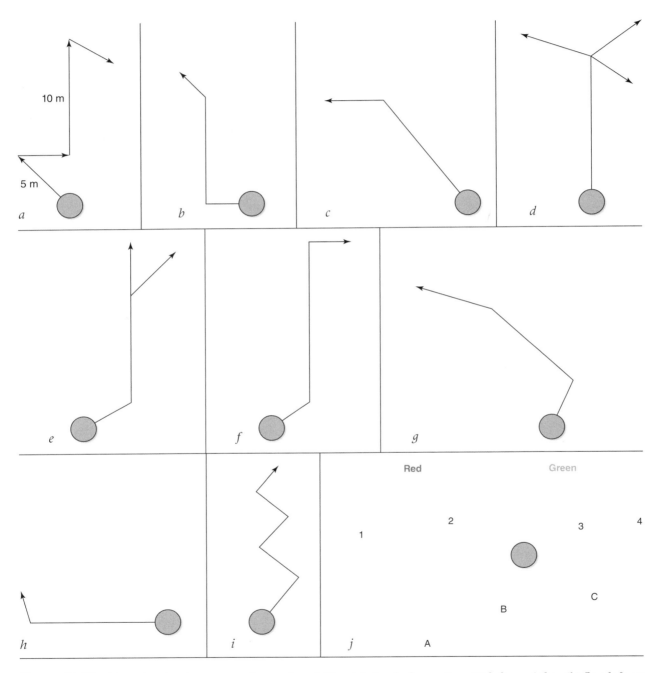

**Figure 11.17**   Running back patterned running drills: *(a)* check down 5 or 10 left or right; *(b)* flag left or right; *(c)* flat left or right; *(d)* options left or right; *(e)* seam left or right; *(f)* out left or right; *(g)* sneak left or right; *(h)* swing left or right; *(i)* zigzag run left or right; *(j)* sequence left or right.

### Dynamic Warm-Up (Monday) for Speed and Direction Change Session

Front lunge × 5, back lunge × 5 and then 20-metre stride (half effort)

Gallop right leg lead

Wide-out × 5 and then 20-metre stride (half effort)

Gallop left leg lead

Single-leg donkey kick × 8 (each leg) and then 20-metre stride (half effort)

20-metre side slide with arm swing turn-in back

Squat thrust alternating heels outside hands, heels inside hands × 10 and then 20-metre stride (half effort)

20-metre side slide with arm swing turn-out back

Single-leg mountain climbers × 10 and then 20-metre stride (three-quarters effort)

Side-lying abductor raise × 5, side-lying adductor raise × 5 each leg

Quadruped hip abduction × 5

Quadruped knee circle forwards and backwards × 5

Scorpion stretch × 10

Single-leg glute bridge × 5 each leg

Supine single-leg hamstring isolated stretch × 10 each leg

Sprint start calf stretch × 10

Horizontal scissors × 5 into rockers to inside hurdle seat stretch × 4 each side

20-metre low walk and then 20-metre low walk backwards

20-metre forwards skip and scoop and then 20-metres backwards skip and scoop

# Summary

This chapter illustrated a fundamental principle of coaching movement skills in an athlete development programme. The objectives of the programme determine the methods used to achieve them. In each case, the athlete is at the centre of the programming considerations, not the needs of the coach or other programme demands.

In reviewing each case study, you should be able to identify key themes and features from previous chapters. All the methods are scientifically based, and an integrated approach is used for programme delivery. In each case, movement skills are improved through a balanced approach to enhancing technique, improving postural control and being able to control and transfer forces. All this is based on a balanced progression that builds from generic movement skill training to sport-specific delivery, based on the athlete's need for challenge to his or her competency. Programmes reflect all the training principles that are central to the development of athletic movement quality.

# References

## Chapter 1

1. Stone, M.H., M. Stone, and W.A. Sands. 2007. *Principles of resistance training.* Champaign, IL: Human Kinetics.

2. Bompa, T.O., and G.G. Haff. 2009. *Periodization: Theory and methodology of training.* 5th ed. Champaign, IL: Human Kinetics.

3. Siff, M.C. 2003. *Supertraining.* 5th ed. Denver, CO: Supertraining Institute.

4. Gallahue, D.L., and F.L. Donnelly. 2003. *Developmental physical education for all children.* 4th ed. Champaign, IL: Human Kinetics.

5. Abbott, A., D. Collins, K. Sowerby, and R. Martindale. 2007. *Developing the potential of young people in sport.* A report for sportscotland by the University of Edinburgh.

6. Jess, M., D. Collins, and L. Burwitz. 1999. The role of children's movement competence as an antecedent of lifelong physical activity. *Health Education Journal,* 1–15.

7. Bailey, R., M. Toms, D. Collins, P. Ford, A. Macnamara, and G. Pearce. 2011. Models of young player development in sport. In *Coaching children in sport,* ed. I. Stafford. Abingdon, UK: Routledge.

8. Stafford, I., ed. 2011. *Coaching children in sport.* Abingdon, UK: Routledge.

## Chapter 2

1. Enoka, R. 2002. *The neuro-mechanics of human movement.* Champaign, IL: Human Kinetics.

2. Kenny, W.L., J. Wilmore, and D. Costill. 2015. *Physiology of sport and exercise.* 6th ed. Champaign, IL: Human Kinetics.

3. Kendall, F.P., E.K. McCreary, P.G. Provance, M.M. Rodgers, and W.I. Romani. 2005. *Muscles: Testing posture and function with posture and pain.* 5th ed. Baltimore: Lippincott, Williams & Wilkins.

4. Semmler, J.G., and R.M. Enoka. 2008. Neural contributions to changes in muscle strength. In *Biomechanics in sport: The scientific basis for performance,* ed. V.M. Zatsiorski, 3–20. Oxford, UK: Blackwell.

5. Coyle, D. 2009. *The talent code.* New York: Random House.

6. Brewer, C. 2008. *Strength and conditioning for sports: A practical guide for coaches.* Leeds, UK: 1st4sport publications.

7. Beachle, T., and R.W. Earle. 2008. *Essentials of strength training and conditioning.* 3rd ed. Champaign, IL: Human Kinetics.

8. Cronin, J.C., and A.J. Blazevich. 2009. Speed. In *Applied anatomy and biomechanics in sport,* 2nd ed., ed. T.R. Ackland, B.C. Elliott, and J. Bloomfield. Champaign, IL: Human Kinetics.

## Chapter 3

1. Bompa, T.O., and G.G. Haff. 2009. *Periodization: Theory and methodology of training.* 5th ed. Champaign, IL: Human Kinetics.

2. Brewer, C. 2013. *Strength and conditioning for sports: A practical guide for coaches.* 2nd ed. Leeds, UK: 1st4sport publications.

3. Viru, A., M. Loko, A. Harro, L. Laaneaots, and M. Viru. 1999. Critical periods in the development of performance capacity during childhood and adolescence. *European Journal of Physical Education* 4 (1): 75–119.

4. Lloyd, R., and J.L. Oliver. 2013. Developing younger athletes. In *High-performance training for sports,* ed. D. Joyce and D. Lewindon, 15–28. Champaign, IL: Human Kinetics.

5. Gallahue, D., and C. Donnelly. 2007. *Developmental physical education for all children.* 2nd ed. Champaign, IL: Human Kinetics.

6. Balyi, I., R. Whey, and C. Higgs. 2013. *Longterm athlete development,* 33–48. Champaign, IL: Human Kinetics.

7. Rumpf, M.C., J.B. Cronin, S.D. Pinder, J. Oliver, and M.G. Hughes. 2012. Effects of different training methods on running sprint times in male youth. *Pediatric Exercise Science* 24 (2): 170–186.

8. Bouvier, M. 1989. The biology and composition of bone. In *Bone mechanics,* ed. S.C. Cronin, 1–14. Boca Raton, FL: CRC Press.

9. Pfeiffer, K.A., F. Lobelo, D.S. Ward, and R.R. Pate. 2008. Endurance trainability of children and youth. In *The young athlete: The encyclopaedia of sports medicine*, ed. O. Bar-or, and H. Hebestreit, 84–95. Oxford, UK: Blackwell.

10. Malina, R.M., C. Bouchard, and O. Bar-Or. 2004. *Growth, maturation and physical activity*. Champaign, IL: Human Kinetics.

11. Behringer, M., A. Vom Heede, M. Matthews, and J. Mester. 2011. Effects of strength training on motor performance skills in children and adolescents. *Pediatric Exercise Science* 23 (2): 186–206.

12. Lloyd, R.S., A.D. Faigenbaum, M.H. Stone, J.L. Oliver, I. Jeffreys, J.A. Moody, C. Brewer, K.C. Pierce, T.M. McCambridge, R. Howard, L. Herrington, B. Hainline, L.J. Micheli, R. Jaques, W.J. Kraemer, M.G. McBride, T.M. Best, D.A. Chu, B.A. Alvar, and G.D. Myer. 2014. Position statement on youth resistance training: The 2014 international consensus. *British Journal of Sports Medicine* 48 (7): 498–505.

13. Verhagen, E., and W. Van Mechelen. 2008. The epidemiology of paediatric sports-related injuries. In *The young athlete: The encyclopaedia of sports medicine*, ed. O. Bar-Or and H. Hebestreit, 141–150. Oxford, UK: Blackwell.

14. Baquet, G., C. Guinhouya, G. Dupont, C. Nourry, and S. Berthoin. 2004. The effects of a short-term interval program on physical fitness in prepubertal children. *Journal of Strength and Conditioning Research* 18 (4): 708–713.

15. French, D. 2014. *Programming and adaptation implications for concurrent training*. UKSCA annual conference, July 2014.

## Chapter 4

1. Whiting, W., and R. Zernicke. 1998. *Biomechanics of musculo-skeletal injury*. Champaign, IL: Human Kinetics.

2. Stone, M.H., M. Stone, and W.A. Sands. 2007. Modes of resistance training. In *Principles and practice of resistance training*, 241–257. Champaign, IL: Human Kinetics.

3. MacIntosh, B.R., and R.J. Holash. 2000. Power output and force–velocity properties of muscle. In *Biomechanics and biology of movement*, ed. B.M. Nigg, B.R. MacIntosh, and J. Mester, 193–210. Champaign, IL: Human Kinetics.

4. Plisk, S. 2008. Speed, agility and speed–endurance development. In *Essentials of strength training and conditioning*, 3rd ed., ed. T.R. Beachle and R.W. Earle, 457–485. Champaign, IL: Human Kinetics.

5. Krzysztof, M., and A. Mer. 2013. A kinematics analysis of three best 100m performances ever. *Journal of Human Kinetics* 36:149–160.

6. Stone, M.H., M. Stone, and W.A. Sands. 2007. Neuromuscular physiology. In *Principles and practice of resistance training*, 15–43. Champaign, IL: Human Kinetics..

## Chapter 5

1. Posture Committee of the American Academy of Orthopedic Surgeons. 1947. Posture and its *relationship to orthopedic disabilities: A report of the Posture Committee of the American Academy of Orthopedic Surgeons*. Evanston, IL: American Academy of Orthopedic Surgeons, p. 1.

2. Wallace, B. 2001. Balance training. In *Therapeutic exercise: Techniques for intervention*, ed. W.D. Bandy and B. Sanders, 239–262. Baltimore: Lippincott, Williams and Wilkins.

3. Enoka, R. 2002. *Neuromechanics of human movement*. 3rd ed., 241–312. Champaign, IL: Human Kinetics.

4. McGill, S. 2004. *Ultimate back fitness and performance*. 3rd ed., 113–124. Ontario, Canada: Backfit Pro.

5. Behnke, R. 2012. *Kinetic anatomy*. 3rd ed. Champaign, IL: Human Kinetics.

6. Enoka, R. 2002. *Neuromechanics of human movement*. 3rd ed., 313–358. Champaign, IL: Human Kinetics.

7. Fisher, L. 2003. *How to dunk a doughnut: The science of everyday life*. New York: Arcade.

8. Hamill, J., and K.L. Knutzen. 2003. *Biomechanical basis of human movement*. 2nd ed., 337–379. Baltimore: Lippincott, Williams and Wilkins..

9. Stone, M.H., M. Stone, and W.A. Sands. 2007. *Principles of resistance training*, 45–60. Champaign, IL: Human Kinetics.

## Chapter 6

1. Watson, A.W.S. 2001. Sports injuries related to flexibility, posture, acceleration, clinical defects, and previous injury in high-level players of body contact sports. *International Journal of Sports Medicine* 22:222–225.

2. Scache, A.G., T.M. Wrigley, R. Baker, and M.G. Pandy. 2009. Biomechanical response to hamstring muscle strain. *Gait & Posture* 29 (2): 332–338.

3. Cook, G. 2003. *Athletic body in balance*. Champaign, IL: Human Kinetics.

4. McDonough, A., and L. Funk. 2014. Can glenohumeral joint isokinetic strength and range of movement predict injury in professional rugby league? *Physical Therapy in Sport* 15:91–96.

5. Watson, A.W.S. 2001. Sports injuries related to flexibility, posture, acceleration, clinical defects, and previous injury in high-level players of body contact sports. *International Journal of Sports Medicine* 22:222, 225.

6. Schmidt-Wiethoff, R., W. Rapp, F. Mauch, T. Schneider, and H.J. Appell. 2004. Shoulder rotation characteristics in professional tennis players. *International Journal of Sports Medicine* 25 (2): 154–158.

7. Kaplan, K.M., N.S. ElAttrache, F.W. Jobe, B.F. Morrey, K.R. Kaufman, and W.J. Hurd. 2010. Comparison of shoulder range of motion, strength, and playing time in injured high school baseball pitchers who reside in warm- and cold-weather climates. *American Journal of Sports Medicine* 39 (2): 320–328.

8. Hewett, T.E., G.D. Myer, K.R. Ford, R.S. Heidt, A.J. Colosimo, S.G. McLean, A.J. Van den Bogert, M.V. Paterno, and P. Succop. 2005. Biomechanical measures of neuromuscular control and valgus loading of the knee predict anterior cruciate ligament injury risk in female athletes: A prospective study. *American Journal of Sports Medicine* 4 (1): 492–501.

9. Hamilton, R.T., S.J. Shultz, R.J. Schmitz, and D.H. Perrin. 2008. Triple-hop distance as a valid predictor of lower limb strength and power. *Journal of Athletic Training* 43 (2): 144–151.

10. Evans, K., K.M. Refshauge, and R. Adams. 2007. Trunk muscle endurance tests: Reliability and gender differences in athletes. *Journal of Science and Medicine in Sport* 10:447–455.

## Chapter 7

1. Eyesenck, M.W. 1994. *The Blackwell dictionary of cognitive psychology*, 284. Oxford, UK: Blackwell.

2. Gholve, P.A., D.M. Scher, S. Khakharia, R.F. Widmann, and D.W. Green. 2007. Osgood Schlatter syndrome. *Current Opinion in Pediatrics* 19 (1): 44–50.

3. Kujala, U.M., M. Kvist, and O. Heinonen. 1985. Osgood-Schlatter's disease in adolescent athletes. Retrospective study of incidence and duration. *American Journal of Sports Medicine* 13 (4): 236–241.

4. Bompa, T.O., and G.G. Haff, 2009. *Periodization: Theory and methodology of training*. 5th ed. Champaign, IL: Human Kinetics.

5. Stone, M.H., M. Stone, and W.A. Sands. 2007. *Principles of resistance training*. Champaign, IL: Human Kinetics.

6. Seefeldt, V., J. Haubenstricker, and S. Reuschlein. 1979. Why physical education in the elementary school curriculum? *Ontario Physical Education & Health Education Association Journal* 5 (1): 21–31.

7. Huber, J. 2013. *Applying educational psychology in coaching athletes*. Champaign, IL: Human Kinetics.

8. Schmidt, R.A., and T.D. Lee. 2011. *Motor control and learning: A behavioural emphasis*. 5th ed. Champaign, IL: Human Kinetics.

9. Schmidt, R.A., and T.D. Lee. 2014. *Motor learning and performance*. 5th ed. Champaign, IL: Human Kinetics.

10. Kirk, D., and A. MacPhail. 2002. Teaching games for understanding and situated learning: Rethinking the Bunker-Thorpe model. *Journal of Teaching in Physical Education* 21 (2): 177–192.

## Chapter 8

1. Buttifant, D., K. Graham, and K. Cross. 2013. Agility and speed in soccer players are 2 different performance parameters. In *Science in football IV*, ed. A. Murphy, T. Reilly, and V. Spinks. Oxford, UK: Routledge.

2. Plisk, S. 2008. Speed, agility and endurance development. In *Essentials of strength training and conditioning*, ed. T.R. Beachle, and R.W. Earle. Champaign, IL: Human Kinetics.

3. Sheppard, J.M., and W.B. Young. 2006. Agility literature review: Classifications, training and testing. *Journal of Sports Science* 24:919–932.

4. Jeffreys, I. 2013. *Developing speed*. Champaign, IL: Human Kinetics.

5. Dawes, J., and M. Roozen, 2013. *Developing agility and quickness*. Champaign, IL: Human Kinetics.

6. Mero, A., P.V. Komi, and R.J. Gregor. 1992. Biomechanics of sprint running. *Sports Medicine* 13 (6): 376–392.

7. Brown, T.D., and J.D. Vescovi. 2012. Maximum speed: Misconceptions of sprinting. *Strength and Conditioning Journal* 34 (2): 37–41.

8. Chelladurai, P. 1976. Manifestations of agility. *Canadian Association of Health, Physical Education, and Recreation* 42: 36–41.

9. Gallahue, D.L., and F.C. Donnelly. 2003. *Developmental physical education for all children*. 4th ed. Champaign, IL: Human Kinetics.

10. Lafortune, M.A., G.A. Valient, and B. McLean. 2000. Biomechanics of running. In *Running*, ed. J.A. Hawley. An IOC medical commission publication, Blackwell.

11. Nimphius, S. 2014. Increasing agility. In *High-performance training for sports*, ed. D. Joyce, and D. Lewindon. Champaign, IL: Human Kinetics.

## Chapter 9

1. Hay, J.G., J.A. Miller, and R.W. Canterna. 1986. The techniques of elite male long jumpers. *Journal of Biomechanics* 19 (10): 855–866.

2. Thompson, P. 2009. *Run, jump, throw: The official IAAF guide to teaching athletics*.

3. Wilt, F. 1978. Plyometrics: What it is and how it works. *Modern Athlete and Coach*, 16.

4. Kilani, H.A., S.S. Palmer, M.J. Adrian, and J.J. Gapsis. 1989. Block of the stretch reflex of vastus lateralis during vertical jump. *Human Movement Science* 75:813–823.

5. Potach, D.H., and D.A. Chu. 2008. Plyometric training. In *Essentials of strength training and conditioning*, 3rd ed., ed. T. Beachle, and R.W. Earle, 413–456. Champaign, IL: Human Kinetics.

6. Maclean, S. 2008. Using deterministic models to evaluate your athlete's performance: What are they and why should I care? Presented at the USOC Training Design Symposium, USOC Training Centre, Colorado Springs, CO, 23 March.

7. Moran, K.A., and Wallace, E.S. 2007. Eccentric loading and range of knee joint motion effects on performance enhancement in vertical jumping. *Human Movement Science* 26 (6): 824–840.

8. Gallahue, D.L., and F.C. Donnelly. 2003. *Developmental physical education for all children*. 4th ed. Champaign, IL: Human Kinetics.

9. Jess, M., D. Collins, and L. Burwitz. 1999. The role of children's movement competence as an antecedent of lifelong physical activity. *Health Education Journal*, 1–15.

10. Allerheiligen, B., and R. Rogers. 1996. Plyometric program design. In *Plyometric and medicine ball training*, ed. by the National Strength and Conditioning Association. Colorado Springs: NSCA. pages 3–8.

11. Wathen, D. 1994. Literature review: Explosive plyometric exercises. In *Position paper & literature review: Explosive exercises and training and explosive plyometric exercises,* ed. by the National Strength and Conditioning Association. Colorado Springs: NSCA. pages 13–16.

12. Lipp, E.J. 1998. Athletic physeal injury in children and adolescents. *Orthopedic Nursing* 17 (2): 17–22.

13. NCAA. 1994. Injury rates for women's basketball increases sharply. *NCAA News* 31 (May 11).

14. Gilchrist, J., B.R. Mandelbaum, H. Melancon, G.W. Ryan, H.J. Silvers, L.Y. Griffin, D.S. Watanabe, R.W. Dick, and J. Dvorak. 2008. A randomized controlled trial to prevent noncontact anterior cruciate ligament injury in female collegiate soccer players. *American Journal of Sports Medicine* 36 (8): 1476–1483.

15. Komi, P., and C. Bosco. 1978. Utilisation of stored elastic energy in leg extensor muscles by men and women. *Medicine and Science in Sports and Exercise* 10 (4): 261–265.

16. Garhammer, J. 1991. A comparison between male and female lifters weightlifters in competition. *International Journal of Sport Biomechanics* 7:3–11.

17. Cormie, P., J.M. McBride, and G.O. McCaulley. 2007. Validation of power measurement techniques in dynamic lower body resistance exercises. *Journal of Applied Biomechanics* 23:103–118.

18. Sale, D.G. 2002. Postactivation potentiation: Role in human performance. *Exercise and Sports Science Reviews* 30 (3): 138–143.

19. Harrison, A.J., S.P. Keane, and J. Coglan. 2004. Force–velocity relationship and stretch-shortening cycle function in sprint and endurance athletes. *Journal of Strength and Conditioning Research* 18 (3): 473–479.

## Chapter 10

1. Stone, M.H., M. Stone, and W.A. Sands. 2007. *Principles and practices of resistance training*. Champaign, IL: Human Kinetics.

2. Laplante, M., and D.M. Sabatini. 2009. mTOR signaling at a glance. *Journal of Cell Science* 122 (Pt 20): 3589–3594.

3. Delavier, F. 2001. *Strength training anatomy*. Champaign, IL: Human Kinetics.

4. Brewer, C., and M. Favre. 2016. Weight lifting for sports performance. In *Strength & conditioning for sports performance*, ed. I. Jeffreys, and J. Moody. Oxford, UK: Routledge.

5. Favre, M.W., and M.D. Peterson. 2012. Teaching the first pull. *Strength and Conditioning Journal* 34 (6): 77–81.

6. Enoka, R.M. 1979. The pull in Olympic weightlifting. *Medicine and Science in Sport* 11 (2): 131–137.

7. Garhammer, J. 2004. USAWUSA Weightlifting Symposium, USOC, Colorado Springs, CO, July.

8. Caterisano, A., R.F. Moss, T.K. Pellinger, K. Woodruff, V.C. Lewis, W. Booth, and T. Khadra. 2002. The effect of back squat depth on the EMG activity of 4 superficial hip and thigh muscles. *Journal of Strength and Conditioning Research* 16 (3): 428–432.

9. Nuzzo, J.L., G.O. McCaulley, P. Cormie, M.J. Cavill, and J.M. McBride. 2008. Trunk muscle activity during stability ball and free weight exercises. *Journal of Strength and Conditioning Research* 8 (1): 95–102.

10. Lloyd, R.S., A.D. Faigenbaum, M.H. Stone, J.L. Oliver, I. Jeffreys, J.A. Moody, C. Brewer, K.C. Pierce, T.M. McCambridge, R. Howard, L. Herrington, B. Hainline, L.J. Micheli, R. Jaques, W.J. Kraemer, M.G. McBride, T.M. Best, D.A. Chu, B.A. Alvar, and G.D. Myer. 2013. Position statement on youth resistance training: The 2014 international consensus. *British Journal of Sports Medicine* 48 (7): 498–505.

11. Hewes, G.W. 1955. World distribution of certain postural habits. *American Anthropologist* 57:231–244.

12. Beachle, T., and R.W. Earle, eds. 2008. *Essentials of strength training and conditioning.* 3rd ed. Champaign, IL: Human Kinetics.

# Chapter 11

1. Bompa, T.O., and Haff, G.G. 2009. *Periodisation: Theory and methodology of training.* 5th ed. Champaign, IL: Human Kinetics.

2. Christmass, M.A., S.E. Richmond, N.T. Cable, and P.E. Hartmann. 1998. A metabolic characterisation of singles tennis. In *Science and racket sports II*, ed. A. Lees, I. Maynard, M. Hughes, and T. Reilly. London: E. and F.N. Spon.

3. Bangsbo, J., M. Iaia, and P. Krustrup. 2008. The yo-yo intermittent recovery test: A useful tool for evaluation of physical performance in intermittent sports. *Sports Medicine* 38 (1): 37–51.

4. Vescovi, J.D. 2012. Sprint profile of professional female soccer players during competitive matches: Female Athletes in Motion (FAiM) study. *Journal of Sports Sciences* 30 (12): 1259–1265.

5. M. Ritschard, and M. Tschopp, eds. 2012. Physical analysis of the FIFA Women's World Cup Germany 2011. *FIFA Technical Study Group.* Switzerland: Aesch/ZH.

6. Stone, M.H., M. Stone, and W.A. Sands. 2007. *Principles and practices of resistance training.* Champaign, IL: Human Kinetics.

7. Plisk, S., and M. Stone. 2003. Periodisation strategies. *Strength and Conditioning Journal* 17:19–37.

# Index

# About the Author

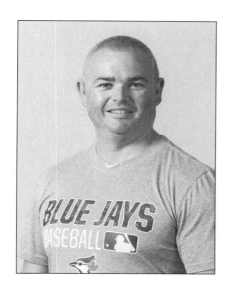

**Clive Brewer** is a world-recognized expert in high-performance sports conditioning, athlete development and applied sports science. He is the assistant director of high performance for the Toronto Blue Jays. He is the human performance consultant for USA Football and has consulted in this capacity with several other organizations around the world, such as Manchester United FC, Wimbledon tennis championships, the UK Strength and Conditioning Association, Scotland National Rugby League, Liverpool Ladies FC, the International Association of Athletics Federations (IAAF) and IMG Academy. As head of strength and conditioning with Widnes Vikings Rugby League Club (2011-2014), he helped them achieve their highest Super League finish while reducing injuries by more than 18% each year. Brewer has also consulted with Sports Med global performance systems, supporting sports performance development for clients worldwide. He has held lead roles as the head of human performance (strength and conditioning, science and medicine) with the Rugby Football League and SportScotland's national program manager for athlete development.

Brewer is accredited by the UK Strength and Conditioning Association (UKSCA), the National Strength and Conditioning Association and the British Association of Sport and Exercise Sciences as a support scientist. He is a chartered scientist with the Science Council in the UK and an original member of the British Olympic Association register of strength and conditioning coaches. In August 2015, he was awarded the fellowship of the UKSCA in recognition of his contribution to the industry.

As the IAAF strength and conditioning expert editor, Brewer was Scotland's first national strength and conditioning coach for track and field. In his 20 year career he has coached sports as diverse as tennis, soccer, rugby and bobsleigh at professional and international levels. From 2007, Brewer worked with other specialists to research the best practice in designing an athlete development framework to underpin the UK coaching model. He has authored several papers and book chapters on applied sport science, training methods, and athletic development coaching and has written two books on training methods for coaches. He has presented at many international conferences, including the pre-Olympic Sports Science Congress, the U.S. Olympic Committee National Coaches Congress, the International Science in Rugby Coaching conference, the National Strength and Conditioning Association national conference and the European Strength and Conditioning conference.

A native of the UK, Brewer lives in the Tampa metropolitan area while working across Canada and the United States with the Toronto Blue Jays baseball organization.

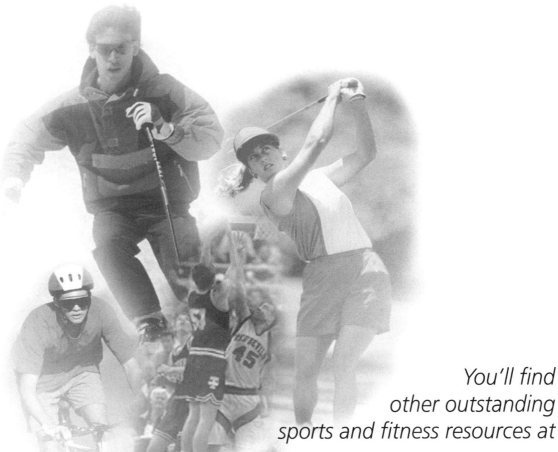